Electricity can now be used to kill bacteria, viruses and parasites in <u>minutes</u>, not days or weeks as antibiotics require.

If you have been suffering from a chronic infection or have cancer, or AIDS, learn to build the electronic device that will stop it immediately. It is safe and without side effects and does not interfere with any treatment you are now on.

The Cure For All Diseases

Published in the United States by:
New Century Press
1055 Bay Blvd., Suite C,
Chula Vista, CA 91911
(619) 476-7400, (800) 519-2465
www.newcenturypress.com

Other books by Dr. Clark available from New Century Press

The Cure For All Cancers
(English, German, Italian, Japanese, Russian)

The Cure For All Diseases
(English, Dutch, French, German, Italian, Polish, Russian, Serbian, Spanish)

The Cure For All Advanced Cancers
(English, German, Italian)

The Cure For HIV And AIDS
(English)

The Syncrometer® Science Laboratory Manual
(English, Spanish)

The Prevention Of All Cancers
(English)

Reprinted 2006

Notice to the Reader:

The opinions and conclusions expressed in this book are mine, and unless expressed otherwise, mine alone. The opinions expressed herein are based on my scientific research and on specific case studies involving my patients. Be advised that every person is unique and may respond differently to the treatments described in this book. On occasion we have provided dosage recommendations where appropriate. Again, remember that we are all different and any new treatment should be applied in a cautious, common sense fashion.

The treatments outlined herein are not intended to be a replacement or substitute for other forms of conventional medical treatment. Please feel free to consult with your physician or other health care provider.

I have indicated throughout this book the existence of pollutants in food and other products. These pollutants were identified using a testing device of my invention known as the Syncrometer.™ Complete instructions for building and using this device are contained in this book. Therefore anyone can repeat the tests described and verify the data.

The Syncrometer is more accurate and versatile than the best existing testing methods. A method for determining the degree of precision is also presented. However at this point it only yields positive or negative results, it does not quantify. The chance of a false positive or a false negative is about 5%, which can be lessened by test repetition.

It is in the public interest to know when a single bottle of a single product tests positive to a serious pollutant. If one does, the safest course is to avoid all bottles of that product entirely, which is what I repeatedly advise. These recommendations should be interpreted as an intent to warn and protect the public, not to provide a statistically significant analysis. It is my fervent hope that manufacturers use the new electronic techniques in this book to make purer products than they ever have before.

Dedication

I would like to dedicate this book to all the persons who visited me professionally, from the very first person in 1963, **Mrs. R. Biehl**, to the present. I learned so much from each of you and I appreciate your confidence, your intelligence and your reluctance to be defeated.

Acknowledgments

I would like to express my gratitude to my son, **Geoffrey**, who always <u>listened</u> to my "crazy ideas" on Sundays, right at supper time. He was patient, kind, helpful and willing to share his expertise in electronics and computers. Without him, this book could not have been written.

A big thank you goes to **Frank Jerome, DDS**. Without the loan of his parasite slide collection many of my discoveries could not have been make, and without his development of metal-free dentistry, many of these patient histories could not have ended happily. Thank you to **Linda Jerome** for nurturing us both with personal interest and patience. And thank you to **Edna Bernstein** for her resourceful assistance.

Contents

Figures

Preface

The sick have been held hostage for their money or intangible assets since time immemorial. Doctors, even primitive and natural healers, surround themselves with mystery as they use herbs or chemicals and incantations or "prognoses" to help the sick recover. Today, the medical industry (doctors and their suppliers and insurers) take a significant amount of the worker's earnings. Wouldn't it be nice if they could all go back to gardening or some other primitive and useful endeavor? Wouldn't it be wonderful if the sick could join them?

The most promising discovery in this book is the effectiveness of electricity to kill viruses, bacteria and parasites. Does this mean you can cancel your appointment with your clinical doctor? No it does not. Killing your invaders does not make you well instantly. But happily, at your next doctor visits she or he will be removing drugs, not adding them.

You might think that such an invention should be quickly patented. That was my universal advice. But I chose not to. It helps me, my children, and my grandchildren, if <u>you</u> are well. The whole world needs to come out of the dark ages of medicine and illness. And to learn the true causes of infection and disease. We must and can usher in the **new age of disease-free living.**

No diabetes, no high blood pressure, no cancer, no HIV/AIDS, no migraines, no lupus and so on!

Not a single disease is left unconquerable with this new understanding!

The Promise

Step into a new world.

A world without chronic diseases.

Step out of your old world.

It has kept you a prisoner.

Try something new.

The prison has no walls. It has only lines. Lines that mark the ground around you. Inside the lines are your old ideas. Outside are new ideas that invite you to step over and escape your prison. Dare to try these new ideas and your illness promises to recede. In a few weeks it can be gone.

If you are very ill or chronically ill you must have asked yourself many times: why have these problems chosen me? Will there never be a way to conquer them?

You may be quite familiar with your doctor's explanation of your illness or your child's illness. A *Coxsackie* virus has entered your child's brain causing inflammation (encephalitis) there. You pray that your child's immunity will overcome it. You may be familiar, but so very helpless against this microscopic invader.

If you had the proverbial 3 wishes they would be: 1) please spare my child's life; 2) please make it so my child doesn't have permanent damage; 3) please bless and guide the wonderful doctors and nurses who are keeping the oxygen tent going, and are watching my child's temperature and vital signs.

What if you could turn a dial and in 3 minutes kill every Coxsackie virus in your child's body?

What if this had no side effects?

What if the virus never came back?

In this book you will learn how to do that. You will also learn why your child got encephalitis or other disease and how to prevent it forever.

If this is too mind boggling, just take it a step at a time: First, learn about the radio-type broadcasting that all living animals do. Second, find the "station frequencies" that your particular invader(s) broadcast at. Third, learn how to "jam" their frequency until they **expire**: it takes only minutes!

Finally, learn how to make your own diagnostic and treatment devices. The instructions are simple enough for anyone. Only by putting this power in your hands will it be safe from government regulation, however well intended.

Only Two Health Problems

No matter how long and confusing is the list of symptoms a person has, from chronic fatigue to infertility to mental problems, I am sure to find only two things wrong: they have in them **pollutants** and/or **parasites**. I never find lack of exercise, vitamin deficiencies, hormone levels or anything else to be a primary causative factor. So the solution to good health is obvious:

Problem	Simplest Cure
Parasites	Electronic and herbal treatment
Pollution	Avoidance

It's a valiant quest: The quest for health. With optimism in one hand and determination in the other, you too can work the miracles for yourself that my clients accomplished in the case histories.

More good news is that it is not expensive. The cost will range from a few hundred dollars to only a few thousand in order to eliminate both problems and cure your chronic diseases.

Be A Health Detective

After curing your own diseases, teach your friends and family how it's done. Families are related and their problems are related. This should make the task easier. Keep a small notebook to become part of the treasured family legacy as much as photographs do. If your aunt, father and brother had diabetes as well as yourself and all were cured after introducing them to this concept and technology, isn't this worthy of notes in your family's history?

Notice what a strong line of inheritance there can be, **not due to sharing genes** but due to sharing a roof, a table, a supermarket, and a dentist!

Many problems can be <u>disinherited</u>. Cure yourself of retinitis pigmentosa, Muscular dystrophy (the "inherited" kind), and break down your family's faith in the gene-concept for these diseases. Bring hope to your family by proving diseases' true etiology. Bring respect back for your loyal genes that bring you hair color, and texture, not hair loss. That bring you eye color, not eye disease. Your genes brought you the good things about your ancestors, not the bad things. Parasites and pollution brought you the bad things.

Killing all your invaders is just the first step, though. It is indeed the life-saving step. But getting well is more than saving your life. Next comes the more tedious task of finding their sources. Where did they come from? Why did they invade you so massively. Why you?

3

The story of your personal pollution unfolds as in a book. Look closely and you see the whole panorama of your numerous tiny invaders being held at bay by your valiant immune system, your white blood cells. You can see what they are fighting besides the invaders. Your ill-chosen diet and lifestyle products!

Your heart may go out to those tiny white blood cells. <u>Never again</u>, you may say, will you give them arsenic and mercury and lead. Never again, cobalt and asbestos and freon.

That great body of wisdom, <u>your body</u>, the same as listened to your three wishes, will reward you over and over as you co-operate with it, until you have had not 3 but 30 wishes granted, each one seemingly as impossible as climbing Mt. Everest.

- Your chronic yeast infection can go away.
- Your hair can stop falling out–might even grow back.
- Your body can become pregnant–when you had already given up.
- Your fatigue can vanish.
- Your insomnia can be gone.
- Your warts can fall off.
- Your sight and hearing can sharpen.
- Your constant hunger can disappear.

Health isn't just being free of sickness. Health is feeling great, feeling like laughing at funny things. Health is feeling grateful to be alive. It is feeling happy to see the sky and to see growing things and to feel confident in human society's progress. Health is remembering the good parts of childhood and believing you still have a lot of them.

The Discovery

What makes me think I can find things in the human body that a blood test can not? What new technology makes this possible? Why is electronic testing superior in many ways to chemical methods? What are my claims of electrically killing parasites based on?

In 1988 I discovered a new way to scan a body organ. It was electronic. We already can "see" an organ with a sonogram, X-rays, computerized tomography (CAT) scan, or with magnetic resonance imagery (MRI). These techniques can identify abnormal shapes in an organ without having to explore or guess. But my new electronic technique can check for viruses, bacteria, fungi, parasites, solvents and toxins, and in addition is simple, cheap, fast and infallible. Electricity can do many magical things; now we can add detecting substances in our body to that list.

The method rests on <u>radio</u> electronic principles.

If you match, very precisely, the capacitance and inductance properties of an external circuit so that its resonant frequency is the same as the emitted frequency coming from somewhere else, the circuit will oscillate. This means there will be positive feedback in an amplifier circuit. You can hear it. Like when a public address system squeals.

The external circuit I use is called an *audio oscillator*, quite easy to build or buy. Your body provides the emitted frequencies. When you combine the audio oscillator circuit with your body, and you hear *resonance*, then you have detected a match! Something in your body matches something in the circuit on the test plate. By putting a laboratory sample of, say, a virus on the test plate, you can determine if your body has that virus by listening for resonance. Hearing resonance is easy if you're a radio

5

technician or musician. Others must patiently practice. The details are given in the Bioelectronics chapter (page 457).

> You do not have to be an expert in anything to learn the electronic detection method. But a keen sense of hearing helps.

In 1988 I learned a way to put anything on my skin, blindfolded, and identify it electronically in a few minutes. I could taste something without flavor and identify it electronically. The system worked fine for detecting things in the skin and tongue. Would it be reliable for internal organs, too?

A whole world of discovery lay ahead of me. I wanted to know what was in my inner ear causing tinnitus, in my eyes causing pain, in my stomach causing indigestion and a thousand other things.

But behind the daily excitement of new discoveries, a gnawing question lingered in my mind. How is this possible without some pretty high frequency energy source, radio frequency in fact, running through my circuit? My audio oscillator was only 1000 Hz (*hertz*, or cycles per second); radio frequency is hundreds of thousands of Hz. And the phenomenon could be produced with an old-fashioned *dermatron*[1], too, that only puts out DC (direct current)–no frequencies at all!

A high frequency energy had to be coming from somewhere. Was it me? *Ridiculous!*

But there was a way to test. If my own body was putting forth the high frequency energy, it could be bled off and diverted into the ground with a correct size capacitor. This should stop the feedback oscillations. This turned out to be true; it was stopped. But *ridiculous* kept ringing in my ears and I tried an-

---

[1]The dermatron was invented decades ago and made famous by Dr. Voll. Establishment science disdained it!

6

other test. If there was indeed radio frequency (RF) running through my circuit I should be able to block it with the right snap-on choke. It did block. I thought of a third test. If this was truly a resonance phenomenon I should be able to add a capacitance to this circuit and see the resonance destroyed. Then add an inductance and see the resonance return. It did just that. I made graphs of the relationship between capacitance and inductance. They were entirely reproducible.

Then why couldn't I see the RF on my RF oscilloscope? Probably because it was <u>high frequency</u> energy, not <u>high energy</u> frequency, and I didn't know how to amplify it above the background noise level. It was nevertheless not convincing. Yet much too tantalizing to ignore.

I thought of yet a fourth test. If I was really producing RF radiation that could be channeled through a circuit, I should be able to interfere with it by adding another RF radiation from an outside source. I added a frequency from my frequency generator, first at 1,000 Hz. Now there was no resonance. It interfered. Did this mean that my body was not producing radiation at 1,000 Hz? Or was my 1,000 Hz radiation being matched and canceled? I raised the frequency gradually, from 1,000 to 10,000 to 100,000 to 1,000,000 Hz. There was no resonance anywhere, and I couldn't draw any conclusions. It was 5 o'clock on Sunday afternoon. Quitting time. But one last look at my generator reminded me that it could reach 2,000,000 Hz and I was just at 1,000,000. One more quick experiment wouldn't take much time. I cranked it to 1,800,000 Hz. And now a resonance screamed out! Was I "hearing things?" No more interference. I did it over and over. Why was it resonating now and not before? Had I arrived at my body's own *bandwidth* (transmission range), and this was the reason it no longer interfered?

I found the lowest frequency that resonated to be 1,562,000 Hz. All frequencies that I checked (about 2,000) from there up to 2,000,000 (my frequency generator would go no higher) also resonated.

A year later I purchased a better frequency generator to search for the upper end of my bandwidth. Any frequency between 1,562,000 and 9,457,000 Hz could be added to the circuit and produce resonance.

It seemed obvious, then, that the human body broadcasts electrically, just like a radio station, but over a wide band of frequencies and very low voltages, which is why it has not been detected and measured until now.

Everything Has A Unique Frequency

It was a busy year, now 1989. I was determined to find a bandwidth for other living things: I found them for flies, beetles, spiders, fleas, ants. They were between 1,000,000 Hz and 1,500,000 Hz; cockroaches were highest amongst insects I tested.

Then came a dismaying finding. A dead insect had a bandwidth too! Much narrower, and near the top end of the same range it had when living, but distinctly present. So it wasn't altogether a living phenomenon.

But if dead things had a resonant bandwidth, then maybe a prepared microscope slide of a dead creature could be used, and my trips to the garden and telephone calls to abattoirs (for meat parasites) could cease. That was a lucky thought. My first slide was of the *human intestinal fluke*, a huge parasite, scourge of humanity. I had just found it to be present in the liver (not intestine) of every cancer sufferer I saw. The (dead) adult parasite had a resonant frequency around 434,000 Hz. Slides of that parasite's redia resonated nearby (432,000 Hz), as did its other stages.

Dead things still resonated! The entire catalog of biological supply companies, hundreds of specimens of viruses, bacteria, parasites, molds, and even toxins, were now available to research with this new technique!

Suddenly an idea bolted out of the blue. If a person were to hold on to the frequency generator while it was generating 434,000 Hz, what would happen to the adult fluke, if you were infected with it?

I tested this plan that same week on myself, not with the fluke but with *Salmonella* bacteria and *Giardia* and *Herpes* that I carried chronically. After a 3 minute treatment, I retested myself. I could no longer find them in my organs! There were no emissions at their characteristic frequencies. I repeated and repeated. Were they really dead? Maybe they were just numbed or were suddenly hiding. But symptoms were gone quickly too. My *Herpes* lesion stopped tingling. It was all too simple and unbelievable.

But was it safe? Within three weeks I had reliable data regarding the necessary level of electrical treatment. It only took 5 volts for three minutes at the specific frequency. It is not as if you had to use house current which would kill you, along with the parasite.

Selective Electrocution

In twenty minutes (three minutes at six different frequencies) a whole family could get rid of this parasite. Cancer cases showed that in a few hours the universal cancer marker, *ortho-phospho-tyrosine* could be banished from their bodies by killing this same parasite.

9

"Incurable" HIV cases lost their virus in a few hours, too. Laboratory retesting for HIV came back negative! Most cases of pain got immediate relief if I could identify the correct "bug" and have its frequency found by the next office visit. This seemed to be absolute proof that living things had an essential high frequency output of some kind of energy.

What was actually happening to the bacteria or parasites? If I could kill something as large as an *Ascaris* worm or intestinal fluke, then perhaps I could kill something even larger, like an earthworm or flea, something I could see with my own eyes instead of having to imagine its demise inside my body.

Ten minutes at a frequency chosen near the top of their broadcast range seemed to anesthetize them. But they didn't die. Later I checked the body bandwidth (the range of frequencies they emit) of each. The earthworms had lost a lot of their bandwidth, both at the top and bottom. The fleas seemed hardier; they had only lost a little. However they did not recover, even weeks later, from this loss.

Could it harm humans to douse them with RF frequencies **in their own bandwidth?** Quite probably, if the voltage were high enough. There was no need to experiment, though, because the parasites we want to kill have characteristic frequencies that **do not overlap** the characteristic frequencies of a human. In fact, they are far away (see the chart on page 17).

So my electronic method attacking illness was born. Find the resonant frequency of a bacterium, virus or parasite using a slide or dead bit. Treat the living invaders inside the human body with this frequency and in a matter of minutes they are no longer transmitting their own bandwidths—they are dead or sick and will be removed by our white blood cells.

It was a worrisome truth. Perhaps the department of defense would use this knowledge and develop super high voltage devices to kill people ("enemies") somewhere in the world. But I couldn't let sick people suffer. Besides, it would probably require a voltage much like lightning to kill people from a distance. Possibly a way could be found to shield yourself from frequencies harmful to humans by wearing a choke (inductor) coil which suppresses these frequencies. Remember, there was no recovery, just a slow death for my experimental animals. It must not happen to humans!

Meanwhile, people must be alerted that they can safely kill their invaders and heal their chronic illnesses. Invaders that have been increasing exponentially due to lowered immunity in recent decades. Possibly this is true for all species on our planet. The pollution of the entire biosphere has been increasing and with it the prospect of acquired immune deficiency syndrome (AIDS) for all of us.

> Remember, though, that the true challenge is not to kill our invaders but to regain our health and immunity.

More than just parasites are making us sick! Pollution is too. Selective electrocution rarely makes people completely well. Sick people always have an environmental factor that must be corrected also.

How do we do that? The ship of "progress", of increasingly complex, processed foods and products, must be turned around and simplicity become our goal. Survival is in simplicity of food intake, simplicity of life habits. Did Ralph Waldo Emerson foresee this when he said "To be simple is to be great"? Or will daily parasite and pathogen electrocution become another crutch that makes us just enough better that we can continue a detrimental lifestyle? Yet another "Band-Aid" treatment for our poisoned planet?

Bioradiation

Strange as it appears, it now seems obvious that every living creature broadcasts its presence like a radio station, the sun, or the stars. I have named it *bioradiation*.

Perhaps it is the same energy as the Asian *chi*; perhaps it is merely related to it. Perhaps it is the energy that runs along the meridians discovered eons ago by Asian practitioners.

Perhaps it is the energy that faith healers and religious teachers know how to harness, perhaps not.

Perhaps it is the energy that psychics perceive and that drives occult phenomena, perhaps not.

What is truly amazing is that ordinary persons have discovered such energy well ahead of scientists. Persons using the "art" of kinesiology, pendulums, radionics, dousing rods and many other forms of "strange energy" have no doubt harnessed a part of this bioradiation. It is a tribute to the generally high intelligence of common people and to their open-mindedness that they discovered this energy, **in spite of** opposition from scientists of today.

Over a century ago the scientists of Europe proposed the existence of a "life force" called "élan vitale." They were scorned out of existence (and out of jobs). Young scientists, (including myself) were systematically taught to scorn this idea. Of course we were also taught that a good scientist was unemotional, does not scorn ideas, has a completely open mind, and does not rule something out until it is disproved to their satisfaction. The youthfulness of college years is so susceptible to prejudices of all kinds, and the desire for acceptance is so great, that special effort needs to be made to teach neutrality. Or at least to distinguish between emotion and fact. Where have these basic pedagogic principles gone? I was indeed inspired with the phrase "search for truth" but then promptly led down the path of "search for acceptance."

I do not know what bioradiation, this electrical broadcast from our cells, is made of. Only its frequency was noticed and caught (modulated) in such a way as to be measurable. And this frequency, 1,520,000 to 9,460,000 Hz (for a human infant) is in the radio frequency (RF) range[2].

Anyone who is experienced with RF knows its strange behavior. Not strange in the "unknown" sense but in the amazing sense. Circuits don't need to be complete or closed for it to travel. Bodies and objects can "pick it up" without being in the circuit. These amazing properties are due to the capacitive and inductive properties of objects all around us, including ourselves.

Zapping Bugs

By *zapping* I mean selectively electrocuting pathogens. For years I used a commercial frequency generator to "zap" one pathogen after another.

First I made a chart of the frequencies for most of the bacteria and viruses in my collection (over 80, see page 561). Then I would test the sick client for each one of these, and hope they did not have one for which I didn't have a sample. Even persons with a simple cold typically had a dozen they tested positive to (not just *Adenovirus*).

Next it was time to tune in the frequency generator to a dozen frequencies for three minutes each. The total process, testing and treatment, would take about two hours. They frequently got immediate relief. But often the relief would be temporary. What I didn't know at that time was that viruses could

---

[2]AM radio broadcasts are from 540,000 Hz to 1,600,000 Hz (slight overlap with lower end of human band), FM is 88,000,000 to 108,000,000 Hz (out of the human range).

infect a larger parasite such as a roundworm. Until you killed your roundworm <u>and</u> your virus, you would keep getting the virus back promptly.

In 1993 my son, Geoffrey, joined me and we tried a new approach. He programmed a computer controlled frequency generator to automatically cover all the frequencies populated by all the parasites, viruses, and bacteria, from 290,000 Hz to 470,000 Hz. It spent about three minutes for every 1000 Hz it covered. This was more efficient, but it meant spending <u>ten hours</u> being zapped.

Again, the results were disappointing. Arthritis pain, eye pain, colds were improved, but not completely cured overnight. Months later I would find that organisms were transmitting as low as 170,000, and as high as 690,000 Hz. My specimen collection was obviously incomplete. To cover this larger range, spending three minutes for every 1000 Hz, would take 26 hours. Still worth doing if it would indeed help all our illnesses. But even this method of zapping was not 100% effective for reasons yet to become clear.

In 1994 my son built a hand held, battery operated, accurate frequency generator. The purpose was to enable everyone to kill the intestinal fluke at 434,000 Hz with a low cost device. Enough benefit would be derived from zapping at various frequencies that I thought everyone should know how to make one. When I tested it on one of my own bacteria, however, **three others at much different frequencies died also!** This had never happened before. When I tested it on others, even though they had dozens of pathogens, all were killed!

Subsequent testing showed it was not due to some unique design, or special wave form produced by the device. It was due to battery operation!

Any positively offset frequency kills all bacteria, viruses and parasites simultaneously

given sufficient voltage (5 to 10 volts), duration (seven minutes), and frequency (anything from 10 Hz to 500,000 Hz).

Before this I had always set my commercial frequency generator to alternate between positive and negative voltage. Now I tried setting it to alternate between positive and zero voltage (*positive offset*). It was just as effective as the battery operated frequency generator my son designed.

Generating positive offset frequencies is the best way to kill all pathogens quickly.

But it takes more than one treatment.

It takes **three treatments** to kill everything. Why? The first zapping kills viruses, bacteria and parasites. But a few minutes later, bacteria and viruses (different ones) often recur. I conclude they had been infecting the parasites, and killing the parasites released them. The second zapping kills the released viruses and bacteria, but soon a few viruses appear <u>again</u>. They must have been infecting some of the last bacteria. After a third zapping I never find any viruses, bacteria or parasites, even hours later.

Why didn't the virus inside the parasite die with the first zapping? It may be because electricity travels on the <u>exterior</u> of things. The body of the parasite shielded the interior. This is why my earlier, promising work spending hours on a frequency generator gave only partial or temporary improvement—it was only done once, not three times. And it explains why a single treatment with a frequency generator or zapper frequently gives you a cold!

Zapping does not kill shielded organisms

such as those that may be in the middle of your stomach or intestines. The electricity travels along the stomach or intestine wall, not through their contents.

So zapping is still not perfect, but can bring such manifest relief that everyone should buy or make one. Parts cost less than $25.00; the plans are in the next chapter.

The Bioradiation Spectrum

Everything emits a characteristic range of frequencies (bandwidth). In general, the more primitive the organism, the lower its bandwidth. Advanced animals have higher frequencies and the range is wider.

BANDWIDTH OF BIORADIATION OF ANIMALS

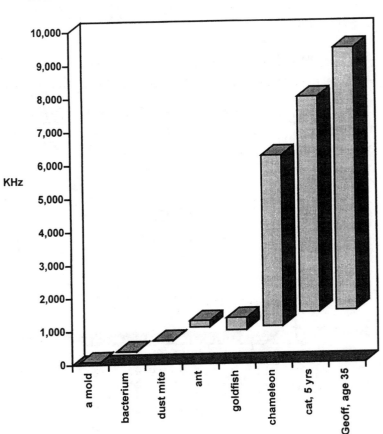

Fig. 1 Selected animal bandwidths.

The human range is from 1520 KHz to 9460 KHz. Pathogens (molds, viruses, bacteria, worms, mites) range from 77 KHz to 900 KHz. Fortunately for us we can work on zapping pathogens in the lower ranges without affecting humans in the upper range.

BIORADIATION OF TYPICAL PATHOGENS

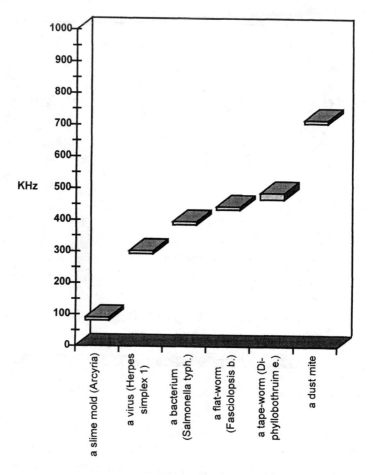

Fig. 2 Selected pathogen bandwidths.

Applying an alternating electrical voltage within an organism's bandwidth injures it. Small organisms with narrow bandwidths are extinguished quite readily (three minutes at five volts).

Positively offset frequencies can kill the <u>entire range</u> of small organisms (viruses, bacteria, parasites) in just seven minutes.

Building A Zapper

Being able to kill your bacteria and other invaders with electricity becomes much more of a panacea when you can do it all in three 7 minute sessions. No need to single out specific frequencies or to sweep through a range of frequencies one KHz at a time. No matter what frequency it is set at (within reason), it kills large and small invaders: flukes, roundworms, mites, bacteria, viruses and fungi. It kills them all at once, in 7 minutes, even at 5 volts.

How does it work? I suppose that a positive voltage applied anywhere on the body attracts negatively charged things such as bacteria. Perhaps the battery voltage tugs at them, pulling them out of their locations in the cell doorways (called *conductance channels*). But doorways can be negatively charged too. Does the voltage tug at them so they disgorge any bacteria stuck in them? How would the positive voltage act to kill a large parasite like a fluke? None of these questions can be answered yet.

Other fascinating possibilities are that the intermittent positive voltage interferes with electron flow in some key metabolic route, or straightens out the ATP molecule disallowing its breakdown. Such biological questions could be answered by studying the effects of positive frequencies on bacteria in a lab.

The most important question, of course, is whether there is a harmful effect on you. I have seen no effects on blood pressure, mental alertness, or body temperatures. It has never produced pain, although it has often stopped pain instantly. This does not prove its safety. Even knowing that the voltage comes from a small 9 volt battery does not prove safety, although it is reassuring. The clotting of red blood cells, platelet aggregation and functions that depend on surface charges on cells need to be investigated. But not before you can use it. Your safety lies in the short period of exposure that is necessary. Viruses and bacteria

19

disappear in 3 minutes; tapeworm stages, flukes, roundworms in 5; and mites in 7. One need not go beyond this time, although no bad effects have been seen at any length of treatment.

The first seven minute zapping is followed by an intermission, lasting 20 to 30 minutes. During this time, bacteria and viruses are released from the dying parasites and start to invade you instead.

The second seven minute session is intended to kill these newly released viruses and bacteria. If you omit it, you could catch a cold, sore throat or something else immediately. Again, viruses are released from the dying bacteria. The third session kills the last viruses released.

Do Not Zap If You Are Pregnant
Or Wearing A Pacemaker.

These situations have not been explored yet. Don't do these experiments yourself. Children as young as 8 months have been zapped with no noticeable ill effects. For them, you should weigh the possible benefits against the unknown risks.

That is all there is to it. Almost all. The zapping current does not reach deep into the eyeball or testicle or bowel contents. It does not reach into your gallstones, or into your living cells where *Herpes* virus lies latent or *Candida* fungus extends its fingers. But by zapping 3 times a day for a week or more you can deplete these populations, too, often to zero.

Killing The Surviving Pathogens

The interior of gallstones may house parasites inaccessible to the zapping. Eliminate this source of reinfection by flushing them out with liver cleanses (page 552).

Although the center of the bowel contents is often unaffected by electric current, which lets bowel bacteria like *Shigella, Escherichia coli (E. coli)* and parasite stages survive, sometimes it is nearly all sterilized by zapping. This results in considerable shrinkage of the bowel movement. Eliminate remaining parasites and bacteria with a single dose (2 tsp.) of Black Walnut Hull Tincture, Extra Strength (see page 543).

There is no way of distinguishing between "good" and "bad" bacteria with either of these methods. However even good bacteria are bad if they come through the intestinal wall, so zapping targets mostly "bad" bacteria. The good news is that perfect bowel habits often result in a few days. Evidently, the good bacteria are benefited by killing the invasive ones. Homemade yogurt and buttermilk (see *Recipes*) are especially good at recolonizing the bowel. But it does not seem wise to culture yourself with special commercial preparations and risk getting parasite stages again when you can become normal so soon anyway. If you do decide to take some *acidophilus* bacteria to replenish your intestinal flora make sure you test for parasites like *Eurytrema* first.

When a large number of parasites, bacteria and viruses are killed, it can leave you fatigued. Try to give yourself a low-stress day after your initial zapping. But there are no significant side effects. I believe this is due to the second and third zapping which mops up bacteria and viruses that would otherwise be able to go on a feeding frenzy with so much dead prey available.

To build your zapper you may take this list of components to any electronics store (Radio Shack part numbers are given for convenience).

Zapper Parts List

Item	Radio Shack Catalog Number
large shoe box	
9 volt battery	

9 volt battery clips	270-325 (set of 5, you need 1)
On-Off toggle switch	275-624A micro mini toggle switch
1 KΩ resistor	271-1321 (set of 5, you need 2)
3.9 KΩ resistor	271-1123 (set of 2, you need 2)
low-current red LED	276-044 or 276-041 or 276-045
.0047 uF capacitor	272-130 (set of 2, you need 1)
.01 uF capacitor	272-1065 (set of 2, you need 1)
555 CMOS timer chip	276-1723 (set of 2, you need 1)
8 pin wire-wrapping socket for the chip	276-1988 (set of 2, you need 1) Note: Radio Shack is discontinuing all wire wrap sockets. Find another parts store or use 276-1995 (but the legs are much shorter and harder to attach clips to).
short (12") alligator clip leads	any electronics shop, get 6
Microclip test jumpers	278-017 (you need 2 packages of 2)
2 bolts, about 1/8" diameter, 2" long, with 4 nuts and 4 washers	hardware store
2 copper pipes, ¾" diameter, 4" long	hardware store
sharp knife, pin, long-nose pliers	

Hints for absolute novices: Don't let unusual vocabulary deter you. A "lead" is just a piece of wire used to make connections. When you remove a component from its package, label it with a piece of tape. A serrated kitchen knife works best as does a large safety pin. Practice using the microclips. If the metal ends are L-shaped bend them into a U with the long-nose pliers so they grab better. Chips and chip holders are very fragile. It is wise to purchase an extra of each in case you break the connections.

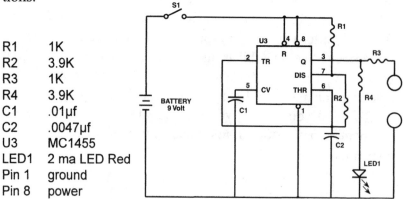

R1   1K
R2   3.9K
R3   1K
R4   3.9K
C1   .01µf
C2   .0047µf
U3   MC1455
LED1 2 ma LED Red
Pin 1 ground
Pin 8 power

Give this to an electronics person or make it yourself in a shoebox by using the following instructions.

Fig. 3 Zapper schematic.

Assembling The Zapper

1. You will be using the lid of the shoe box to mount the components. Save the box to enclose the finished project.

2. Pierce two holes near the ends of the lid. Enlarge the holes with a pen or pencil until the bolts would fit through. Mount the bolts on the outside about half way through the holes so there is a washer and nut holding it in place on both sides. Tighten. Label one hole "grounding bolt" on the inside and outside.

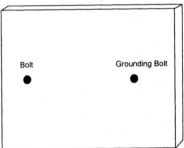

3. Mount the 555 chip in the wire wrap socket. Find the "top end" of the chip by searching the outside surface carefully for a cookie-shaped bite or hole taken out of it. Align the chip with the socket and very gently squeeze the pins of the chip into the socket until they click in place.

4. Make 8 pinholes to fit the wire wrap socket. Enlarge them slightly with a sharp pencil. Mount it on the outside. Write in the numbers of the pins (connections) on both the outside and inside, starting with number one to the left of the "cookie bite" as seen from outside. After number 4, cross over to number 5 and continue. Number 8 will be across from number 1.

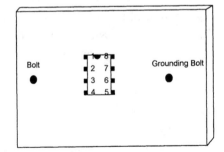

5. Pierce two holes ½ inch apart very near to pins 5, 6, 7, and 8. They should be less than 1/8 inch away. (Or, one end of each component can <u>share</u> a hole with the 555 chip.) Mount the .01 uF ca-

23

pacitor near pin 5 on the outside. On the inside connect pin 5 to one end of this capacitor by simply twisting them together. Loop the capacitor

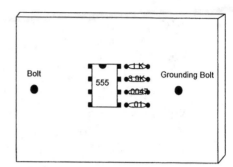

wire around the pin first; then twist with the long-nose pliers until you have made a tight connection. Bend the other wire from the capacitor flat against the inside of the shoe box lid. Label it .01 on the outside and inside. Mount the .0047 uF capacitor near pin 6. On the inside twist the capacitor wire around the pin. Flatten the wire from the other end and label it .0047. Mount the 3.9 KΩ resistor near pin 7, connecting it on the inside to the pin. Flatten the wire on the other end and label it 3.9. Mount the 1 KΩ resistor and connect it similarly to pin 8 and label it 1K.

6. Pierce two holes ½ inch apart next to pin 3 (again, you can share the hole for pin 3 if you wish), in the direction of the bolt. Mount the other 1 KΩ resistor and label inside and outside. Twist the connections together and flatten the remaining wire. This resistor protects the circuit if you should accidentally short the terminals. Mount the 3.9KΩ resistor downward. One end can go in the same hole as the 1K resistor near pin 3. Twist that end around pin 3 which already has the 1K resistor attached to it. Flatten the far end. Label.

7. Next to the 3.9KΩ resistor pierce two holes ¼ inch apart for the LED. No-

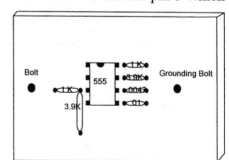

tice that the LED has a positive and negative connection. The longer wire is the anode (positive). Mount the LED on the outside and bend back the wires, labeling them + and - on the in-side.

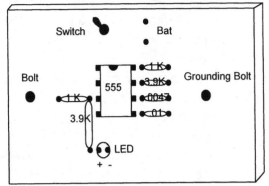

8. Near the top pierce a hole for the toggle switch. Enlarge it until the shaft fits through from the inside. Remove nut and washer from switch before mounting. You may need to trim away some paper with a serrated knife before replacing washer and nut on the outside. Tighten.

9. Next to the switch pierce two holes for the wires from the battery holder and poke them through. Attach the battery and tape it to the outside.

NOW TO CONNECT EVERYTHING

First, make holes at the corners of the lid with a pencil. Slit each corner to the hole. They will accommodate extra loops of wire that you get from using the clip leads to make connections. After each connection gently tuck away the excess wire.

1. Twist the free ends of the two capacitors (.01 and .0047) together. Connect this to the grounding bolt using an alligator clip.

2. Bend the top ends of pin 2 and pin 6 (which already has a connection) inward towards each other in an L shape. Catch them both with a alligator clip and attach the other end of the alligator clip to the free end of the 3.9KΩ resistor by pin 7.

3. Using an alligator clip connect pin 7 to the free end of the 1KΩ resistor attached to pin 8.

4. Using two microclips connect pin 8 to one end of the switch, and pin 4 to the same end of the switch. (Put one hook inside the hole and the other hook around the whole connection. Check to make sure they are securely connected.)

5. Use an alligator clip to connect the free end of the other 1KΩ resistor (by pin 3) to the bolt.

6. Twist the free end of the 3.9KΩ resistor around the plus end of the LED. Connect the minus end of the LED to the grounding bolt using an alligator clip.

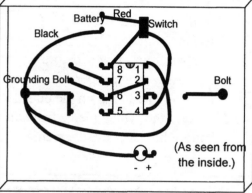

7. Connect pin number 1 on the chip to the grounding bolt with an alligator clip.

8. Attach an alligator clip to the outside of one of the bolts. Attach the other end to a handhold (copper pipe). Do the same for the other bolt and handhold.

9. Connect the minus end of the battery (black wire) to the grounding bolt with an alligator clip.

10. Connect the plus end of the battery (red wire) to the free end of the switch using a microclip lead. If the LED lights up you know the switch is ON. If it does not, flip the switch and see if the LED lights. Label the switch clearly. If you cannot get the LED to light in either switch position, you must double-check all of your connections, and make sure you have a fresh battery.

11. Finally replace the lid on the box, loosely, and slip a couple of rubber bands around the box to keep it securely shut.

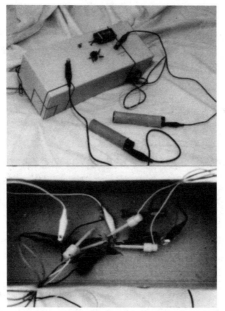

Fig. 4 Finished zapper, outside and inside.

- Optional: measure the frequency of your zapper by connecting an oscilloscope or frequency counter to the handholds. Any electronics shop can do this. It should read between 20 and 40 kHz.
- Optional: measure the voltage output by connecting it to an oscilloscope. It should be about 8 to 9 volts. **Note: a voltage meter will only read 4 to 5 volts.**
- Optional: measure the current that flows through you when you are getting zapped. You will need a 1 KΩ resistor and oscilloscope. Connect the grounding bolt on the zapper to one end of the resistor. Connect the other end of the resistor to a handhold. (Adding this resistor to the circuit decreases the current slightly, but not significantly.)

The other handhold is attached to the other bolt. Connect the scope ground wire to one end of the resistor. Connect the scope probe to the other end of the resistor. Turn the zapper ON and grasp the handholds. Read the voltage on the scope. It will read about 3.5 volts. Calculate current by dividing voltage by resistance. 3.5 volts divided by 1 KΩ is 3.5 ma (milliamperes).

Using The Zapper

1. Wrap handholds in one layer of wet paper towel before using. Grasp securely and turn the switch on to zap.
2. Zap for 7 minutes, let go of the handholds, turn off the zapper, and rest for 20 minutes. Then 7 minutes on, 20 minutes rest, and a final 7 minutes on.

Trying the zapper on an illness to see "if it works" is not useful. Your symptoms may be due to a non-parasite. Or you may reinfect within hours of zapping. The best way to test your device is to find a few invaders that you currently have (see Lesson Twelve, page 492, or Lesson Twenty Seven, page 509). This gives you a starting point. Then zap yourself. After the triple zapping, none of these invaders should be present.

Simple Pulser

If you are ill or want a reliable zapping, make the first model. However, there is another way to make a zapper if you can not afford to build the first model.

An ordinary battery is a source of positive voltage. It is the positive voltage that eliminates so many parasites at once, not a specific frequency. So although the zapper's frequency is about 30 kHz (thirty thousand "zaps" per second), even 5 Hz (five "zaps" per second), **about as fast as you can tap the battery with your hand, is moderately effective!**

You must be connected to both terminals. One will be marked + (positive) and the other − (negative). If you simply touch these terminals with your wet fingers, nothing much happens. That is because your resistance to the current starts going up right away, so less and less current passes through you.

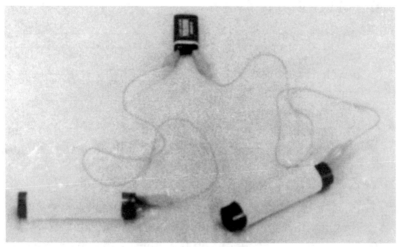

Fig. 5 Simple pulser.

However if you <u>tap</u> the positive terminal with your wet hand, and tap it at a fairly high rate, your body's capacitors come into play. Capacitors only take part in the flow of electricity when they are charged and discharged. Tapping the terminal starts and stops the voltage so capacitors charge and discharge. This kind of resistance to current flow is much smaller.

The faster you tap, the greater the frequency of current pulses and the lower this kind of resistance becomes. Now you can have a considerable sustained current flow through your body.

If you can tap even twice per second (2 Hz) for ten minutes without interruption you can give yourself a zapping that is moderately effective. Remember to take an intermission of twenty minutes and then repeat to avoid catching new viruses. After a second twenty minute intermission repeat zapping a third time.

Using The Simple Pulser

1. Wrap each handhold with one layer of wet paper towel. Place each on a non-conductive surface, like a plastic bag.

9 volt battery
2 short (12") alligator clip leads (from any electronics shop)
2 copper pipes, ¾" diameter, 4" long (from a hardware store)

2. Connect the positive battery terminal to one handhold and the negative terminal to the other handhold using alligator clip leads.
3. Don't let the handholds touch.
4. Place a clock in front of you to time yourself.
5. Pick up the right handhold with your right hand.
6. Leave the left handhold on the table. Tap it with your left hand, preferably the fleshy part of the palm. You may brace yourself with your fingers on the plastic. Keep up a steady pace as fast as you are able.
7. When you get tired pick up the left handhold with your left hand and tap with your right hand. Keep changing off with the least interruption.
8. Repeat a second time 20 minutes later, and a third time 20 minutes after that.

A single 9 volt battery will wear out rather quickly used this way. Put two together, in parallel, for longer lasting power. This requires two more short alligator clips. Connect positive terminals of the batteries to each other, and the negatives also.

Parasites & Pollution

The word "parasites" is used in two senses. Everything living on you or in you, not just to perch, but to take its food from you is a *parasite*. No matter what its size, it can be called a parasite.

But in some way the big worms need to be distinguished from the medium-sized amoebae, the even smaller bacteria and the smallest of all—viruses. So often the term parasite is reserved for the bigger things, from amoebae on up. In this book, the word parasite will be used in both ways as usual. You can easily guess what is meant.

Parasitic worms are divided into *roundworms* and *flatworms*. Roundworms are round like earthworms even though they may be as thin as hairs (threadworms, *filaria*) or microscopically small (like *Trichinella*). Flatworms are more like leeches. They have a way to attach themselves sometimes with the head (*scolex*) like *tapeworms,* sometimes with a special sucker like *flukes.*

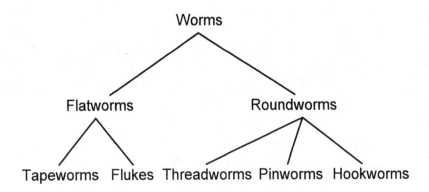

Worm parasites go through stages of development that can look very, very different from the adult.

Roundworms like *Ascaris* (common cat and dog round-worm), are simplest. The **eggs** are swallowed by licking or eating a bit of filth. They hatch into a tiny **larva**. The larva treks to the lungs. You cough it up and swallow it. Meanwhile it has molted a few times. It then crawls to the intestine where it becomes an adult, shedding eggs in your stool.

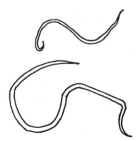

Fig. 6 Ascaris.

Worms usually have preferred locations. The favorite organ for *Dirofilaria* (dog heartworm) is the heart (even human heart). Sometimes the rules can be broken. My tests show *Dirofilaria* can live in other organs, too, if they are sufficiently polluted with solvents, metals and other toxins.

Flatworms like **tapeworms** are much more complicated in their life history. You could eat the eggs accidentally with dirt. After hatching, the tiny larva burrows into its favorite organ. Your body encases it with a cyst. The white blood cells have been taught never to attack your body...and the cyst case is your body! So the tapeworm stage has safe residence for some time. If you are a meat eater, you could eat such a cyst if it happens to be lodged in the meat you are eating! Your teeth break it apart as you crunch. The little larva is swallowed and tries to attach itself to your intestine with its head. Then it grows longer by making segment after segment. The segments with their eggs leave with the bowel contents. I often see dog tapeworm of the small variety in their human family.

Flatworms like **flukes** are also very complicated. The eggs, passed out with bowel contents were not meant to be eaten as such. They were meant to hatch in a pond where snails and minnows eat them. The larva grows up in these new

32

"secondary" hosts. Later, the snail sheds them and they attach themselves to foliage near the pond. They over-winter in a tough *metacercarial* cyst. An unsuspecting browsing animal now eats them. They come out of their metacercarial cyst as a small adult and quickly attach themselves to the intestine with a sucker. They now have "safe haven" and can go about maturing and laying eggs.

Four common flukes are: **human intestinal fluke, human liver fluke, sheep liver fluke, pancreatic fluke of cattle.** Don't let the terms <u>sheep</u> and <u>cattle</u> mislead you. They are all found in humans.

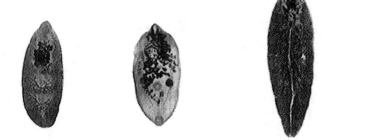

Fig. 7 (L to R) Human intestinal fluke, pancreatic fluke, sheep liver fluke, and human liver fluke.

The Worst Parasite

Fasciolopsis buskii is the fluke (flatworm) that I find in <u>every</u> case of cancer, HIV infection, Alzheimer's, Crohn's disease, Kaposi's, endometriosis, and in many people without these diseases. Its life cycle involves <u>six</u> different stages:

Stage	Normal Life Cycle	
1 Egg	Expelled with bowel movement onto soil. Washed by rain into ponds.	
2 Miracidia	Hatches from egg in water. Has cilia, can swim vigorously and must find intermediate snail host in one to two hours or may be too exhausted to invade.	
3 Redia	Develop inside miracidia as little balls until expelled. Those are "mother" redia, and each one bears "daughter" redia for up to 8 months, all still inside the snail, and living on the fluids in the lymphatic spaces. Similarly, daughter redia are continually developing cercaria.	
4 Cercaria	Have a tail, use it to exit from snail and swim to a plant. If the snail is feeding on a plant, cercaria can latch onto plant with sucker mouth and start to encyst (form a "cocoon") within minutes. Tail breaks off and swims away to dissolve.	
5 Metacercaria	Two-walled cyst. The outer wall is very sticky. But as you eat the plant it is stuck to, the least pressure will break it, leaving the cyst in the mouth. The "almost unbreakable" inner cyst wall protects it from chewing, and the keratin-like coat prevents digestion by stomach juices. However when it reaches the duodenum, contact with intestinal juices dissolves away the cyst-wall and frees it. It then fastens itself to the intestinal lining and begins to develop into an adult.	

6 Adult	Lives in your intestine and can pro-duce 1000 eggs per bowel movement and live many <u>years</u>.	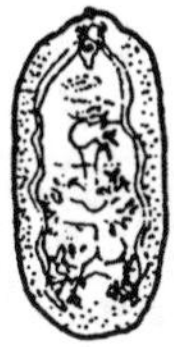

Fig. 8 Fasciolopsis' normal life cycle.

Note that the adult is the <u>only</u> stage that "normally" lives in the human (and then only in the intestine). *Fasciolopsis* depends on a snail, called a *secondary host*, for part of its life cycle. **But when your body has solvents in it, the other five stages can develop in you!**

If **propyl alcohol** is the solvent, the intestinal fluke is invited to use another organ as a secondary host—this organ will become cancerous. If **benzene** is the solvent, the intestinal fluke uses the thymus for its secondary host, setting the stage for AIDS. **Wood alcohol** invites pancreatic flukes to use the pancreas as a secondary host. This leads to pancreatic dysfunction which we call *diabetes*. If **xylene** (or **toluene**) are the solvents, I typically see any of four flukes using the brain as a secondary host. If **methyl ethyl ketone** (MEK) or **methyl butyl ketone** (MBK) are the solvents, the uterus becomes a secondary host and endometriosis a likely result.

This is a new kind of parasitism, based on pollution. I call the diseases caused by fluke stages in inappropriate locations **Fluke Disease**; it is discussed in more detail later (page 249).

Are tapeworms and roundworms affected by solvents this way, too? This is a fascinating and very important question. Search for the answer and help others search for the answer. I do not know yet.

Pollution

Pollutants are all the dead things around us that should not get into your body because they interfere with its work. As long as they don't penetrate your tissues, they won't interfere, like plastic eyeglasses and clothing. But if they are invasive, your body must fight to remove them.

Pollutants can invade your body via the air you breath, the foods and beverages you eat, and the products you put on your skin.

> **The biggest tragedy is not recognizing when a pollutant is harming you.**

Two people can use the same face cream. One develops a rash, the other does not. The one who did not assumes the cream is not harmful to them...that they are like a bank vault, impregnable to that product. A better assumption is that the face cream is somewhat toxic, as evidenced by the rash that can develop, and they escaped the rash only because they had a stronger immune system. The immune system is like money, paid out of the bank vault, for every toxic invasion. When the money is gone, the bank (your health) fails.

Solvent Pollution

Solvents are compounds that dissolve things. Water is a useful, life giving solvent. Most other solvents dissolve fats and are life threatening, because fats form the membrane wall around each of our cells, especially our nerve cells.

The solvent that does the most harm is **benzene**. It goes to the thymus, ruins our immune system, and causes AIDS. The next worst solvent is **propyl alcohol**. It goes to the liver and causes cancer in some distant organ. Other major culprits of disease are **xylene, toluene, wood alcohol, methylene chloride,** and **trichloroethane** (TCE). I'll discuss each one later, with the ailment it's associated with.

Metal Pollution

Biochemists know that a mineral in raw element form always inhibits the enzyme using that mineral. Copper from the meat and vegetables you eat is essential. Inorganic copper, like you would get from a copper bottomed kettle or copper plumbing, is carcinogenic[3]. Unfortunately, the inorganic form of metals is what pervades our environment. We put metal jewelry on our skin, eat bread baked in metal pans, and drink water from metal plumbing.

Another obvious metallic threat is tooth fillings. **Mercury amalgam fillings**, despite the assurances of the American Dental Association, are <u>not</u> safe. And sometimes the mercury is polluted with **thallium**, even more toxic than mercury! **Gold** and **silver** seem to have fewer harmful effects, but <u>no one should have any pure metal in or on their body.</u>

Other prevalent toxic metals include **lead** and **cadmium** from soldered and galvanized plumbing, **nickel** and **chromium** from dentalware and cosmetics, and **aluminum** from food and drink cans, and cooking pots.

---

[3]Haleem J. Issaq, <u>The Role of Metals in Tumor Development and Inhibition</u>. From *Carcinogenicity and Metal Ions*, volume 10, page 61, of a series called *Metal Ions in Biological Systems*, edited by Helmut Sigel, 1980.

Mycotoxins

Molds produce some of the most toxic substances known, called *mycotoxins*. One small moldy fruit or vegetable can pollute a huge batch of juice, jam or other product. Although molds are alive, and can be killed by zapping, mycotoxins are not, and must be detoxified by your liver.

But because mycotoxins are so extremely poisonous, a tiny amount can incapacitate a part of the liver for days!

Aflatoxin is the most common mycotoxin I detect. It is produced by molds that grow on quite a variety of plants. For that reason I am always cautioning people to eat only perfect citrus fruit, and never drink commercial fruit juice. Of the thousands of oranges that go into the batch of orange juice you drink, one is sure to be moldy, and that is all it takes to give your liver a setback.

A heavy dose of vitamin C helps the liver recover quickly. It also helps get rid of aflatoxin <u>before</u> it is consumed, right in the food container. So keep a plastic shaker of vitamin C powder handy and use it like salt on all your food.

There are thirteen other mycotoxins I have searched for in our foods. They are described in the section on moldy food (page 381).

Physical Toxins

Breathing in dust is quite bad for you so your body rejects it by sneezing, coughing, spitting up and out. Imagine breathing in broken glass particles. They cut into the lungs in a thousand places and couldn't be coughed up. They would travel. Imagine swallowing a needle or open pin. If the tip was blunt it could move through the intestine. But because it is sharp it gets caught in your tissue, then works its way deeper and deeper.

Would we ever knowingly breathe in broken glass? We are justifiably afraid of it in our food or under our bare feet. We are unaware that it fills our homes when **fiberglass** insulation is left imperfectly sealed off. Any hole made through the ceiling or wall, even if covered with cloth, lets swarms of broken glass bits into the house air. Air currents flow inward, into your living space. So all holes leading to the attic or insulated spaces must be sealed airtight. Of course, fiberglass should never be used in home construction, draperies, or around water heaters. The best advice is to have it all removed while you are away and then vacuum and dust.

Occasional exposures by house builders working outdoors does much less harm. Chronic exposure from a single small hole in the ceiling does a lot of harm, leading to cyst formation. And that cyst is a perfect place for parasites and bacteria to settle and multiply. When the intestinal fluke settles there it becomes malignant!

Cancer patients with *solid tumors* have either fiberglass or asbestos in them.

Asbestos is another tiny bit, sharp as glass, that moves through your body like a swordfish, impaling your cells until it, too, gets routed into a cyst.

We have been led to believe that we no longer have asbestos in our homes because we have outlawed the fireproofing materials it was used in. While that may be true, the source I find most often is all too prevalent: the clothes dryer belt. As it gets hot the belt releases a blast of asbestos particles that are forced through the seams of your dryer, and also openings in your exhaust hose, by the high pressure formed inside. It is now in your air.

Chemical Toxins

Chlorofluorocarbons (CFCs) or **freon** is the refrigerant in your air conditioner and refrigerator coils. CFCs are suspected of causing the ozone hole above the South Pole. All cancer sufferers test positive for CFCs in their cancerous organ! I have preliminary evidence that it is CFCs that attract other pollutants–fiberglass, metals, PCBs–to form a growing tumor instead of allowing their excretion. This would make it a "super carcinogen.". How could you detect CFCs leaking in your home? By the time your air conditioner or refrigerator needs recharging, you have been exposed for a long time. We desperately need an inexpensive, in-home test for this unsuspected killer.

Arsenic is used in pesticide. Why would we poison ourselves along with the cockroaches? Is it because we can't see it happening? Just as we couldn't see the fiberglass floating in the air? Our diligent scientists have studied the mechanism of arsenic poisoning in great detail. Then why are we allowed to put it on our lawns to be carried into our carpets via shoes?

Polychlorinated biphenyls (PCBs), oily compounds with wonderfully useful electrical properties, were originally used in transformers until their inability to break down into less toxic substances in our environment was spotlighted. Banned from use, I find them in most commercial soap and detergents! Is transformer oil being disposed of by selling it to soap makers?

Formaldehyde is used to cure foam. As a result, foam furniture, pillows and mattresses give off formaldehyde for about two years after manufacturing. If you sleep with your nose buried in a new foam pillow all night, you are risking major lung problems.

Every cleanser in your house probably has a toxic warning on its label. Every fluid your automobile uses is toxic. Every pesticide, herbicide and fertilizer you put on your lawn is probably toxic. Every paint, varnish, wax, lubricant, bleach and detergent will send you to the hospital if even a small amount is ingested. Why do we keep them around? See *Recipes* (page 513) for safe, old-fashioned, alternatives.

If you are ill even after zapping, it is toxins still at work. Getting rid of them is a major step toward being well.

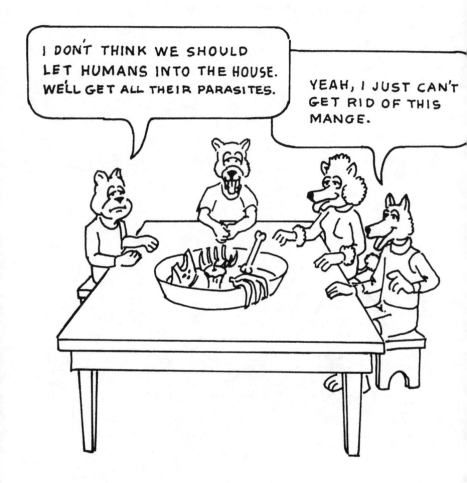

How We Really Get Sick

What if you invented a device that could search people for the presence of mycotoxins (extremely toxic substances made by food molds)? And what if you found that although many people had them, those who were sick with a cold <u>always</u> had at least one of them. Would you ask whether a sudden buildup of mycotoxins is what really lets colds develop? Why do some people in the same family get the cold while others do not?

- What if you found everyone with **cancer** had the human intestinal fluke in their liver, and no one else did?
- What if you found everyone with **diabetes** had the pancreatic fluke of cattle in their pancreas, and few others did?
- What if you found everyone with **environmental illness** tested positive for *Fasciola* (sheep liver fluke) in their liver?
- What if you found everyone with **asthma** tested positive for *Ascaris* in their lungs?

What if you <u>always</u> found <u>every</u> mysteriously ill person had some unsuspected <u>parasite</u> or <u>pollutant</u>?

The device is the Syncrometer™, and these "what ifs" are all true. They forced me to alter my entire outlook on what really causes some of our "incurable", mysterious diseases.

We used to believe that diabetes was caused by over consumption of sugars, a cold by a virus you caught from somebody, cancer from carcinogen exposure, depression from poor parenting. This multicausal concept is what made the study of medicine so difficult that only a few could undertake it. And every year new syndromes are added to the list of human illnesses.

But these diagnoses are based on a description of what is happening at a particular place in your body. This is like calling a mosquito bite behind the ears by one name and a mosquito bite behind the knee by another name. If you never see the true cause, a mosquito at work, this system could be excused as somewhat sensible.

And, until now, the profession of medicine has made some sense. The new truths, however, make the old descriptive system obsolete. You can now find the true causes of all your illnesses. And you can find them yourself by building the electronic diagnostic circuit (page 457)!

Once you have seen a mosquito at work on your body you no longer need to go to the doctor for a red, itchy bump. You don't need to search for the correct diagnosis and an appropriate drug. **You put up screen doors and windows!**

Once you have seen how common house dust is implicated in the common cold you get rid of the house dust. Once you have seen the mold in your food facilitate the cold virus you throw out that moldy food. But only seeing is believing. Nothing is left to faith. The electronic resonance method described in this book will let you see all these things for yourself.

You are not a hapless pawn attacked by bacteria and viruses that dart at you from nowhere to make you ill. You are not at the mercy of diseases all around you, hoping, by chance, to escape, like a soldier hoping to come home from the war. Nature and your body make good sense.

There is no disease that can outwit you if you know enough about it. Not even Lou Gehrig's disease! Nor asthma or diabetes. Read how the people in the case histories made themselves well. Read why some people failed. You have an advantage they did not have. Their instructions were hard to carry out because they had to have <u>faith</u> in them. You don't. You can replace <u>faith</u> with your own hard headed observations by building the diagnostic circuit (Syncrometer). The great convincer is seeing it yourself. When you personally find the mold in your peanut butter, or *Shigella* in your cheese, you have the knowledge, not faith, that convinces and guides you.

All illness comes from two causes, PARASITES and POLLUTANTS.

Only two causes! This is what simplifies the picture to make it possible for you to cure yourself.

We have been taught that illness is largely our own fault. That it is due to "catching something", not eating what we should, like roughage or vitamins, or not doing what we should, like dressing properly, exercising or going to bed on time. Somehow, it's our own fault. Either by doing something we shouldn't or not doing something we should. When absolutely no fault can be found we are told it's in our genes! True inherited diseases are extremely rare. Our genes have evolved over millions of years to produce healthy humans. Nor are genes that mutate during your lifetime at fault. Pollutants, which are known to be mutagens, are the real culprits.

Neither the parasites nor the pollutants in you are "your fault". Notice that other people all around us are doing the same things or not doing the same things, and even share our genes <u>and don't have our illness</u>. The current concepts on disease causation blaming our actions and our genes are simply not logical.

But until now they appeared logical. Suppose 1000 people were bitten by a mosquito or flea, it would always be in a dif-

45

ferent place, and if you were using the <u>location and effect system</u> to diagnose the problem you could have a thousand diagnoses listed for them, including a defective gene. Could you be persuaded to accept a gene replacement for your red itchy bumps? The new gene might be for antihistamine production so the welts don't become large, red and hot, or lead to impetigo. If you were the research doctor, you might be tempted to alleviate a thousand persons' distress with a new gene. Fortunately, you are not and only need to solve your own problems. You can be more logical.

After you have found the parasite interlopers hiding in your body you can kill them electronically. And after you have identified the pollutants stuck in your organs you can stop eating them, breathing them or putting them on yourself. In response, your body will begin to heal, just as surely as a mosquito bite heals.

Heal from multiple sclerosis, emphysema, myasthenia? Yes!! Some healing will be swift. Some healing will be slow. Healing is not understood. It is much faster in young persons. But fast or slow you know it has begun. It will be an exciting adventure to watch yourself lose your symptoms and get stronger.

Self Health

The entire purpose of this book is to enable you to diagnose and treat <u>yourself</u> for any disease. You have three new approaches that make this wish a reality: the understanding that only pollution and parasites make you sick, the quick and inexpensive diagnostic circuit that lets you find which pollutants and parasites they are, and the zapper or herbal recipe that kills the parasites.

Wouldn't it be nice not to have to go to the doctor for your aches and pains? And not to be dependent on the doctor to diagnose and treat you?

Self health means <u>keeping yourself healthy</u>. Doing it **yourself**.

Suppose your doctor has already diagnosed you as having "Atypical Lateral Sclerosis" or "Shoulder-Hip Girdle Metastable Aplasia." Could you re-diagnose this for yourself so as to treat and cure it? And be successful? Why not? You have already succeeded in many enterprises. You learned to talk, walk, read, get along with people. These skills took a few years to master. Learning to keep well is a new skill. It may take a few years too. After you have learned these skills you may pass them on to your children. And so a new gift is given to humanity, like the gift of music or the art of cooking.

How To Heal

Your body has been trying to rid itself of its parasites and pollutants all your life! It had its own ways. It made stones, it made mucus secretions, it made itself toxic dumpsites. These were good tactics but now of course, they are no longer necessary. Can you help your body get rid of these accumulations and sweep itself clean again?

Sweeping your liver clean is the most powerful way of helping your body to heal itself after the parasites are gone. There are thousands of bits of "trash" accumulated in the liver bile ducts. They will turn into stones (gallstones) if left in place.

The kidney, too, has made numerous small stones in its effort to keep your body clear of lead, cadmium, mercury and other impassable pollutants. You can assist the kidney to expel all these.

In days, not weeks or months, you can feel the healing effects of clearing gallstones and kidney stones from your body. But there are miles of bile ducts (50,000 ducts) in the liver; the herbal recipes that do this are used over and over, patiently, until all the "trash" is removed. This can take several years.

So, although you can stop your disease very quickly from progressing, the healing process may not be complete for years.

Nevertheless, you are healthy again. This means your pains are either gone or greatly reduced. Your organs are functioning better. You have a new sense of well being. Your energy is up. Your desire to live and accomplish something is back.

Organs that have been damaged beyond the ability of our simple methods to reverse can be treated with the magic of modern surgery. Cataracts, bunions, old injuries are examples. Possibly, these too, are "stone" formations. But no recipe has been found to clear them up simply and in a useful time frame.

Killing parasites, removing pollutants and clearing gallstones and kidney stones from your body is a powerful combination of treatments. It is so powerful you can change yourself into a new person in half a year. And then go on improving for years more.

Should you stop taking your prescription medicine while you are treating yourself? NO. Wait until you have cured yourself of the condition that required the medicine. Reduce your medicine and eventually go off it. Will your doctor approve? Find one that will. Remember that the medicine is buying you the time to cure yourself, something to be grateful for.

The Road To Wellness

To review our new understanding of health vs. disease:

- We have only two problems: parasites and pollutants. Parasites are things that live on us, using up our food and giving us their wastes. Pollutants are toxic things in us making it difficult for our organs to do their work. These two things are responsible for all our other problems.

- Our bodies have been trying to rid us of these by making stones, making secretions, giving us swellings, inflammations and benign tumors. We develop deficiencies and disabilities.

- Finally, some permanent damage is done. Our hair turns gray, we develop cataracts, the spine bends, nerves and muscles die. We weaken.

Our strategy to undo all this will be a logical one.

First, we will kill all parasites, bacteria, viruses and fungi.

Second, we will remove the toxic molds, metals and chemicals in our foods and body products.

Third, we will clear away and wash away the stones, secretions and debris already formed, that hinder healing.

Fourth, we will use herbs and special food factors to hasten healing, being very careful to use pure products. (These act more quickly when given intravenously but the emphasis in this book will be on oral consumption.)

Finally, for repairs that are beyond our abilities, we will seek help from health and medical professionals.

What could be more exciting than finding the tremor is out of your arm or the pain is out of your shoulder? Won't it be admirable to correct your pulse and your high blood pressure, by yourself? What an adventure it could be to get rid of all your warts.

But getting rid of pain seems like a first priority to me, since pain often undermines our morale, our initiative to do things, even our interest in getting well!

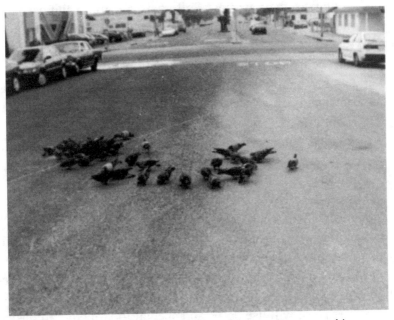

Many of our illnesses are caused by unsuspected sources. I have found pigeon tapeworm in humans, for instance.
Fig. 9 Feed animals out of your yard and away from where children play. Their wastes contain pathogens.

Pain From Toe To Head

I would rather die than endure excruciating, unrelievable pain. That puts **pain** at the very top of my priority list.

Fortunately for us, pain killers are at hand to get us through it and buy us the time it takes to solve the real problem behind it.

The pain killing industry also brought us the addiction industry. As we turn to electrical pain killing the need for addicting drugs should decline. There are other very useful pain killers: acupuncture, massage, listening to music, feedback devices, contemplation, hypnotism, and prayer.

But we will focus on getting rid of the <u>cause of pain</u> and healing the organs that are in pain so none of these methods are needed.

I am not talking about the pain of a broken bone, twisted ankle, bee sting or sunburn. I am not talking about the pain of a misaligned vertebra or stretch trauma in your leg muscles or arm muscles. I am referring to pain that is in one of your organs and refuses to go away. For example, arthritis. Other pains are headache, foot pain, elbow pain, hip pain, chest pain. All of these may have special names like rheumatoid arthritis, cluster headache, fibromyalgia, bursitis, tennis elbow and so on, but they are all the same phenomenon.

Knowing that parasites and pollutants are the real culprits, let us get right down to the job of finding out which they are, where they come from, and how to get rid of them.

The parasites that cause pain are not the large ones, like worms or amoebas. Nor are they the very tiny viruses. They are *bacteria*. Bacteria are the right size to get into the doorways of our cells. Our cells try to keep their doorways tight-shut but, of course, they have to open to let food in, or hormones, or other life-signals. If bacteria are swarming around the outside of cells, some will manage to slip into a doorway while it is open. A battle begins. The cells refuse to let the bacteria in. The bacteria refuse to let go of the door latch. There is probably a specific electrical attraction between them and an exact physical fit. The body's extra forces, the immune system, are called in to help quell the invasion. The bacteria multiply as fast as they can. There is swelling. There is heat produced. There is pressure against other organs. All together it is called inflammation and infection.

The answer is not to deinflame with drugs (like the cortisone variety). The answer is not to reduce swelling or body temperature. **The answer is certainly not pain killer.** The answer is to kill the bacteria. (Even this is not the <u>ultimate</u> answer. We must stop the <u>source</u> of the bacteria and your body's <u>invitation</u> to be <u>invaded</u>. We will get to this later.)

So **Step One** is to search for the bacteria nibbling at our painful regions and identify them. This gives us the clue to finding their source. **Step Two** is to exterminate them electrically. Within minutes they fall out of the doorways to our cells. Your white blood cells are waiting for them, and will gobble them up in a grand feast.

But, remember, there is another cause of pain, pollutants. **Step Three** is to find the pollutants and identify them because this gives us a clue as to <u>their</u> source. **Step Four** is to eliminate our pollution sources. **And the job is done. Pain is gone.**

An intriguing question will pop into your head as you search your organs for parasites and pollutants. Which came first? Pollutants can jam their way into your cell's doorways too. Does this allow the bacteria to swim in? Or do the bacteria come first, jamming open the doorways so the pollutants can enter? Both seem possible. Maybe both events go on simultaneously. Perhaps that is why bacteria and pollutants are <u>always</u> seen together. Viruses can land on your cell's doorways, too, and cause viral diseases, but they are not as often pain producing.

You will also notice something, as you keep testing and watching over your health. **Your body is very good at killing bacteria and viruses.** Your body kills them faster than a wave of a magic wand! The only ones that get away are those that are stuck in doorways and channels with pollutants in them! This seems like evidence that pollutants do the gate-opening. But it isn't proof and we must keep all possibilities in mind.

Fortunately we do not have to know exactly how parasites and pollution make us sick in order to get well.

Searching For Bacteria

In order to find which organs have the bacteria and which bacteria are present you will need to learn the new technology that makes all of this possible. This technology is a simple electronic circuit that is capable of trapping frequencies in such a way that you can hear them. Your body's frequencies, the frequencies of bacteria, viruses and parasites are all different and can be heard as distinctly as a **mooo**, **baah**, **tweet**, or **oink** coming from a farm yard.

But do you have to do all that?

No! You don't. You could simply electrocute all these tiny invaders. But how would you know what to avoid in the future? If your pain returned how would you know if it was the same old bacteria or a new one?

Learning to test takes the guesswork out of diagnosis.

My hope is that you will find it all so intriguing, so absolutely fascinating, that in spite of some chronic pain, you will feel compelled to make the searches yourself. Find someone willing to help. Trade your information. It is less difficult than learning to use a computer.

What You Will Find

First we will study and cure pains of all kinds, starting with the toes and working our way up the body. We don't need to be very specific about the location of the pain since bacteria and toxins flow over to nearby locations anyway.

For each kind of pain, we will look into the causes so you can eliminate them. Pain could come back in an hour if you didn't know the bacteria were coming from cheese and you had a cheese sandwich after *zapping* (killing parasites electrically). In fact, the pain may not have had time to go away before the next onslaught begins and you might conclude, wrongly, that this method doesn't work.

Parasites might also come back to your specially painful place from a few far away places that are hard to reach by your zapper's electrical current. The inside of your eyeball, the testicle, the interior of gallstones, the middle of a tooth abscess or the bowel contents are such places. Your zapper current, because it is high frequency, prefers to "go around" these items, rather than through them. But with repeated zapping, and herbal parasite treatment, you can decimate them, too, and stop reinfecting the rest of your body.

In fact, it is such knowledge about reinfection and sources of our pollutants that is the most important contribution of the case histories.

After dealing with pains we will turn our attention to the diseases that aren't pain producing, like diabetes, myasthenia gravis, and so on.

Toe Pain

The ends of your feet get the poorest "service" from your blood supply. They are the furthest away. The blood here has the most accumulated acid and the least oxygen supply. The body produces quite a bit of *uric acid* and this should, of course, be excreted into the bladder by the kidneys. But if the kidneys are doing a poor job of this, levels in the body and blood stream rise. The blood can only hold so much. It holds even less in acid conditions such as the ends of your feet experience. Uric acid begins to settle out or <u>precipitate</u> at our feet.

Hippuric acid, too, is found where pain is found. Hippuric acid is made in large amounts (about 1 gram/day) by the liver because it is a detoxification product. It makes no sense to consume *benzoic acid*, the common preservative, since this is what the body detoxifies into hippuric acid. Read all labels on food you buy. Don't buy any beverages or baked goods preserved with benzoic acid. *Citric acid* is fine. The joints of the big toes are favorite places for pain to develop. This is made even worse when circulation is poor. <u>Take a *cayenne* capsule with each meal to improve circulation.</u> If you cannot find your pulse just below your inner ankle your circulation is poor.

The accumulation of uric and hippuric acid invites bacteria to feed on them. As bacteria multiply the tissue fights back with

inflammation. Now the stage has been set for **pain**. Some people do not have pain although these acids and other deposits are present making their joints knobby and unbending. Bacteria have not found them yet or haven't multiplied sufficiently in them to invade your tissues. Perhaps there are other reasons as well.

If you have **toe pain** your course of action is this:

1. Kill all bacteria possible with your zapper. Repeat daily until no further benefit is seen.
2. Dissolve the deposits away. An herbal recipe, quite elaborate, is capable of doing this. It is called the Kidney Cleanse (page 549). Toe deposits are made of the same crystals as kidney stones, which is why the Kidney Cleanse works for toe pain. But because these deposits are far away from the kidney, it takes longer than merely cleaning up kidneys. It may take six months to make a significant dent on these deposits. This will at the same time remove kidney crystals so that these are no longer a source of bacteria.
3. Get teeth cavitations cleaned (cavitations are bone infections in the jaw where a tooth was pulled; it never healed; see Dental Cleanup page 409). This can "magically" stop the toe pain the same day as they are cleaned. The effect lasts for days afterward showing it is not the dental anesthetic that is responsible. It also teaches you that the bacteria in the toes can come from the teeth. But pain may return as other bacteria find the deposits.
4. Clean the liver of stones using the Liver Cleanse (page 552). This, too, can give immediate pain relief in the toes showing you they are a source for bacteria. Liver cleaning may take you two years to complete! Meanwhile your toe pain is receding. And, of course, this pays extra dividends in health for your body.

5. Reduce the acidity in your toes. First, check your acidity with pH paper meant for testing urinary pH, called Nitrazine™ paper. Ordinary pH paper, as for fish tanks, is almost as accurate and will serve as well. Tear a ½ inch piece and hold it in the urine stream. Early morning is the time your urine is most acid. If this reads below 5.5 your feet must have been even lower in the night (lower is more acid).

Once deposits start, it is hard to stop them. If they start forming at 2 a.m., they are likely to continue for several hours even if the pH goes back up to normal. Your tactic will be to <u>go to bed with an alkalizing action</u>. Taking a calcium and magnesium supplement at bedtime, drinking milk at bedtime, using baking soda at bedtime are all remedies to be tried. They should raise your urinary pH to 6 in the morning.

Balance Your pH

Most persons with painful deposits anywhere in their feet have a morning urine pH of 4.5! At 4.5 it is safe to guess that a lot has precipitated again in the night. During the day, your body's pH swings back and forth. The urine gets quite alkaline right after a meal; this is called the *alkaline tide*. Three meals a day would bring you three alkaline tides. During these periods, lasting about an hour, you have an opportunity to dissolve some of your foot deposits. But if you allow your pH to drop too low in the night you put the deposits back again. The net effect decides whether your deposits grow or shrink.

To alkalinize yourself at bedtime, choose one of these options:

1. Two oyster shell tablets, equaling 750 mg. of calcium plus a magnesium oxide tablet, 300 mg (see *Sources*). The magnesium helps the calcium dissolve and stay in solu-

tion. Taking more calcium at one time is not advised because it cannot be dissolved and absorbed anyway and might constipate you. For the elderly only one calcium tablet is advised. Take calcium tablets with vitamin C or lemon water to help dissolve (¼ tsp. vitamin C powder; adding honey is fine).

2. One cup of sterilized milk or buttermilk, drunk hot or cold, plus 1 magnesium oxide tablet, 300 mg. (adding cinnamon is fine).

   If these two remedies work for you, your morning urinary pH will come up to 6.0 but if for some reason they don't, you need to take more drastic measures. Take the supplements and milk earlier in the day and reserve bedtime for:

3. ½ tsp. baking soda in water. This is *sodium bicarbonate*. But don't use baking soda from a store because most brands I have tested are polluted with benzene! (See *Sources* for safe baking soda.) Using a combination of sodium and potassium bicarbonate in a ratio of 2:1 is actually a much more healthful potion. You can make your own or ask a pharmacist to make it for you. Mix two parts baking soda and one part potassium bicarbonate (see *Sources*) in a jar. Keep tightly closed. Label it **sodium potassium bicarbonate alkalizer** (this potion is also very useful in allergic reactions of all kinds). Take 1 level tsp. in water at bedtime. If your pH reaches 6 in the morning continue each night at this dose. If it does not, take 1½ tsp. Keep watching your pH, since it will gradually normalize and you will require less and less. If you are using plain baking soda, instead of the mixture, watch your pH each morning, also, so you can cut back when the pH goes higher than 6.

Persons with a limit on their daily sodium intake must carefully count the grams of baking soda consumed in this way.

Each tsp. weighs about 2 grams, of which half (1 gram or 1000 milligrams) is sodium. The sodium/potassium mixture would only give you half as much sodium (½ gram per tsp.). By comparison, the usual daily intake of sodium is about 5 gm., although salt eaters consume twice that amount.

You have done five things to pull the rug out from under the bacteria living in and around the deposits in your toes. Now when you kill bacteria with your zapper, you can expect the pain to go away and stay away.

Locations at the base of toes may be painful due to a *neuroma*. Deposits and bacteria here are even more painful because this is the location of nerve centers. If the build-up is large, you may prefer some surgical help or a cortisone shot rather than wait several years for solid relief.

Foot Pain

This kind of pain does not involve as much deposits as toe pain and is therefore easier to clear up. But trauma to the foot is more important. First, even though your shoes are comfortable, change them. Get wider shoes, longer shoes, lower heels. Alternate two pairs of shoes in a single day. In your home take shoes off.

Keep feet very warm. Wear natural fiber socks, not synthetics. If your circulation is poor, take a *cayenne* capsule with each meal. When circulation is moderately poor, your feet get cold easily. When circulation is very poor, the heart pulse cannot be felt in your feet (take your pulse just below your inner ankle). Again:

- Get teeth cavitations cleaned (Dental Cleanup, page 409).
- Do the herbal Kidney Cleanse (page 549).
- Kill parasites and bacteria with a zapper.

- Then clean the liver (page 552).
- Check body pH in the morning upon rising using Nitrazine™ or other pH paper. Correct it as discussed in Toe Pain. If the urinary pH is 7 or higher, it means you have a bladder infection. Treat it immediately (page 101).

If there is any swelling around the foot or ankle, you are "holding water." It may be called *edema*. This is due to poor adrenal and kidney function. The adrenals are located on top of the kidneys and together they regulate how much salt and water stays in your body. Because they are situated so close together, they share their parasites and pollution. When the kidneys form *kidney crystals* the flow through the kidney tubes is hindered, and less water and salt can leave the body. It stays in your tissues as edema.

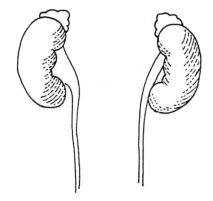

The kidney herb recipe will dissolve the crystals. But you must remove toxins such as metal from tooth fillings and kill parasites. Continue doing the Kidney Cleanse after the original six weeks is up until all foot pain and edema are gone. Continue killing your tiny

Fig. 10 Your kidneys with the adrenal glands sitting like hats on top. The ureters lead to the bladder.

invaders with a zapper twice a week. You may need to cleanse the liver several times, too, before all the pain and edema are gone.

The supplement, *pantothenic acid* (see *Sources*), is particularly good for feet. Take 500 mg three times a day for several weeks to see if it helps. Massage and reflexology are also good for them.

Heel Pain

Sometimes heel pain is due to heel spurs, sometimes it is not. Heel spurs are due to deposits. The usual heel deposits are *uric acid* and various *phosphates*. Uric acid deposits become a breeding ground for bacteria. The phosphates give the deposits a rigid structure that is hard to dissolve. You may have to choose a pain killer, get specially built "orthopedic" shoes, or stop your daily walks to get relief from the piercing pains. These will not cure the problem but may "buy you some time" while you make basic changes in your lifestyle.

Stop drinking tea and cocoa because they contain *oxalic acid*. Stop drinking coffee, decafs, fruit juice and soda pop because they are contaminated with solvents. All of these must be detoxified by your body and eliminated by your kidneys. We should spare the kidneys these extra tasks when we wish them to clean up heel spur deposits. You must first dissolve the deposits, then help the kidneys eliminate them.

To dissolve them, you alkalinize your body's pH, watching over it carefully with pH paper or Nitrazine paper. To help kidneys eliminate them, use the Kidney Cleanse and drink <u>lots</u> of water. Only water, not a beverage, helps the kidneys to eliminate.

Drink a pint of water upon rising in the morning, and a pint of water between meals.

Do not buy "special" water. Use your cold tap water only. If you don't like the taste of your own tap water, get it from somebody else's tap. Use only glass or reused polyethylene jugs. Polyethylene is opaque, not clear. It has already lost its plasticizer into the water that stood in it earlier. (Somebody drank it!) Purchased water has traces of solvents from machinery and sterilizing equipment used in its bottling. Your own tap water is not pure (indeed it may have 500 toxic elements), but it never contains solvents in amounts I can detect.

> Traces of solvents are worse than traces of other toxins.

Water filters are not the solution. They trap the pollutants and then allow a tiny amount to enter the water on a daily basis. Chronic toxin consumption is much worse for your health than periodic surges of toxins. You can use a small filter, that gets changed every month without much risk. This would dechlorinate the water, at least, and improve the flavor. The pitcher variety (it should be made of hard, inflexible plastic) and the faucet variety are listed in *Sources*.

Bottled water is popular,

and tasty, and has appealing advertising, but it is just not safe.

Why is it easier for everyone to spend dollars per day, for the rest of their life, buying water instead of insisting that their water pipes are metal-free?

Another reason not to drink water from bottles, however convenient, is that it is stagnant and is soon contaminated with our own bacteria from contact with mouth or hands. *Staphylococcus (Staph)* and *E. coli* are commonly seen. The solution is not to add still more chemical disinfectants, the solution is to drink from a flowing source, such as our faucets. If you must carry water, use glass containers; plastic is porous and much more difficult to wash clean (sterilizing in a dishwasher is effective, though).

By drinking a total of four pints of water in a day, the kidneys will notice the assistance. (Any single herb tea without added salt or sweetener counts as water.) The urine will stop having any odor and will become very light colored. This is especially important while you are dissolving the heel deposits since your body is now carrying these in the circulation.

Killing bacteria with a zapper may give you instant pain relief and is, of course, beneficial to your body. But you can't expect the pain to stay away until the deposits are gone and the source of bacteria is also removed. Go after the usual sources: teeth and stones. Another source is dairy food contaminated with *Salmonella* and *Shigella* bacteria. Sterilize all of it by boiling. Even the amount put on cereal in the morning or used in scrambled eggs is enough to reinfect you! Butter and heavy whipping cream also need boiling. Stop eating yogurt and cheese which can't be boiled.

Phosphate deposits are a mixture of three phosphates: *monocalcium phosphate* ($CaH_2 PO_4$), *dicalcium phosphate* ($Ca_2H PO_4$) and *tricalcium phosphate* ($Ca_3 PO_4$). They are formed by eating too much (way too much) phosphate relative to calcium.

Our high phosphate foods are meats, carbonated beverages and grain products like rice, cereals, breads, pastas and nuts.

The body's normal elimination tactic for phosphate is to combine it with calcium and magnesium in order to neutralize it first. Unneutralized phosphate is very acidic and would burn the delicate kidneys. But where shall the calcium and magnesium be taken from? Magnesium is often in very short supply since it comes from green vegetables in the diet and is not stored up in any special organ. So it falls on calcium to be used for this purpose since it is stored up (in your bones and teeth).

The acid condition created by phosphates dissolves your bones and allows large amounts of bone structure to be washed out with the urine: this can be directly seen with an analysis of urine (you can ask your doctor to order this at a lab). If you catch all the urine in a 24 hour period you can measure all the calcium you have wasted. You should not lose more than 150 mg calcium in a day because this is all you can absorb in a day![4] If you do lose more than 150 mg in a day, you are dissolving your bones at a fast clip. This also means there is too much calcium in your blood and lymph, from dissolving so much bone so quickly.

Once you have dissolved your bones it is not so easy to put the calcium back into them. Your body will try to put it back as soon as possible—as soon as your acid condition is gone. But your bones can't do this without *vitamin D*. Vitamin D may "come from" sunshine and from vitamin D in milk but it isn't that simple. Vitamin D must be <u>activated</u> by your kidneys before it can go to work! Remember, though, it was the kidneys that had a problem in the first place, allowing deposits to form! With old kidneys, clogged with crystals, hampered by heavy metal and mold toxins, and beleaguered by bacteria and parasites, is it any wonder that sunshine and vitamin D fortified milk don't supply large amounts of activated vitamin D? It takes <u>large</u> amounts to put back into your bones the large amount of calcium that dissolved out during the acid state you put yourself in by over consuming phosphate food.

If you can't put the calcium back into your bones promptly where is it to go? It may attach itself to tissues that were never meant to be used this way. Your arteries fill with "scale," your

---

[4]You absorb 5 to 10% of what you eat. If you eat 1 gram (1000 mg) you absorb 50 to 100 mg. But you absorb 25-40% if it comes from milk!

kidneys form calcium phosphate crystals, heels form spurs, joints become knobby with deposits.

Young persons and children, with healthy unclogged kidneys, make–that is, activate–ample vitamin D, so even if they consume too much phosphate and develop an acid condition that dissolves their teeth and bones, **they can put the dissolved calcium back in its proper place.** They don't develop hardened arteries, heel spurs, and knobby joints, at least not at first. Their bodies can take a considerable amount of abuse without showing it.

In general, people eat way too much phosphate. Meat eaters eat too much meat. Vegetarians eat too much grain. Most everyone drinks phosphated beverages. In this way we set the stage for hardened arteries, joint disease, calcified tissues that no longer have flexibility. We all get kidney crystals that become stones. This is *aging.* All these deposits invite bacteria to live in them and on them, creating pain.

Old age and pain go together as if they were true partners. Yet it is just the result of bad food choices.

Try to undo as much of this false aging as possible.

1. Reduce your meat consumption. Switch to fish which supplies calcium in the tiny bones. It is true, these bones are made of calcium phosphate and one might expect, logically, to be getting a less effective calcium source. Logic isn't necessarily biologically correct. The bones of fish work nicely as a calcium source and their phosphate content is not too great. Such a diet has worked for many primitive societies. Further, I have never seen a case of mercury toxicity from eating fish; amalgam tooth fillings are our truly significant source.

2. Reduce your grain consumption. Instead of cereal for breakfast, add fruit and reduce the cereal to half. Cut bread consumption in half. Cut pasta consumption in half. Cut rice and corn consumption in half. Eat more bananas and other fruits. Eat more vegetables; always choose potato (not potato chips) instead of rice or macaroni. Always choose a leafy salad instead of pasta salad. At any restaurant or salad bar ask yourself: is this wheat, rice or corn? If so, choose potatoes or other vegetables. Choose coleslaw. Choose mixed fruit. You don't need to go off the grains, only reduce them to improve your condition.

3. Take vitamin D as a supplement. Nothing less than 40,000 units has any real impact by the time there are problems. This strength is available by prescription only (usually 50,000 units, which is close enough). To avoid getting a polluted product, ask your pharmacist to follow the recipe on page 560. (In the past some cases of poisoning by overdosing resulted in this regulation. If you overdose you will get joint and muscle pain and nausea but it is reversible.) Take one a day (not more), for the first three weeks, then two a week forever after.

4. Finally, toss the carbonated beverages right out of your diet or make your own (see *Recipes*). It is not the carbonation that is harmful, it is the added phosphate. Drink water, herb teas, homemade fruit and vegetable juices, milk or buttermilk.

Milk, like fish, is full of calcium in the form of calcium phosphate. Again, logic might speak against the effectiveness of this form of calcium. Again, logic is wrong. Evidently, the calcium and phosphate story must be much more complex than I am depicting here.

Milk works best as a calcium source, in spite of its phosphate content. Possibly the *lactose* and other complexities of its composition contribute to this. My recommendation when deposits have formed anywhere in the body, such as heel, toe, arteries, joints, is to switch to milk as a beverage. Compare the calcium level of your urine before and after the switch (allowing several weeks first). Also compare calcium levels in your blood serum. It should move towards normal. This means **up** if it is too low (below 9.2). It means **down** if it is too high (10). If you are monitoring the effectiveness of the kidney herb recipe in dissolving away your phosphate crystals, notice that drinking milk keeps them from reforming. Taking calcium tablets does not! Taking nothing lets them reform the quickest.

> The milk must be 2% or higher in butter fat to be effective.

With your body fluids at their proper acid level, with your kidneys able to flush out acids, with heavy metal toxins no longer settling in, with your bone-dissolving stopped, your heel deposits can shrink. Bacteria have no place to feed and breed. You can kill them several times more with your zapper to catch stragglers. And your heel pain becomes history. Be careful not to bruise the sensitive tissue with too much walking or running immediately after the pain is gone. Wear cushioning socks and well cushioned shoes.

> Names in the case histories have been changed to ones of the same sex, picked at random from a telephone directory. Other facts may have been altered in non-essential ways.

Walter Jones, a man of 67, was diabetic for 14 years. His feet and upper legs hurt so much for the past 13 years he could barely shuffle along now. They were also cold and clammy. The herb, juniper berry was added to the Kidney Cleanse recipe to make it even more effective for him and he was advised to stop smoking, using alcohol, and caffeine. He also started the parasite killing program (at that time an herbal parasite program was being used instead of a zapper) and a liver cleanse that yielded several hundred small gallstones. Three months from his first visit his legs were better and feet OK, although he still had some trouble walking due to pain in upper thighs.

Dinah Sagun, a minister's wife, had a lot of walking and standing to do besides traveling a lot. She had knee surgery 15 years ago to remove deposits but now they were getting bad again. Also her heels were sore. My tests showed she had phosphate and oxalate deposits in her kidneys. She was started on the Kidney Cleanse followed by the parasite program. She stopped using benzene polluted items, especially her Chap Stick™. Her diet was changed to include milk and leave out store-bought beverages. In 4½ months her heel pain was gone along with the bad headaches we had not even started to work on.

Julie Fernandez came with a list of 10 serious problems including foot pain and ankle swelling. Her urinalysis showed crystals. My test showed they were uric acid crystals. Her parasites included *Trichinella*. There was a house cat. Her toxic metal test showed tellurium and platinum accumulation from metal dentalware, and arsenic from pesticide. She was to start on a Kidney Cleanse and add the parasite program two weeks later. She was to remove all roach hives and other pest killers from her house and arrange for dental metal replacement. At her third visit, four weeks later, she could walk without pain although she still had *Trichinella* and arsenic problems. Two months later she was aching all over again and her kidneys hurt. She still had *Trichinella* and some dental work to do. She was to do a 5-day high dose parasite treatment and treat the cat also and repeat the kidney cleanse. This relieved her pain.

Dorothy Shelley had numerous pains including foot pain in the arch, lower back pain and cramps with her period. She had oxalate and uric acid crystals in the kidneys so was started on kidney herbs. Three weeks later her foot pain and low back pain were gone.

Paul Longtin had toe cramps, calf cramps, and heel pain. After cutting down on smoking, quitting caffeine and soda pop and taking niacin (250 mg time release; 1 capsule each meal and upon rising in morning) and doing a kidney cleanse, all in three weeks, he was much improved and didn't even need his arch supports.

68

Juan Onley, age 58, came for his gout in both feet and one hand. He could hardly walk, in spite of soft shoes and pain killer. It started 7 years ago. He also had prostate pain and couldn't sit comfortably. My tests showed his kidneys were full of uric acid, oxalate and cystine stones. His prostate was full of *Gardnerella* and *Campylobacter* bacteria. His wisdom teeth were harboring *plantar wart #4 virus* and *Coxsackie B4* virus. *Gardnerella* often comes with fluke parasites and indeed he had intestinal flukes in his kidney! He began with the kidney herb program, then the parasite killing program. It took five months to clear them all. Then he could walk and sit without pain.

Leg Pain In Children

It is commonly accepted as normal(!) in children to have pain in the shins or calves of the leg. They may even be called "growing pains." Children may cry with the pain and never tell anyone the reason for crying. It happens mostly after napping. This may be caused by cramping of the leg or spasms of the blood vessels. *Lead toxicity* is a common cause of both. Test for the presence of both **lead** and **cadmium** in the tap water. Only your own electronic tests are helpful. Water department tests are much too crude.

If either poison is

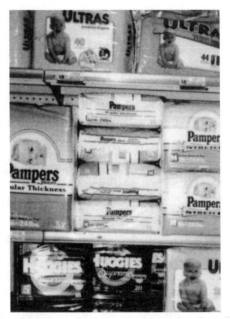

Fig. 11 All disposable diapers I tested had mercury and thallium! These toxins can be absorbed through babies' skin.

69

found, test the water supply from each faucet in the house, in the morning, before it has been run. Find the offending sources, change the water pipes to polyvinyl chloride (PVC).

Also search for thallium or mercury in the child's saliva. If it is there, remove all dental metal. Stop using all commercial disposable diapers, dental floss, cotton swabs and bandages; they are polluted with mercury and thallium probably from manufacturing them in foreign countries where it is legal to sterilize with mercuric chloride. Test again, several times, after plumbing or dental work has been completed. To relieve pain:

- immerse legs in warm water
- massage legs gently
- give 25-50 mg niacin, not time-release, to dilate blood vessels.

Leg Pain In Adults

Leg pain in adults is usually associated with *cadmium* or *thallium*. Cadmium is present in tap water that runs through corroded galvanized pipes. The cadmium is probably a contaminant of the zinc used for galvanizing. Test the water, electronically, for cadmium. If you have all copper pipes but there is cadmium in the water, there must be a short piece (a **Y** or a **T** joint) made of old galvanized pipe lurking somewhere. Track it down by testing water from all your faucets.

Cadmium causes the blood vessels to spasm and it is made worse by smoking, that's why the condition is sometimes called **Smoker's Leg**. But extremely painful legs are due to chronic thallium poisoning more than any other cause!

It is very important to know exactly how toxic thallium is. Read the clipping on page 417 right now!

Where would you ever get thallium? From your very own mouth! The mercury in fillings is often itself polluted with thallium! Replace your amalgam fillings with composite.

Bandages

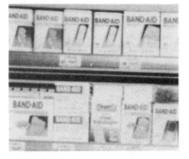

Sanitary napkins and tampons

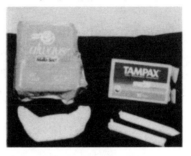

Cotton swabs

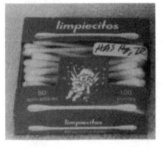

Cotton balls

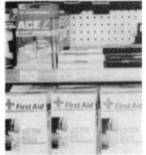

Floss

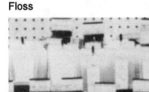

Toothpicks (the one on the right is ten years old and had no mercury or thallium)

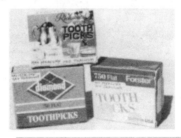

Fig. 12 Do not use any commercial personal products, the risk of pollution is too great.

Thallium has another source: it is riding along as a pollutant in cotton swabs, cotton balls, commercial bandages, toothpicks, floss, gauze, sanitary napkins, tampons, disposable diapers, and paper towels. Evidently these are being sterilized with mercuric chloride which, in turn, has thallium pollution.

- Line **disposable diapers** with a tissue
- Line **sanitary napkins** and pads with a tissue
- Use the **polyester puff** in the top of vitamin bottles in place of cotton balls. Twirl some around a plastic stirrer for a swab.
- Use pieces of **tissue and masking tape** for bandages.

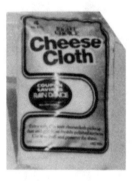

Use cheesecloth in place of gauze.

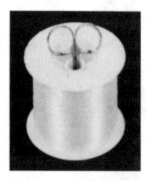

Use monofilament fish line (2 or 4 lb. test) for floss

Fig. 13 Safe substitutes for personal products.

If you do have thallium in your white blood cells and you haven't used toothpicks, etc. earlier in the day, then it is in your tooth fillings and **you have no higher priority than getting the**

amalgams out. Find a dentist <u>immediately</u> who will remove them, drilling deeply and widely not to miss a speck of it, thereby getting the thallium out, too. You cannot cure your leg pains without removing thallium.

Leg Pain Protocol

1. Stop smoking.
2. Repair plumbing.
3. Do dental cleanup and chelate out the mercury and thallium that has gotten into your tissues with EDTA (see *Sources*). You will need to find a chelating doctor; ask a friendly chiropractor to help you locate one. Or at least take thioctic acid 100 mg, (2 three times a day) and vitamin C (5 gm or one teaspoon) daily for a month.
4. Take magnesium oxide 300 mg (take 1 twice a day).
5. Take niacin, as much as you tolerate—time release varieties are less effective. Try 50 mg with each meal.
6. Change your diet to reduce phosphate and include milk (sterilized).
7. Do the herbal Kidney Cleanse (page 549) followed by a Liver Cleanse (page 552).
8. Zap yourself on alternate days at bedtime. If this zapping makes no difference whatever, your problem is purely spasms. But if you get relief, even if it's very short lived, you must have killed something. Bacteria must come from somewhere. Concentrate your efforts on dental health and better diet.

Jean Booth, age 30, had sore, tired legs and severe three-day headaches. She would get stabbing pains in back of her thighs. After we found thallium and mercury in her kidneys she did a Kidney Cleanse and got all her metal tooth fillings replaced. She then felt fine for one year. Suddenly she got fatigue and heavy legs again with stabbing pain at the outer thigh. She had seen a neurologist. Her chiropractor suggested it was leftover mercury so she came back to us. Indeed, she was toxic with lead, mercury, thallium, but her dentist could not find the leftover metal in her mouth. Three cavitations were cleaned; she was put on thioctic acid; eight varieties of bacteria and viruses were killed with a frequency generator and her legs became well again. Our test showed thallium at 4 teeth, but it was not a big enough deposit to show up on dental X-ray. She may eventually choose to have these redrilled.

Charlie Snelling was a picture of pain: pain in arms, elbows, shoulders, wrist, hands, chest, low back, legs, knees, and feet. He was started on kidney herbs and a few pains were reduced. He was toxic with cadmium so he changed his plumbing to plastic. However, he continued to be toxic with cadmium and thallium throwing suspicion on his numerous old tooth fillings. He got them all replaced and cavitations cleaned. He used our frequency generator to kill beta *Streptococcus*, *Pseudomonas*, *Troglodytella* and *Staphylococcus aureus* all of which were under one tooth (#15). A year later he still had bouts of leg pain. He still had numerous bacteria under his

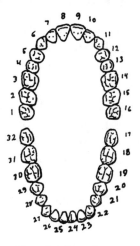

Fig. 14 Tooth numbering system.

teeth because the jaw bone was not healing. He had not been taking vitamin D, nor magnesium nor drinking milk for the necessary calcium. But he had improved enough to go back to work full time.

Victor Abhay, age 16, could no longer play in high school sports because of knee pain. It began "with a virus" and high temperature two years ago. His knee started to bother him after that. He had *cysteine* kidney crystals and four parasites: *Cryptocotyl*, human liver fluke, *Echinococcus granulosus* cyst and *Echinostomum revolutum* in his white blood cells. He was to start the kidney herb recipe and follow this with the parasite program. Five months later, when we next saw him, his knee was fine.

Kim Murphy, 45, had painful legs, feet and knees. They also were swollen and itched. She was parasitized by *Trichuris*, (dog whipworm). She also had tapeworm stages (*Taenia pisiformis*) and intestinal fluke in the intestine. She started on the kidney herbs, followed by the parasite program. She stopped using zirconium-containing products (deodorant) and barium (lipstick). She stayed out of bus exhaust. (She knew she was allergic to diesel exhaust.) In one month her leg pain and itching were gone; slight swelling remained.

Nancy Tong, 80's, had edematous legs. In fact she could get no stockings on. They appeared like pillars with no taper at all. She was on diuretic medicine from her doctor. It kept her blood pressure down but she was losing ground with water excretion. This raised her general toxicity (blood BUN[5]) which made her feel bad most of the time. Yet she drank enough water, curtailed her salt, used no caffeine and had no really bad habits. She had to wear several pads for incontinence. We found she was toxic with cadmium and lead, which were probably responsible for her huge accumulation of kidney stones. The metals were in her tap water and she was unable to resolve this problem since she lived in a senior citizen center. We advised her to move, or to have her tap water carried in, but she could do none of these. Although the situation was hopeless, she did the kidney cleanse, parasite killing program and changed her metal rimmed glasses and wrist watch to plastic. She gained enough ground from these improvements to be able to wear elastic hose and thereby give some physical assistance to her body. This encouraged her to do a liver cleanse. She had a headache with the cleanse but immediately afterwards she fit into a smaller size "Keds" (elasticized stockings). A half a year from the beginning, her legs had taper to them; she didn't even mind wearing a dress.

Fibromyositis and Fibromyalgia

When pain is widespread, not just in joints or legs but in many muscles and soft tissues of your body your doctor may call it *fibromyositis* or *fibromyalgia*.

---

[5]BUN stands for blood urea nitrogen. It is a body waste and is normally kept low by the kidneys.

For bacteria to get all over your body, they must be riding along with parasites that get all over your body. Microscopically tiny roundworms can do this.

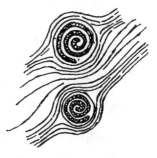

Trichinella is the most common cause of these diseases, but sometimes *Ascaris* larvae or *hookworms* or *strongyle* larvae are the main culprits. These wormlets bring hosts of **bacteria** with them, mainly "*Streps*" (*Streptococcus* varieties) and "*Staphs*" (*Staphylococcus* varieties), but also "*Clostridiums*" (*Clostridium* varieties) and "*Campyls*" (*Campylobacter* varieties). The bacteria are probably the pain causers. By killing all bacteria—*Staphs, Streps, Clostridiums* and *Campyls*—using a zapper, you may get relief for <u>one hour</u>!

Fig. 15 Trichinella larvae settled in muscles.

By killing *Trichinella* and *Ancylostomas* (worms) <u>first,</u> followed by the bacteria, you may get relief for <u>several hours</u>. By killing the parasites and bacteria <u>in every household member and the pets</u> at the same time and by <u>never</u> putting your fingers to your mouth, you can expect <u>permanent</u> pain relief. It is interesting to speculate why the other family members, who are also infected with these tiny roundworms <u>don't</u> develop *fibromyalgia*. Perhaps the larvae stay in the intestine or go to the diaphragm (causing coughing) or the eyes (causing "lazy" eye muscles). Perhaps they merely cause **anemia**. *Trichinella*, hookworms and *strongyles* are extremely difficult to get rid of in a family.

These roundworm larvae undoubtedly cross the placenta into the unborn child during pregnancy, too. So they can be "inherited." Try to clear up the whole family before the next pregnancy.

Clearing up pets of these parasites is even harder. The best advice is to give your pets away. They will continue to harbor them even though they are on a pet parasite program. It is impossible to stay free of the parasites your pets have: they will move to your soft tissues immediately, giving you the bacteria and inflammation again.

The next most important advice is to <u>keep fingers out of your mouth</u> (read Hands, page 397). None of these parasites enter through your skin (this is in spite of teachings that hookworms enter this way), you must put them into your mouth somehow! Consider your mouth off limits to anything but food and kissing.

Finally, if there is a baby in diapers in the family, be patient. When diapering days are over you will have less bowel contact, giving you an opportunity to finish your own treatment. Meanwhile, wash fingernails in Skin Sanitizer (see *Recipes*) after cleaning up children's bowel movements, diapers and yourself. Use borax liquid for soap to leave an antibacterial residue on the skin.

Try to identify your parasites before killing them so you can be on the lookout for them in the future. Get slides or dead cultures of various pathogens and search in your white blood cells. If you can't do this, at least save a saliva sample of your own; keep it frozen or preserved. Also make a saliva sample for your pet. This gives you specimens to test yourself for later. You won't know which parasite is in this saliva specimen, but if you ever test positive for it again you will know you got it back. Then zap yourself.

Brenda Byrd was diagnosed with myofibrositis two years earlier at the age of 36. Her blood test showed triglycerides slightly high (152 mg./DL), indicating the beginnings of urinary tract problems. Her urinalysis stated "hazy" (hazy with bacteria or crystals) instead of clear urine. It also listed white blood cells, red blood cells, and a few bacteria present in her urine. Our tests revealed mercury and numerous other heavy metals distributed in her thyroid, stomach, kidney, lungs, bones and bone marrow. She was also full of beryllium (usually from "coal oil") contained in the hurricane lamps she kept in every room. She had numerous parasites, including *Strongyloides* and hookworms spread through her body tissues. She was thrilled to learn how to get her health back and started with the dental problem.

Marcia Cochran, 36, had muscles twitching all over her body. It was diagnosed as fibromyalgia. Her joints were tender and her chest felt "tight." She had bronchitis twice a year. She was on Amytryptaline™ for muscle twitching and Bentyl™ to calm the intestine (spastic colon). She had depression with it and was on medicine for that. It all started with fever and chills that she thought was the flu but after they went away, she was left with a tremor. Sometimes she felt that little electric shocks were going through her. She had *Ascaris* and hookworm larvae widespread in her body. She had sheep liver flukes in her liver. She was started on the parasite program. She was also toxic with PVC and tellurium (dental metal). The PVC was traced to plastic storm windows applied to the <u>inside</u> of the window and to new shower curtains. Two months passed and she had not solved any of her problems. Then she did her first liver cleanse and got over 100 stones out. This instantly reduced her fibromyalgia to occasional attacks. She was so encouraged she decided to go ahead with dental cleanup.

Joint Pain or Arthritis

Two main kinds of arthritis are recognized clinically, *osteoarthritis* and *rheumatoid arthritis*. In osteoarthritis the joints have bacteria living on the deposits left there. In rheumatoid arthritis the bacteria come from larger parasites—wormlets actually living in these joints. The worms are the common little roundworms whose eggs hatch into microscopic wormlets that travel.

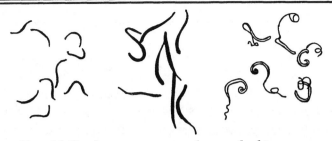

Fig. 16 Hookworms, strongyles, and whipworms.

We have four common roundworms: *Ascaris, hookworm, Strongyloides, Trichinella*. Their life cycle normally directs them to travel to the lungs but in some people they travel through the entire body, including brain, muscles and joints. More research is necessary to explain this. My suspicion is that there are toxins, like **mercury, thallium, cadmium, lead,** as well as **solvents,** distributed through the body, lowering immunity and allowing the tiny larvae to reside there. Once the pathway (routing) to these organs has been established, it continues to be used by other parasites as well. Soon a variety of parasites, their bacteria and viruses, and pollutants are all headed toward these organs.

Osteo or Common Arthritis

When joints are painful it is a simple matter to kill the bacteria with an electronic zapper. Treat yourself with a zapper daily until the pain is gone. Maybe it will stay away, but chances are the bacteria have a steady source.

The most common source for *Staphs* and *Streps* are small abscesses in the jaw bone, under and beside old extractions, root canals and mercury fillings. You may get immediate pain relief just from a dental cleanup, and again disappointment may follow. *Staphs* and *Streps* are such ubiquitous bacteria, they may come not only from jaw bone infections but from gallstones, kidney stones and other parasites. The correct treatment for arthritis is a complete overhaul of body health: a diet cleanup, a body cleanup, and environmental cleanup.

Start with the herbal parasite program and zapping. Follow this with a kidney cleanse, then liver cleanse. If any toxin is overlooked, especially asbestos and fiberglass, it is sure to find your joints and permit bacteria to return and cause pain. Make sure to correct your body acid levels after doing pH measurements of the urine (page 57).

Arthritic deposits contain a large amount of phosphates combined with calcium. This calcium came from some other bone, such as the base of your spine or the wrist. Here the bones are getting weaker due to this calcium loss. Calcium was taken out of your bones for the simple purpose of neutralizing the excess phosphate in your diet. Reduce phosphate consumption (meats, soda pop, grains) by half, eating fish, milk, vegetables and fruit instead. Drink three cups of milk a day. If you are allergic to milk, do several liver cleanses, switch brands of milk, use milk digestant, and use it in cooking and baking. Cheese and cottage cheese are not substitutes for milk (the calcium stayed in the whey). Dairy products must be boiled before consuming and should be no less than 2% butter fat. It takes <u>bile</u> to make calcium absorbable, yet milk with less than 2% butterfat does not trigger the gallbladder to empty it's bile at mealtime.

If you are not used to dairy products, start slowly and work up gradually to the 3 cups a day needed.

Carol Lachance was diagnosed with arthritis of her back and knees. (She had spurs in both places.) She was positive for *Trichinella*, *Ascaris* and *Dirofilaria* (she also had pain over the heart). They had an outdoor dog. Her blood test showed a high phosphate and alkaline phosphatase level showing she was dissolving her bones. After changing her diet to include milk, extra oyster shell calcium (one a day), magnesium oxide and vitamin B_6, and reducing her meat and grain consumption her phosphate level went down to normal (below 4). She did the kidney cleanse and liver cleanse as well as parasite program but still had pain. A toxic element test

80

revealed lead in her bones. It was traced to a drugstore variety multivitamin tablet she had taken daily for years. When she stopped these and added prescription vitamin D (50,000 units) for three weeks to help her bones heal she got relief.

Gail Hildebrand, age 62, had painful arthritic hands and gum disease. She had 12 parasites free-loading on her and was toxic with asbestos. This was traced to her clothes dryer. Four months later, after killing parasites, her hand pain and gums were much better. She had the dryer vent taped up tighter and this got rid of her asbestos problem. She started on kidney herbs and in one month saw that her enlarged knuckles were beginning to go down.

Norma Littrell, age 53, came in for her severe arthritis of six years. Her knees, shoulders and hands were painful. I explained to her that painful shoulders did not belong to the arthritis picture but had a gallstone etiology which she could easily fix in a single night at a later time (liver cleanse). She also had mid-back, upper back and lower back pain; again the upper back pain belonged to the liver problem. She had tricalcium phosphate kidney crystals as well as uric acid crystals. She was told to go off coffee (no decaf either), decrease her meat and grain consumption (phosphate) and increase milk and use stone ground cornmeal products (genuine stone ground tortillas as well as pickled pigs' feet are high in utilizable calcium). She started on the kidney herbs. In 33 days her low back pain had improved a lot, she could wash her own hair again and she could sit down and get up from her living room floor without pain. She was elated but we recommended less stress than such exercises for her joints.

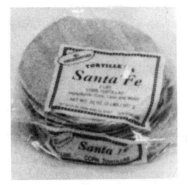

Fig. 17 Stone ground corn tortillas, high in calcium.

Patricia Robinson, age 76, had pain in her knees, feet, lower back, hands and wrists. Also in her shoulders and upper back which is not part of the arthritis

81

picture. <u>She had swollen puffy eyelids which is a telltale sign of</u> <u>Ascaris</u>. She had heartburn, cold feet and insomnia as well as high blood pressure. She was on several medicines. We started her on the kidney recipe and ornithine (four to eight as needed at bedtime) for sleep. We hoped she could stop her Ativan™ drug soon. She was to go off coffee, tea and decafs. Her hands were knotted and misshapen at the joints, also tender. Two months later there was little change; her doctor had put her on Prozac™ and she hoped that would do a lot for her (so she stopped the kidney herbs) but it didn't. The parasite test still showed *Ascaris* and she was started on the parasite program. We also found fluoride (from toothpaste), iridium, samarium and palladium, all from her tooth implants. She was to remove as much metal as the dentist could replace, clean cavitations, and take thioctic acid, 2 a day, to help clear metal from her body. In four weeks the sharp pain in her back was gone and in three more weeks the pain in her hands was gone.

Lynne Snyder, 72, had pain in every joint and had to be on pain medicine to keep moving. Her potassium level was very low (3.6—an adrenal/kidney problem), and she was started on kidney herbs, carrot juice, vegetable juice and bananas. In ten days she could feel some new energy but her pains were terrible, especially her knees. She was taken off tomato juice, cranberry juice, citrus, pepper (she was using a lot), and given buttermilk as a beverage which she enjoyed. After three weeks of kidney herbs she was started on parasite killing herbs. In another month her arthritis was much better. She was not on any pain medicine and could get to sleep without it. She thought it was mostly going off pepper that helped.

Rheumatoid Arthritis

When inflammation and swelling affect your joints, besides pain, it is called *rheumatoid arthritis*. In addition, a blood test may reveal "rheumatoid factor" to be present. In this case, the common tiny round worms have invaded your joints. These are *Ascaris, Ancylostomas, Strongyloides*, and *Trichinella*. Their eggs are everywhere around us, in dust and dirt and the filth under fingernails and our own bowel movements.

Superior sanitation is your first defense. Rinse fingernails in alcohol after cleaning up bowel movements or changing diapers. Never, never, tolerate long fingernails in any family member. If this discipline can't be enforced, do not allow food preparation by "long nails" unless gloves are worn. He or she may not be getting ill (yet) from the family parasites, but you are. Of course, you can kill them with a zapper (internally, not the ones under the nails) but that is after you have been infected. They are easily picked up again. It would be wise to zap for roundworms every week, just in case.

Make sure your pet is treated with parasite herbs or by zapper as well. A pet that goes outdoors will quickly (the very next day) bring these roundworms into the house again. Give away your pets if possible.

Check for dental problems. Do the Dental Clean-Up (page 409). Then do a Kidney Cleanse and Liver Cleanse.

You may relieve your pain and begin to heal immediately after zapping but it is wise to do all the health programs, anyway. Change your diet. Reduce phosphate, start using sterilized milk for calcium. Switch to fish from meats. Drink much more water. Use only harmless beverages (see *Recipes*) and foods. Switch to toxin-free body products. Live in a non-toxic house. Stay on a maintenance parasite program of herbs, and zap regularly. Stay on the kidney cleanse for three to six weeks and repeat a one-week session every few months to keep removing deposits which may also choose these sick joints to settle in. Knees are a favorite location for rheumatoid arthritis. Knees are very dependent on kidneys.

To summarize, do everything as for osteoarthritis, emphasizing the roundworm parasites for elimination.

Allergic Arthritis

A prominent food toxin that is said to affect knees is *piperine*, found in the pepper family which includes black and white pepper (not cayenne). The *Solanaceae* family of plants (potatoes, tomatoes, eggplant, tobacco!) also has a common "allergen" that produces joint pain. Try going off these for two weeks to see if it helps. Two more chemicals that can trigger arthritis -like pain are *hippuric acid* and *phenylisothiocyanate* (PIT).

Your body makes large amounts of hippuric acid, up to a gram a day. It is the product of benzoic acid detoxification by the liver. Quite a few fruits contain natural benzoic acid. But we can easily triple and quadruple our benzoic acid intake by consuming commercial beverages and pastries where benzoic acid is used as a preservative. It is indeed a "natural" preservative. All of it must be detoxified, though, and this gives us way too much hippuric acid. The kidneys are unable to excrete such overloads of hippuric acid, so it distributes itself in our organs. I suspect a simple mechanism could explain its pain-triggering action: hippuric acid molecules could attach themselves to our cell's conductance channels keeping the gates jammed open. This might invite bacteria and viruses to enter there. But there are also hippuric acid-loving bacteria that feed on it. Perhaps hippuric acid can cause pain without the help of bacteria. This requires further study. It is only sensible for persons with chronic pain not to consume benzoic acid (or benzoate) preserved foods.

PIT is a food chemical found especially in chicken, eggs, the cabbage family, peas. PIT is also part of the body's own chemistry, taking place in the liver, and involving detoxification of *cyanide*-containing foods. Many vegetables, notably the cabbage family, contain such cyanides, giving them protection from insects, disease, and grazing animals. It can take the liver a

84

week to detoxify a meal full of these cyanides: in the meantime, PIT levels are higher in the body. PIT is very reactive. In fact, it is <u>the</u> chemical used as a general reactant with amino acids in the well known **Edman degradation** reaction. But now, your body is the reaction flask, supplying the amino acids. Since all organs supply amino acids, it is no wonder they can all react to PIT, giving you multiple allergic reactions and pains.

If you have any kind of arthritis, stop eating the high-PIT foods and clean the liver until you are free of all allergies you are aware of. This suggests that the liver is capable, again, of detoxifying the cyanides for you in a reasonable time and you may eat them again. These foods do have many benefits, of course.

Joint pain, or arthritis, was known in antiquity long before dogs and cats were household pets and giving us their parasites. Pigs and horses harbor these roundworms too and may have been the source at that time.

Herbs and treatments that help arthritis are, therefore, plentiful. Maybe they act by killing roundworms, bacteria, and viruses, or help metabolize hippuric acid and PIT. Homeopathic treatments, as well as massage, heat and electronic devices also help. With this wide range of effective treatments dating to the distant past, why is none of them a permanent cure? The answer is simple. The common roundworms are everywhere about us, sanitation is poor, and our civilized lifestyle leads to deposit formation that invites bacteria. But knowing this, you can stop your pain and remove the causes to become one of the first humans to achieve a permanent cure.

Verna Plumb, age 46, was diagnosed with rheumatoid arthritis four years earlier. Since then she had been continuously on methotrexate™ and prednisone.™ This had caused her to gain a lot of weight from water retention. The drugs were no longer effective and she would need to do something else very soon. She had the typical causes: her body was toxic with mercury and nickel from tooth fillings. Her kidneys were full of five kinds of stones. She had numerous roundworm parasites including two kinds of *Ascaris*, two kinds of hookworm, *Strongyloides* and *Trichinella*. She would have to clean everything up to get relief. She started on the kidney herbs, killed parasites with a frequency generator and in two months noticed her swelling was receding.

Camille Franklin had hands that were swollen and hot and painful. She also had "arthritis" in shoulders and knees. We explained that shoulders were not part of the arthritis picture. She could deal with that in a single evening, soon. She also had bone spurs at sinuses which needed surgical removal. Her kidneys revealed tricalcium phosphate crystals. She was given a diet change; onto milk, fruits and vegetables, off other beverages, less meat and grains. She was started on kidney herbs. In five weeks all the swelling and redness and heat was out of her finger joints.

Thigh Pain

Inner thigh pain often stems from the *sciatic nerve* which is suffering pressure at the lower back. If this is so, chiropractic adjustments should help. The correct treatment, after killing bacteria electronically, is to clean up the entire kidney area using the kidney herb recipe.

If this is not the correct explanation, (and you're not getting pain relief) you may have a trauma—perhaps you overstretched your leg in some exercise. The minor trauma invited bacteria to settle there and give you pain.

If the pain recurs after clearing it several times, there must be a chronic source of bacteria. Since the kidneys are already cleaned, consider the teeth, as well as recurring parasites, and the liver. Clean the liver every two weeks until 2000 or more stones have appeared and no more appear. This could take 1-2 years. Be patient. Do a dental clean up. Keep killing the bacteria so they can't spread. And, of course, let the painful leg rest.

Hip Pain

Hip pain is <u>always</u> due to bacteria. In fact, these bacteria regularly come from two sources: the kidneys and the teeth. This simplifies the treatment since neither of these places takes a long time to clear.

Start yourself immediately on the kidney cleanse (page 549) to clean your kidneys. <u>Continue on the recipe until the dental cleanup has been completed</u>. Both must be clean <u>together</u> to stop exporting bacteria to the hip.

The dental cleanup could take several weeks if extensive work is required. During this time, kill all parasites electronically. Keep killing bacteria, especially *Staphs, Streps, Clostridia, Campyls*.

The dental problem is not always on the same side as the hip pain. The jaw may be very fragile and porous, full of invading bacteria. Cleaning these cavitations may give immediate pain relief in the hip (proving the bacterial source). But getting the jaw bone to heal by taking up calcium again is not guaranteed by the cleaning process.

Give your jaw bone every chance to heal:

- Start taking vitamin D (40,000 to 50,000 u.), every day for three weeks from the day of the dental work or before. After this, take it twice a week forever. **Do not take more.**
- Take vitamin C (1+ gm a day) and B$_6$ (250-500 mg a day) for healthy gums.
- Get one gram of usable calcium in your daily diet.

Bone Strengthening

Vegetable calcium can't be dissolved by our stomachs (*ruminants,* like cows, can dissolve it—they have an extra stomach loaded with special bacteria who do the actual retrieving of calcium). Tablet-form calcium can't be dissolved well either, especially as we age. We need predissolved calcium if a little is to go a long way.

Primitive people who lived on fish or stone-ground meal ate 4-6 grams of calcium a day.[6] Even if only 20% of this got dissolved, they would still have about 1 gram of utilizable calcium for themselves. Chances are good they dissolved even more, since they were young (life expectancy was less than 50 years). Their skull remains show beautiful, cavity-free teeth. They lived outdoors, mainly, so getting enough sunshine-derived vitamin D was not a problem. Their natural diet supplied enough vitamin B_2 to protect them from UV (ultraviolet) damage from sunshine exposure.

But these are civilized times. Our lives are stretched into old age, when our stomachs no longer produce enough acid to kill bacteria, nor to dissolve the minerals in our food. So they need to be dissolved for us. Milk is a beverage where the calcium has already been dissolved by the other ingredients. The lactic acid in milk formed during digestion gives the calcium the correct chelated structure for absorption by the intestine. Even the bile participates in calcium absorption. Milk also contains phosphate, but not too much to be useful. I recommend milk as a calcium-source to heal the jaw bone after and before dental work. You need 1+ grams a day. One quart of milk has 1 gm (1000 mg) of utilizable calcium. You absorb only 250-400 mg. The rest is excreted and eliminated. Only the absorbed calcium can heal your jaw bone. Use milk in cooking as well as a beverage. The calcium in it is indestructible.

Bones are not made of calcium alone. **Magnesium** is essential. Since magnesium is more soluble and easy to assimilate than calcium, the tablet form (magnesium oxide, 300 mg, see

---

[6] Read Nutrition and Physical Degeneration by Weston A. Price, DDS first published in 1939. At least, gaze at the pictures. Ask your library to buy a copy, available from Price-Pottenger Nutrition Foundation, (800) 366-3748.

Sources) will do. If you are not absorbing the magnesium it will stay in your intestine and act as a laxative. If this happens acidify your stomach during meals: always add fresh lemon, vinegar, or vitamin C to your food or drink to help digest milk and dissolve minerals for you. **Boron** (3 mg. once a day) and **manganese** (15 mg. once a day) are additional bone hardeners.

When your diet is improved, your dental problem is cleared, and your kidneys are clean, your hip pain will stay away and you can stop thinking about hip replacement surgery.

Mary Hammond, 48, had two painful hips. She was diabetic and drinking five cups of coffee a day. She had *Staphylococcus aureus* infections under three teeth that she no longer had. After going off caffeine (caffeine may spread bacteria by making tissues more permeable) and getting some dental work done, her right hip stopped hurting. When cavitations were cleaned, her left hip stopped hurting too, but after a week the pain returned. She still had parasites and their bacteria to kill. She had solvents to eliminate and a kidney cleanse to do but she was quite enthusiastic and enjoyed showing off how well she walked.

Groin Pain

Lymph nodes are situated here, as well as in armpits and around the neck. Lymph nodes are your best friends. They are hives of activity. Your white blood cells "nest" here. Lymph nodes sample your body fluids (lymph) at these locations, much like the water department and health department sample our milk and water, making sure they are pure and sterile. Of course, they never really are. But your white blood cells <u>keep working at it.</u> They are busy removing impurities like zirconium and titanium and pathogens like bacteria and viruses.

When an especially challenging dose of parasite or pollution arrives at the node, it enlarges, in order to handle the bigger sized task. This enlargement can be felt. It may press against other organs and you feel the pain of pressure in the groin. This should alert you, of course, to the danger. Kill the parasites and pathogens immediately with your zapper. Start the kidney cleanse. Stop using toxic products and eating toxic food. If you are being effective, the lymph nodes will begin to shrink in a few days, relieving the groin pain. If it does not come back, you probably eliminated the main cause. But if it recurs, try to diagnose it accurately. Test yourself for HIV and AIDS and then to pet saliva,

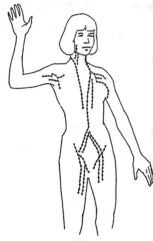

Fig. 18 Your lymph nodes are your best friends.

dairy products and other disease specimens. Stop reinfecting from humans or pets or dairy food. Assist your body by cleaning up your dentalware, and environment. Check all supplements for toxins before using them on a daily basis. (If they show up in your white blood cells a few minutes after eating them, there is a toxin.) If your groin pain doesn't go away, you probably missed something!

There are other causes of groin pain, though, such as **hernia**. A physician will help you identify it. Have it surgically repaired. The Shouldice Hospital[7] has the best surgical record and will disclose their statistics! You won't even need full anesthesia there.

Pain from the **ovaries** is often felt near the groin. Sometimes a large cyst in the ovary puts pressure on the sensitive nearby

---

[7]Shouldice Hospital, 7750 Bayview Ave. Box 370, Thornhill, Ontario, Canada L3T-4A3, telephone (905) 889-1125.

organs. The formation of cysts, *cystic ovaries*, is a common condition of cats, too. Obviously, something is not right in the ovaries.

Ovaries make hormones: **progesterone** and **estrogen**. If bacteria (like *Gardnerella, syphilis, gonorrhea*) are living there, the ovaries are handicapped and may under-produce or over-produce some hormone. The first treatment should be to kill parasites, especially the flukes. Then kill all other parasites and bacteria, especially *Gardnerella* and enteric bacteria which can migrate easily from intestine to ovary. In spite of all this, the cyst may not shrink. In order to shrink the cyst you must determine <u>what is filling the cyst</u>. Then <u>stop</u> filling it. The cyst will eliminate itself and shrink.

Many kinds of pollution can fill an ovarian cyst. Test for CFCs and PCBs. Gold is another favorite. Particulate pollutants like asbestos and fiberglass are often put into cysts by your body. Your body is <u>wise</u>. If these can't be eliminated through the kidneys or bile, it will at least keep them all together (in the form of a cyst) the same way a toxic dump spares the rest of the landscape. As long as you are adding to it, it cannot get smaller. Fortunately, your loyal white blood cells are trucking toxins <u>away</u> from your cysts every minute of every day and night. All you need to do is <u>stop adding</u>. Remove dental mental, clean up your body, diet, and environment.

You will notice shrinking of cysts in three weeks. What you actually notice is absence of pain, implying shrinkage. Meanwhile pain relief by killing bacteria, herbal ovarian assistance (try wild yam), chiropractic, pain killers are all useful. Decongest the area by means of a kidney cleanse. If your cyst does not shrink you have missed the pollutants. After it does shrink, stay on a regular program of parasite killing, herbal or electronic, and improved lifestyle.

Ovaries may be giving you pain even without a cyst present. By cleaning up parasites and pollutants you can eliminate it quickly; much more quickly than when a cyst has formed.

Synthetic hormones (Provera,™ Premarin,™ Ogen,™ etc.) are often used to clear up ovary problems of various kinds. Don't continue to use them when the need no longer exists. Although they have low toxicity, there are disadvantages such as the need for liver detoxification, and risk of heavy metal pollutants. Cancer acceleration has been seen when taking estrogens.

Low Back Pain

We have been told that lower back pain originates in an inherited weakness of the spine at its base because we humans walk upright instead of on four legs. And we have been told that the bony hooks that keep the spine aligned are flatter in some families, making it harder for them to hold the spine together. We are also told that "proper exercises" could have kept this part of our bodies strong so lower back pain could be avoided.

These theories become obsolete when, without surgery or exercise or change in posture, lower back pain can be made to disappear quickly and permanently.

Acupressure massage and chiropractic can bring "miraculous" relief. The most severely crippled lower back pain sufferer can shuffle lamely into a chiropractor's office and walk out normally, without pain or painkiller after treatments. So although there has been slippage of disc or spine, apparently it goes back into place rather easily.

If muscle relaxation is the clue, we must ask why these muscles spasm so easily. Any muscle spasms if you irritate or injure it suddenly. In fact, your whole body spasms and flinches if a sliver or bit of broken glass is in your shoe. If you remove these objects, the leg can walk normally.

Oxalic acid crystals are as sharp as broken glass. Use the kidney cleanse (page 549) to dissolve them and other stones. <u>All lower back pain can be cured by removing the sharp crystals in the kidneys</u>. It takes about three weeks to dissolve them. In some very severe cases, it may take six weeks.

Whether you have suffered a year or 20 years, the permanent cure is only weeks away.

Our bodies make eight or more different kinds of kidney "stones." The oxalic acid variety is associated with sharp stabbing pains. In its effort to eliminate this extremely vicious acid your body neutralizes it with calcium first to make calcium oxalate. Your kidneys can keep a <u>bit</u> of calcium oxalate in solution but not a <u>lot</u>. The excess hardens into crystals. A glass of regular or iced tea (not herb tea or green tea) has about 20 mg[8] of oxalic acid—way too much for kidneys to excrete. Tea is a toxic drink, not to be considered a beverage. Chocolate is very high in oxalate, too, and should not be used as a beverage (as cocoa).

Children should never drink tea or cocoa. Their delicate kidneys should not be faced with the daily burden of excreting large amounts of oxalic acid. And calcium used to neutralize

---

[8]Taken from Food Values 14th ed. by Pennington and Church, 1985.

oxalic acid is wasted. Calcium is a precious nutrient. It should be conserved for children's bone development.

It isn't necessary to find which variety of kidney crystals are causing your muscle spasms. Different herbs dissolve different kinds. And by combining them into a grand herbal mixture you can be dissolving all varieties at the same time.

Wherever oxalate crystals have formed, a particular bacterium, *Proteus vulgaris*, can be found. Does that bacterium somehow thrive on oxalate crystals? Or even help them form? Does *Proteus* itself contribute to lower back pain? Is lower back pain in reality two pains in one—the sharp jabbing of glass-like particles plus the inflammatory effect of bacteria? Fortunately, you can kill *Proteus vulgaris* electronically.

By using your new diagnostic skills, you can test your kidneys for crystals. The kidney stone varieties I have tested for are: **calcium oxalate, uric acid, cysteine, cystine, monocalcium phosphate, dicalcium phosphate, tricalcium phosphate.** All these varieties can be dissolved by the herbal mixture. But all can be formed again in a week!

To prevent **oxalate** formation stop drinking oxalic acid (eating oxalate rich vegetables is not significant—spinach, chard, rhubarb and sorrel all have their place in the diet). Also take magnesium and B_6 supplements (as directed in the kidney cleanse).

To prevent **phosphate** crystals from forming, reduce phosphate consumption and drink milk as a calcium source. Keep your kidneys squeaky clean with herbs and copious water drinking. After drinking one quart of sterilized milk, two pints of water, one-half glass of homemade fruit juice and one-half glass of vegetable juice, there is little desire for additional beverages.

I have no understanding of what may cause **cysteine** or **cystine** stones (the genetic theory does not explain them either, considering that people without *cystinuria* make these stones).

94

Since they are sulfur-containing, and I have seen them appear after taking sulfa-drugs, it may be wise to avoid use of sulfa-drugs if you have a choice, or go on the kidney cleanse afterward.

If you have severe lower back pain you probably have several kinds of stones. Some persons have all seven kinds!

Rosie Zakar, age 30, came to see us because her mother was cured of lower back pain so severe she could do no housework for 30 years. Rosie had the usual crystals in her kidneys: oxalate, urate and phosphates. She was started on the kidney herb recipe. In three weeks she was so much better she would have missed her appointment if she had not wanted to cure her digestive problem and fatigue too.

Vera Vigneault, age 32, came mainly for help in getting pregnant but she already had lower back pain and mid-back pain. If she had gotten pregnant before clearing this up, she might have developed eclampsia and high blood pressure which are kidney-related disorders. She was started on kidney herbs for these. She chewed gum a lot and had bleeding gums. She stated her bad teeth were hereditary (meaning other family members had bad teeth also). For this she was instructed to stop chewing gum, start drinking three glasses of 2% milk a day and take a vitamin A&D perle. She was to floss her teeth once a day. (All floss varieties are polluted with mercury and thallium. Use monofilament fish line, 2 to 4 lb. weight.) Immediately after flossing she was to brush them with a new very soft toothbrush with five drops of 17½% food grade hydrogen peroxide. She was to avoid brushing teeth with metal fillings to reduce erosion. She was to brush them a second time without flossing first, this time with five drops of white iodine (potassium iodide) made up by the pharmacist, again avoiding the metal. She had only oxalate kidney stones and was to stop drinking regular tea, replacing it with single-herb teas. In five weeks her gums were better although she was still chewing a little gum and the "peroxy" had been too painful for her to use. Her low back and mid-back pains were gone too.

Gerhard Rogers, age 39, came for his lower back pain and leg cramps. He had mono, di, and tricalcium phosphate crystals in his kidneys. His diet was changed to reduce phosphate (meat, cereal, breads, pasta, carbonated beverage) and increase calcium and minerals. He was to drink three glasses of 2% milk a day and to start the kidney herb recipe. In 25 days he had only minor improvement. He still had phosphate crystals. He was afraid to drink milk because he had heard so many bad things about it. He was told to boil it first to eliminate these "bad things". A toxic element test showed a buildup of copper, arsenic, cobalt, cadmium, lead, thallium, vanadium and radon. This could easily explain his leg cramps, headaches and sleep problem, too. The arsenic came from pesticide, cobalt from detergent, thallium and copper from tooth fillings. The vanadium was fixed by having the gas pipes tightened, and radon could be reduced by improving ventilation under the house. He was thankful for the information and set about cleaning up his body and environment.

Alberta Mellos, age 52, came in for lower back pain and upper back pain. It was explained to her that lower back pain was simply due to tiny stones cutting into her tissues but upper back pain was due to gallstones. She could clear her low back pain first. The kidney test showed she had oxalate and cysteine crystals. She was started on the kidney herb recipe. Nineteen days later she arrived with a cold but stated that her low back pain was gone.

Glenn Dirk, age 62, called on the telephone to say his urination had stopped, probably due to kidney stones. This had happened once before and now he was in a panic. He started our kidney herb recipe the same day and passed 117 stones the same night without bleeding or enough pain to need painkiller. After this, he could focus on his prostate enlargement and pain with sitting. He had intestinal flukes and other stages in his prostate gland as well as in his intestine. He also had *Clonorchis* (human liver flukes and their eggs) in his prostate. He had carbon tetrachloride, methyl butyl ketone and TC Ethylene from food pollution accumulated there too. After stopping grocery store beverages and killing parasites with a frequency generator, he could urinate normally, freely and without pain.

Lower Abdominal Pain

The lower abdomen on the left side has the sigmoid colon as it comes down and bends. This is a favorite location for larger parasites to settle permanently. Flukes, roundworms, parasites of all kinds and their attendant bacteria and viruses can be felt if they produce gas and pain. Sometimes they live perfectly quietly, seemingly in harmony with us.

Moving the bowel more frequently expels them repeatedly and prevents their numbers from getting very high. Nature may help you with this by setting up diarrhea. Diarrhea is your clue that intestinal freeloaders are present.

The small intestine leads into the colon at your lower abdomen on the right side. At the junction is the ileocaecal valve that prevents backwash, and the appendix. The ascending colon goes up your right side then becomes the transverse colon that crosses your abdomen at the belly button level. The colon descends on your left side, leading into the sigmoid.

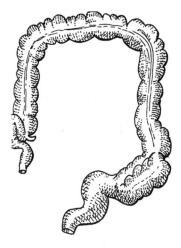

Fig. 19 Colon.

E. coli and *Salmonella* and *Shigella* are "enteric" (they live in your bowel) bacteria that can give you severe abdominal distress and pain. In fact, you can become a <u>chronic</u> sufferer. They can live on hands and under your fingernails, so reinfection from yourself is the most important source. Never, never touch your fingers to your lips. Most importantly, don't try to stop your frequent bowel movements. They will stop on a dime when your parasites and bacteria are dead and gone.

Other sources of *E. coli* are personal water bottles, other people's hands, hands that have changed baby diapers or cleaned bathrooms.

Hands do everything. To eliminate their threat of reinfection, cut out the section on hands (page 397) and paste it on your refrigerator.

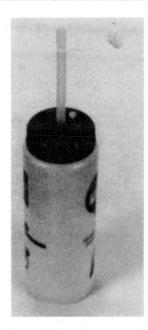

Stomach Pain

Fig. 20 Keep personal water bottles sterile.

Our dairy foods are polluted with *Salmonella* and *Shigella* bacteria. It is impossible to operate a dairy without getting some cow manure into the milk. Although udder wash contains antiseptic it does not kill all manure bacteria. Later, when milk is pasteurized, many heat sensitive bacteria are killed like the "friendly" *streps* and *staphs*, but not all the harmful *Salmonellas* and *Shigellas*. Some survive to colonize the milk, then later infect the consumer. Only milk that is sterilized is safe. A commercial source of sterilized (safe) milk can sometimes be found on the shelf (unrefrigerated). If it had any bacteria, it would not survive shelf life for more than one day!

You may not notice any discomfort from drinking milk, buttermilk, or eating yogurt without sterilizing it. Your stomach acids may be strong enough to kill them, or your liver able to strain them out of your body fluids and dump them, dead, into your bile ducts. Or they may live quietly in some part of the bowel where you feel no effects. Sterilize all your dairy foods by heating at the boiling point for 10 seconds, even if you have no symptoms.

If you are intolerant of milk it doesn't mean that you are lactase deficient, but that you are unable to kill any *Salmonellas* and *Shigellas*. These, in turn, can make you lactase deficient via frequent diarrheas. You can correct this situation by not eating any more bacteria. Give your body clean food, as intended by nature. Don't eat any deli foods, don't eat salad bar food or restaurant food unless it has been baked or cooked. Never eat chicken or red meat at restaurants. They are not thoroughly cooked.

As soon as a new abdominal pain or discomfort, or a gassy condition appears, zap bacteria and try to eliminate your bowel contents. Use the herb, *Cascara sagrada* (follow directions on label) as a laxative, or Epsom salts if necessary. Also start the Bowel Program (page 546).

If you have chronic abdominal problems, make sure you eliminate the bowel contents two or three times a day. There are herbs that can kill enteric bacteria, known to our ancestors of various cultures. **Echinacea** was a treasured herb of American Indians. **Goldenseal** is another favorite. **Turmeric** can kill *E. coli* and some *Shigellas*. **Fennel** can also kill some. But a single dose of Black Walnut Tincture Extra Strength seems to do the most. Make it yourself if possible (see *Recipes*, page 543).

If your body has lost its ability to kill *Salmonellas* and *Shigellas*, all the antibiotics and herbs and good bowel habits cannot protect you from these ubiquitous bacteria. You could ask how you lost your natural protection from them. There is evidence that common **antibiotics** that kill *Streptococcus* and *Staphylococcus* varieties are responsible.

A fraction of your bowel bacteria should be the friendly *Strep. lactis* and *Staph. epidermidis*. After repeated doses of penicillin-like antibiotics (that you may be taking for your strep throat) they are eradicated along with the "bad" *Strep. pneumoniae* bug. No amount of acidophilus culture (which contains active *Lactobacillus*) can replace these *Streps* or *Staphs*.

In mice, it takes a <u>million</u> Salmonella bacteria to start an infection. After giving them streptomycin, it only took <u>10</u> bacteria to infect them![9] Your intestines are similarly handicapped after antibiotics, and allow even very small amounts of *Salmonella* and *Shigella* to escape and multiply!

Try to get some natural killing power back. This means improving the stomach's ability to produce acid and the liver's ability to make bile. In turn, this means getting the toxins out of the stomach and cleaning the liver. Certain toxins accumulate in the stomach when the liver and kidneys can't keep up with elimination. Arsenic is a prominent stomach toxin. Get all sources of arsenic removed. Freon is another stomach toxin. Switch to a non-Freon containing refrigerator.

The metals from dentalware: mercury, silver, copper, thallium, first are swallowed and then land in the stomach. Clean up your dentalware. Toxins you inhale such as asbestos, formaldehyde, fiberglass, also are coughed up and swallowed to accumulate in the stomach. Test for them and clean up your environment. Any stomach can recover a significant part of its function by cleaning it up. Even though you regain your tolerance toward minute bits of filth in dairy products, do not go back to unsterilized milk products.

Appendicitis

The lower abdomen on the right side has the valve that separates the small intestine (*ileum*) from the large intestine

---

[9]Sherwood L. Gorbach, M.D., <u>Perturbation of Intestinal Microflora</u>, Vet Human Toxicol 35 (Supplement 1) 1993.

(*caecum*) called the *ileocaecal valve*. It is a common trouble spot because large parasites can attach themselves behind it and keep themselves safe from elimination. (A parasite's biggest worry is your elimination.) It is a favorite location for pinworms in children. It is near this point where the appendix attaches and this, too, is a favorite location of pinworms. With an appendix full of pinworms and their bacteria, is it any wonder when it gets inflamed and causes pain?

Appendicitis refers to inflammation of the appendix. Often, the pain isn't felt over the appendix but over the navel (this is an example of pain being caused at one location but felt at another; it is called *referred pain*). If there are any suspicions of appendicitis, zap pinworms and all enteric parasites and bacteria immediately. Because the current does not penetrate the bowel contents very well, zap every day for two weeks and take 2 tsp. (½ tsp. for children) Black Walnut Hull Tincture Extra Strength one time. Make sure bowel movements are regular after this (see the Bowel Program, page 546, for hints) and hands are washed after bathroom use and before eating. Keep fingernails short for the whole family.

If appendicitis does not clear up it can lead to a burst appendix, spewing the dreadful contents into the abdomen. Kill pinworms and roundworms and enteric parasites regularly (once a week) in children. Keep pets on a regular diet of parasite-killing herbs.

Urinary Tract Pain

Urinary tract infections, including bladder, kidney, and urethral infections, are easier to clear up than to test for. Start by drinking a half gallon of water a day. Put yourself on the kidney herb recipe (page 549). This will dissolve the tiny crystals where bacteria hide and multiply.

Common urinary tract pathogens are *Gardnerella*, *Proteus*, *Trichomonas*, *Campylobacters*, *E. coli*, and *Salmonellas*. Sex will give you an instant dose of your partner's urinary tract bacteria. Make sure both of you clean up the urinary tract by zapping and doing the Kidney Cleanse.

Irritable Bowel Syndrome(IBS), Colitis, and Spastic Colon

are all conditions that combine parasite and bacterial problems plus an allergic trigger. If dairy foods trigger yours, you can guess it is not allergic at all but simply *Salmonella* or *Shigella* infection. Boil all dairy foods, stop eating ice cream, cheese and yogurt which you cannot boil. If eating lettuce triggers your intestinal attack, but other roughage does not, it may be a true allergen and cleaning the liver will eventually cure it. Apples, cinnamon and other "allergic" foods can be salvaged the same way. Wheat "allergy" is due to the pancreas being full of pancreatic flukes, wood alcohol, Kojic acid (a mycotoxin), and gold.

All these bowel diseases are quite easily cured by killing all parasites, bacteria, and viruses. Since reinfection is such a big problem, give your pet away until you are completely cured. Have your pet on the herbal parasite program before bringing it back. Clean up your diet, dentalware and environment. Your abdomen will be happy once more and grateful to you for your kind attention. Remember that zapping does not penetrate into the bowel contents. It kills only the outside layer of pathogens. For this reason you should zap daily for several weeks. For this reason, too, I recommend the Bowel Program (page 546) and Black Walnut Hull Tincture Extra Strength even though you may have gotten immediate relief from zapping alone.

Crohn's Disease

is somewhat more serious because the sores are higher up in the digestive tract. This is because sheep liver fluke and pancreatic fluke are commonly the main parasites and these live in the pancreas and liver. They often spill over into the upper intestine. *Salmonella* and *Shigella* are always part of the picture, too, as are various amoebae and fungi. The treatment is the same, kill all parasites and remove all pollutants, especially wood alcohol in commercial beverages. Healing of the digestive tract is very quick, often in a week. Reinfection is very quick too, if the rule about cooking dairy foods is not observed. Keep up meticulous hand sanitation.

Michelle Whorton had stomach pain at the middle of her abdomen, not related to eating. She had occasional very bad diarrhea and also daily headaches. She was started on the kidney herbs for other reasons. Her diarrhea disappeared! We found she had *Ascaris* (probably in her stomach where they cause indigestion and inflammation). She zapped them with a frequency generator set to 408 KHz for three minutes at 10 volts. She was to be very careful with sanitation since they owned a number of farm dogs. Next seen after six weeks, she stated that all her previous problems were gone but she had a different pain in the mid-lower abdomen that got worse during her period and sent pain shooting down both legs.

This turned out to be uterine in origin, but not endometriosis. Her uterus was full of asbestos, arsenic, gold, silver, titanium, propyl alcohol, benzene, styrene, toluene and carbon tetrachloride. This would invite any bacteria toward it!

Mark Lippman, age 51, came in for his irritable bowel syndrome, hoping we would find *Giardia* and put an end to it quickly. Actually, he had intestinal flukes, beginning to invade the liver. He also had propyl alcohol built up in his body giving him a precancerous condition that needed immediate attention. The flukes were killed in twenty minutes, along with *Ascaris* (he had swollen eyelids). He was allergic to milk as could be expected with so much interference with digestion. He was immediately better and did not need to come back.

Billy Henry, a 9-year-old boy, had diarrhea daily and stomach aches. He also wet the bed. There was an indoor pet dog and a bird. Electronic testing showed he had two kinds of *Ascaris* and pinworms. His young body also had a buildup of benzene, moth balls and carbon tetrachloride that he was eating, drinking, and breathing. His bed wetting stopped after killing parasites with the herbal program. His other problems recurred until he was older and could stop licking his fingers when eating.

Tom Ochs, age 36, had chronic stomach problems, alternating constipation and diarrhea, was labeled "lactose intolerant" after an elaborate test, and finally had been diagnosed with irritable bowel syndrome. Actually, he had *Ascaris*, besides other smaller parasites. He was also toxic with cesium from drinking beverages out of clear plastic bottles. This frequently causes depression and he was happy to understand his mood changes. After changing to purer food and products and killing his parasites, he did not need to come back. Five months later he was able to drink all the milk he wanted, no longer had sinus problems and lost his IBS.

Rex Callahan, age 5, had dark circles under his eyes, numerous ear infections until tonsils were removed and tubes put in, and many strep throat infections. Clinically, he was found allergic to dust mites, pollens, and animal dander. His skin got "rashy" if he drank too much fruit juice. He had frequent diarrhea. We found he had *Ascaris* parasites. They were not difficult to clear and he was soon a new person.

David Falls, age 52, had stomach pain and numerous health problems stemming, no doubt, from his diagnosed Crohn's disease. He became allergic to the sulfa drugs commonly used in this disease. We found he had sheep liver flukes and all their developmental stages in his blood and intestine. He was put on the herbal parasite program which he found difficult to follow. Nevertheless, in three months his bowel was nearly normal and the pain in his intestine much less.

Edward Marsili, age 7, had bouts of stomach pain. He had intestinal flukes and a build-up of benzene in his body. This would seriously lower his immunity and ability to fight off tiny parasites. He was using a product containing an herbal oil that was polluted with benzene. His parasites were quickly killed with a frequency generator and he was put on the herbal parasite program. One month later his stomach felt much better, but he still had an occasional stomach ache. Testing showed hookworm and rabbit fluke. His benzene was now gone so the tendency to "pick up everything" was gone too. Staying on a child's maintenance parasite program would protect him.

Kim Johnson, almost two years old, had lots of ear infections. It started at eight months so the mother took her off cow's milk and wheat. This stopped her ear infections until mid-winter. She had to be back on antibiotics and a few months ago the doctor began discussing tube implants with her since she was still on antibiotics (six months). Another ear, nose and throat doctor agreed with this opinion, but was willing to wait until Autumn. The baby had been passing a lot of undigested food and was unhappy. They were vegetarians. The baby nursed. Our test showed pancreatic fluke infestation; this would easily lead to bad digestion, especially of milk and gluten in wheat. Fortunately, she was nursed throughout, in spite of going to daycare. Simply killing the parasites (in both mother and baby) solved both problems and she did not need to come back. The ear infections were probably caused by bacteria and viruses brought in by the parasites.

Cynthia Prout, age 36, brought her three children because of their poor health. They all, including herself, had stomach problems, a lot of allergies, asthma, ear infections, and milk intolerance. One boy, age 8; was intolerant of both milk and wheat and hadn't had them for years. He was infested with two kinds of *Ascaris* and pancreatic flukes. His sister, Nola, had itching legs and headaches besides; she was toxic with bismuth and antimony (from shampoo fragrance and laundry fragrance). She also showed a build up of vanadium, implying a gas leak in the home. The youngest, age 5, had frequent stomach aches and vomiting. It was a simple matter to kill *Ascaris* electronically at 408 KHz and the pancreatic fluke with all its stages (421 through 434) after which the children did fine.

Sofia Sobel had extreme ulcerative colitis although she came for her headache. She had been on Prednisone for a month with no relief. We found she had the three large flukes plus *Chilomastix*, dog whip worm, and amoebas in her intestine (but not in body organs).

There were several house dogs. Her stomach and intestines were much too sensitive to accept parasite herbs, or in fact, anything— anything except slippery elm powder. This herb (1 tbs. made into a paste first with water and then drunk as a beverage three times a day) paved the way for acceptance of two oyster shell calcium, one magnesium and one zinc tablet. Her blood test showed high phosphate levels since she was dissolving her bones to get calcium. She added sodium alginate (¼ tsp. to a cup of vegetable broth soup) twice a day to help her tolerate the parasite killing herbs. Her children were given VMF (vermifuge or parasite killing) syrup. By the 12th day of the parasite program she no longer needed colitis medicine; her bowel movements were down to twice a day, soft and formed, but still with a little blood streaking. She loved the alginate mixed with slippery elm. She was able to eat fruits and vegetables but agreed to stay off wheat and corn until her liver was cleansed. In another week she was free from all abdominal complaints except a heaviness over the uterus, possibly due to two missed periods. The thought of pregnancy put her in a panic. She was instructed to induce her period (Emmenagogue, see *Recipes*). She was sure she wanted her period, not a pregnancy and this seemed to be her God-given right. Three weeks later she had a flare up of colitis due to *Salmonella* in food; it also gave her a urinary tract infection. This time she took Quassia herb to kill invaders in addition to the maintenance parasite program which she had begun to neglect. She had been very busy, had lots of energy and wasn't on medications. She treated her urinary tract infection with betaine-hydrochloride (to acidify the stomach), began using plastic utensils to reduce her nickel intake (see Prostate Pain, page 124)) and drank a lot of water. This experience taught her valuable lessons that she was eager to learn, benefiting her family and herself immensely.

Rebecca Goetz, age 53, had ulcerative colitis and her husband had Crohn's disease. She had been on Azulfidine™ and Flagyl™ frequently. Her parasites were only intestinal flukes and their stages, and *Endolimax*, an amoeba. It was a simple task for her to clear her problems by killing them and by sterilizing her dairy foods. Wes, her husband, had three surgeries to remove sections of bowel due to Crohn's disease. He now had a colostomy but was on Advil™ for pain in the rectal area. He could hardly sit. He had been tried on anti parasitic medicine (Cypril™ and Flagyl™) but they did no good. He had intestinal flukes and all their reproductive stages in his body, also pancreatic flukes, *Capillaria* roundworm, and *Diphyllobothrium erinacea* scolex. We interrupted his testing at that point. His kidneys were full of phosphate crystals—he ate no dairy products. He was started on half-doses of kidney herbs and only part of the parasite program in view of his colostomy and possible diarrhea. Two weeks later we continued testing, finding pinworms, *Haemonchus*, *Leishmania tropica*, *Paragonimus*, *Sarcocystis*, *Stephanuris* and *Trichuris* (whip worm.) Quassia was added and doses increased. His blood test showed a high thyroid hormone level (T4), contributory to over activity of his bowel He was started on goat milk, vitamin C (3 gm. daily) and B_{12} shots. He was given magnets to sit on for pain. He was toxic with cadmium, from his old tooth fillings. But in five weeks he could sit comfortably without pain pills. There was less blood in the stool. Dental work would bring him his next big improvement.

Benito Villamar, a middle age man, had severe side pain for several weeks. He was also gassy. He had sheep liver fluke and stages in his thymus and intestine. The thymus is under the top of the breastbone and is a very important organ of immune function. It is easily damaged by benzene. He did, indeed, have benzene accumulated there. He was given a list of benzene-polluted products to avoid and was started on the parasite killing herbs after killing the flukes instantly with the frequency generator. Two weeks later his side was very much better, his benzene was gone and he was eager to rid himself of lower back pain, which he also had.

Al Vickers, age 9, had stomach aches, headaches, a constantly runny nose and asthma. He was on Slo-Bid™ medicine and allergy treatment. He had a sleep problem. He also had two dogs, one rat and two hamsters. The dogs and he had high levels of *Ascaris*. He was zapped for *Ascaris* and the four common flukes (without testing). He was put on vermifuge syrup and Rascal capsules. This ended his problems and began a new chapter of better care for his health by his parents.

Tim Melton, age 16, had several colitis attacks yearly, requiring hospitalization, from third grade to the present. He also drooled constantly, needing to spit a lot. (This is due to mercury toxicity from amalgam fillings. It is better to spit out the mercury than to swal-

107

low it.) He had intestinal flukes at a high level for which he was started on the parasite program. One month later he was very much better. He had only one diarrhea session since the last visit. But he still had sharp pains under both buttocks (probably due to kidney stones). He had been an iced tea drinker and had numerous oxalate and cysteine crystals deposited. He was appalled that a common beverage could be so harmful.

Central Abdominal Pain

can be coming from the uterus, bladder, or bowel. It is difficult to tell which is the source. The first step is to simply kill enteric (bowel) free-loaders and get into good bowel habits. Gas and bloating should be gone. If this isn't the solution to the pain there may be special bladder parasites with their bacteria. *Schistosomes* prefer to invade the bladder wall. In fact, very many parasites temporarily invade the bladder because the body is trying to excrete many of them. The whole family should be cleared of these same parasites. Kill them by zapping. Pets should not be kept indoors since they have many of these parasites, too, and they are easily transmitted to us.

Interstitial Cystitis

is one of the most painful conditions described by clients. *Schistosomes* are the real perpetrators but after the bladder wall is weakened, other parasites and their bacteria and viruses accumulate here too. To regain your bladder's health all toxins must be cleared as well. Dental metal, environmental toxins, including radon, asbestos, formaldehyde, must be cleaned up. The diet, body products and home should be carefully searched for toxins. *Schistosomes* are easily zapped but easily picked up

108

off toilet seats and doorknobs. Always wash hands after toileting: a single droplet reinfects you!

Uterine Pain

Endometriosis

Many a woman's dreams have been shattered by her inability to have a child. Endometriosis is often the cause. It starts with painful cramps at period times. They get worse and worse until pain killers are necessary just to get out of bed and move about the house. There are flukes in the uterus! Large intestinal flukes in a rather small organ! Did they migrate to the uterus from the intestine or did they develop there from eggs?

Sometimes sheep liver fluke is seen there. Once an avenue to the uterus is established, numerous other parasites move in the same direction: *Clonorchis*, the human <u>liver</u> fluke and even *Eurytrema*, the <u>pancreatic</u> fluke, can invade the uterus wall. Why have they taken up so abnormal a living place? Because the uterus has solvents in it! This is the green light for flukes. This disarms your organs so they are left helpless against fluke stages left there by the blood and lymph. Stop eating solvent-polluted foods. There are solvents in <u>all</u> cold cereals. Make cooked cereal. There are solvents in purchased drinking water. Drink from your cold kitchen faucet. There are solvents in grocery store bread, grocery baked goods and cholesterol-reduced foods. Eat <u>none</u> of these. Buy baked goods and bread at your local bakery. Stay away from "low cholesterol" foods. There are solvents in decaffeinated and other powdered mixes for beverages. Drink <u>nothing</u> except milk from the grocery store (sterilize it). Milk does not have solvent pollution. The hormones, antibiotics and udder wash can be tolerated—solvents cannot.

Beverages and powdered mixtures sold at health food stores are <u>no</u> exception. Use <u>no</u> powdered mixture intended for weight loss or weight gain, nor vitality supports, nor dietary supplements. They are <u>all</u> polluted. Some solvents (I often see methyl ethyl ketone and methyl butyl ketone) <u>choose</u> the uterus to accumulate in. This sets the stage for endometriosis and fertility problems. Where there are large parasites, smaller ones soon crowd in. All bring their own bacteria and viruses. *Gardnerella*, especially, is found in cases of endometriosis, ovarian cysts and menstrual problems. The flukes evidently travel from the uterus to other parts of your body cavity, distributing bits of the uterine lining as they go. Once this distribution has occurred, can the bleeding (regular menstrual bleeding) at these extra sites ever be stopped?

> It stops <u>immediately</u> when the flukes are dead!

Your body knows how to clean up after dead flukes and does the job perfectly. You can be free of pain in time for your next period. Zap to kill the four common flukes, *Gardnerella*, all other common parasites, and urinary tract bacteria (common ones include *Proteus*, *Salmonella*, *Campylobacter*, *Chlamydia*, *Trichomonas*). Avoid reinfection by avoiding solvents! It is impossible <u>not</u> to pick up parasites. If your uterus has solvent in it, they <u>will</u> find their way to it <u>in a day</u>. Without solvent, they will not.

The solvents will leave by themselves. Help your body get rid of them with vitamin C and B_2 (3 grams and 300 mg. respectively, daily, see *Sources*).

To heal the uterus so it no longer attracts parasites, clear up its internal pollution besides solvents. This means mainly the dental metal that has piled up and environmental toxins such as asbestos, arsenic, fiberglass, and formaldehyde. Gold and silver are especially attracted to the uterus. Don't wear gold rings or any metal jewelry touching your skin anymore, and, of course, get all metal out of your teeth. Never try to get pregnant before you have cleared up endometriosis.

The advice given by obstetricians to get pregnant to solve your pain problem is most unwise. Indeed, pregnancy changes your body's metabolism and without periods you get pain relief. But it seems much too risky to grow a baby in an infested, polluted uterus. Fear of birth defects is an intelligent fear. Be careful not to get pregnant while you are killing parasites and getting mercury removed from your teeth.

> Healing starts as soon as all the parasites and pollutants are gone.

Joanne Biro, age 22, had severe cramping pain with her periods, diagnosed as endometriosis. She had adult intestinal flukes and the *cercaria* stage in her uterus. She had a xylene (solvent) buildup in both her brain(cerebrum and cerebellum) and uterus. She was started on the herbal parasite program following the kidney cleanse. Her next period was pain free. A check up showed she was free of flukes but had thallium in her immune system. Dental cleanup was next on her agenda.

Denise Leyva, 22, was on birth control pills to control the growth of endometrial tissue. She had laser surgery previously. She had hexanedione and methyl butyl ketone buildup in her uterus supporting the intestinal fluke and its eggs in the uterus. There were also some sheep liver flukes and human liver fluke stages there! She was advised to stop eating cold cereals and commercial beverages and kill the parasites immediately. She had no recurrence.

Anita Pierce, age 32, had numerous surgeries for her endometriosis. She also had chronic fatigue syndrome, and several allergies. She had two beautiful poodles in her home. She could not part with them so she gave them the pet parasite herbs faithfully. She had intestinal flukes, tapeworm stages, *Ascaris* and various other

111

flukes in the uterus. She had all her dental metal removed and home detoxified. Her body was teeming with *Nocardia* and Epstein Barre Virus (EBV). In spite of repeatedly killing the flukes and bacteria with a frequency generator and making herculean efforts she was no better off eight months later. She was unable to solve the problem of reinfection from her dogs.

Christine Solton, age 27, had extremely heavy and painful periods and didn't stop bleeding between periods. A large cyst had been seen by X-ray in the uterine wall. She also had constant bladder pain. Both problems kept her in the bathroom most of the time (90 visits/day). She had the intestinal fluke in her uterus (probable cause of cyst) and *Schistosoma haematobium* (bladder parasite) throughout her body. She was started on the parasite program and in one week her bladder pain was under control but bleeding (from the cyst in uterine wall) continued. *Schistosomes* are very contagious, probably even from toilet seats and the house dust of an infected person. She had them again three weeks later. This time she zapped them and got instant relief. Her bladder and uterus were both full of propyl alcohol, tooth metal, fluoride, cobalt, zirconium, aluminum, antimony, cadmium, and formaldehyde. She was delighted, though, to understand her problem and made the dental appointment.

Contraception

There is an excellent pamphlet available at health food stores, called Wild Yam for Birth Control Without Fear[10] that informs that 3 capsules taken two times a day provides reliable (perfect) contraception <u>provided</u> you give it a two month head start. Also, an emmenagogue recipe is on page 546.

The Silent Cervix

The cervix is a big "trouble spot" for women just as the prostate is for men. It seldom lets you know with pain, however,

---

[10]Willa Shaffer, published by Woodland Health Books, PO Box 1422, Provo, Utah 84603.

that bacteria or parasites or toxins are present. Sometimes a brief needle-like pain does alert you to something going on there, but it is easy to miss. The cervix is constantly secreting a little bit of mucous and this helps it stay clean but why give it mercury and copper and gold to secrete? Many a fertility problem has been solved by stopping the toxic pollution of uterus, ovaries, and cervix. Clean up your dentalware and clean up your diet and environment.

Kill parasites and bacteria regularly, every week, with the herbal recipe or by zapping. You should have no pain with menstruation, no bloating, fatigue or headaches. A PAP smear test should always be "good". If it isn't, hurry to the rescue of your cervix.

Menopausal Symptoms, Hot Flushes, PMS

Insomnia, irritability, PMS (pre-menstrual syndrome), depression, anxiety, nervousness, are all not to be expected at and after menopause. They may certainly be caused by hormone imbalances. It is these imbalances that are not normal.

NO menopausal symptoms are normal

After the ovaries are done with their cycles of estrogen and progesterone production, the **adrenal glands'** hormone production was meant to "kick in" and make up any deficit.

During your fertile years, you were meant to have a peak of 100 picograms/milliliter (pg./ml) of estrogen on day 9 and day 22 of your cycle. Progesterone, on the other hand, only peaks once, on day 22, and it should reach a level 20 to 100 times as high as estrogen! After this ends, your adrenals can still keep your hormone levels regulated. Typical values are 20 pg./ml

113

estrogen and, again, 20 to 100 times as much progesterone. Keeping these two hormones in balance is just as important as the actual amounts. **20 pg./ml estrogen is enough to prevent menopausal symptoms** including hot flushes, and to give you heart protection and bone density protection. Taking synthetic hormones usually gives you exactly such levels. But if your own adrenal glands can supply them, surely it is a better approach. (A blood test can tell you your levels; do it on day 21, 22 or 23 before menopause, after menopause the day is not critical.)

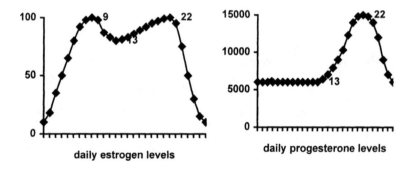

Fig. 21 Estrogen and progesterone levels (pg./ml).

Why aren't your adrenals producing them? Because they are hampered by parasites and pollutants! Kill all the parasites, bacteria and viruses, especially *Gardnerella, Proteus, Chlamydia, Campylobacter, Neisseria, Treponema, Salmonella.* Use the zapper.

Notice that these are also the favorite urinary tract bacteria! This makes good sense, because the adrenal glands sit right on the kidneys and would be geographically close to the kidney bacteria. To avoid getting them back, do a kidney cleanse (page 549) to remove all crystals where they might hide.

After this, hot flushes can be suddenly gone. If not, continue the cleanse. Meanwhile, do some permanent lifestyle improvement. Start drinking two pints of water between meals plus water and milk (sterilized) at mealtime.

Don't drink cranberry juice with its copious *hippuric acid* and its solvent pollutants. You won't need such insufficient help after cleaning up your body, dentalware, and environment. Besides giving you a better hormone supply, your newly revitalized adrenals will get you through stress in better shape and keep your blood pressure normal.

If bacteria are not kept down they will begin to invade other organs. *Gardnerella* goes to ovaries to feast on the corpus luteum after ovulation. This keeps the corpus luteum from making enough progesterone and PMS results.

Menstrual problems and PMS, in general, although they may not be pain-causers, are a sign that all is not well with the uterus and ovaries. Go on a cleanup program. Kill your invaders with herbs or the zapper. Clear up your toxic accumulations from dental metal and environmental sources.

Don't be surprised by a pregnancy! This is not the time to get pregnant, though. If you wish to get pregnant, clean up your body first, being very careful to <u>prevent</u> pregnancy during this time. If this is not under your control do your <u>dental work first</u>. Since every cleanup job increases your fertility, it is best to get the mercury, thallium, copper and nickel out of your body before your risk of conception is raised further by making other improvements. Many an amalgam replacement job had to be halted in the middle due to pregnancy! Couples just couldn't believe they could have a child as a result of cleaning up their bodies so they were careless in spite of my warnings! **A dentist will not take out mercury during pregnancy.**

Nicole Truett, 40ish, had PMS before her periods. She was a returning student and couldn't afford to feel emotionally upset. She also had recurrent yeast infections, *Herpes* and panic attacks. She complained that her thinking was weird, although she was an excellent student (she got her birth date wrong on our office forms!) She had high levels of mercury and we suggested dental work immediately. Two months later she was feeling much better and had all metal removed but was experiencing a slight return of symptoms which panicked her. She still had *E. coli* and *Bacillus anthracus* at four tooth locations, giving her chronic sinus symptoms. She needed her cavitations cleaned. Four weeks later she described how she had gotten immediate <u>emotional</u> relief after two cavitations were done. Our solvent test showed methyl butyl ketone, benzene and carbon tetrachloride (which we found in her Mountain Valley Arkansas Spring Water). They were lowering her immunity giving recurrent Herpes and yeast problems. These disappeared in a week. She was so happy to find the <u>cause</u> of her problems and yet so angry at the nature of the cause that she planned to write to the water company. We need more such environmental activists.

Monica Koziol was on Ibuprofen™ for menstrual cramps. She also got a severe sugar craving and minor depression and headache with her period. She was toxic with silver, copper, platinum, mercury and lead. She also had hookworms, pinworms, human liver fluke and cat liver flukes infesting her. A hormone test showed very low estrogen (57.6 pg/ml) probably due to all these interfering factors. She had all the metal from her fillings replaced and killed parasites with the herbal recipe. This gave her regular normal periods for several months. She decided to get pregnant but couldn't. A follow-up showed she was full of parasites again. She had stopped the maintenance parasite program. She resumed it and began kidney and liver cleanses to get longer lasting benefits.

Barbara Ashby, age 43, had suffered for 1½ years from menstrual pain. She had oxalate crystals in her kidneys and was started on the kidney cleanse. She followed this with the parasite program and dental metal replacement. Then she cleaned her liver and after three cleanses (she got over 1,000 stones the first time!) she said she felt <u>great</u> again.

Terri Entzminger, age 16, had a long list of health problems including painful ovaries and painful periods for which she was put on birth control pills by her doctor. She had several bacteria in her genital tract: *Neisseria gonorrhea, Plasmodium cyano, Staphylococcus*

116

aureus (also at tooth #28 which had a plastic filling), *Streptococcus pyogenes* (also at tooth #28). A parasite test showed intestinal fluke adults in the uterus, not in the intestine or liver. There were also fluke *cercaria* here. She was started on the parasite herbs. Three weeks later there was no improvement. She had a rabbit, a dog and a hamster. She was to get them all onto the pet parasite program. Her diet was changed to exclude solvents. Six weeks later her periods were "great", she did not need the pill and she was keeping the whole household on a maintenance program killing parasites. Three weeks later she had cramps again. This time it was sheep liver fluke in the uterus. She probably got them from the snails in her fish tanks. She was off the maintenance program and drinking caffeine free cola again. This would fill her with solvents that make fluke disease possible. She killed them all with a frequency generator and decided to be more vigilant over parasites as long as she was such an ardent animal lover.

Azar Moya, 57, was on Premarin™ and Provera™ for hot flushes and emotional extremes, Synthroid™ for the thyroid, Xanax™ for nerves and sleep problems, something for diarrhea and something for depression. In five months she needed none of it. She had done a liver cleanse by then and got a commode-full of stones (about 1,000), she had changed her plumbing, got rid of the water softener, killed parasites and cleansed her kidneys. She still had sinus problems and some arthritis and was planning dental metal replacement and cavitation cleaning to clear them up too.

Infertility

An ominous sign in any species, infertility is not just another disease or "problem."

When birds' eggs don't hatch their species is doomed. So we learned from the DDT experiment humans did with birds in the 1960's. The DDT changed the thickness of their egg shells so they cracked when the mother bird sat on them. All changes are experiments whether intentional or unintentional. Nature by itself produces sweeping changes, too, such as droughts, wind storms, fires, ice ages, but usually living things had time or mobility to adapt to them. When there wasn't time, and they couldn't run away, the species went extinct.

Are we humans an exception to this rule of adapt or perish? Nobody feels more helpless and hopeless than the infertile couple. They can not run away, time is limited, and obviously adaptation is not occurring. More likely their lineage will perish. The couples' only wish is "Give us one child, now." Surely, it is their birthright, as it is any living creatures', to reproduce.

Can we relax with the assurance that our intelligence, through the arm of science, will always rescue us? Are test tube fertilizations, fertility drugs, Cesarean sections, incubators for premature babies all triumphs for science? No, they are signs of reproductive <u>failure</u> for the human species.

When the concern is overpopulation of this planet, reproductive failure might seem less ominous. Maybe it's no worse than the natural way any species curbs its growth rate. Maybe only those who can survive parasitism, pollution and immune deficiency <u>should</u> survive in order to strengthen the species. But when reproductive intervention becomes a necessity, not an option, surely the danger signal is present as it was for the DDT'd birds who saw cracks develop in their eggs. The solution to our reproductive failure is <u>not</u> to find ever more artificial ways to conceive, to give birth, and to care for damaged babies. The solution is to fix the old fashioned way; to safeguard the natural way.

If you are unable to conceive or to provide viable sperms use an intelligent approach. Remove the obstacles. **The obstacles are parasites and pollutants, the same enemies of health we have seen before.**

Kill all large and small parasites with a zapper and the herbal parasite killing program. Don't <u>try</u> to keep a pet parasite free, give it away. Living close to another species is a luxury you can't afford at present. The pet can live with its parasites, you can't. Remember to kill bacteria and viruses too, especially *Gardnerella, Neisseria, Treponema,* the ancient enemies of human reproduction.

Is it safe to kill parasites if you might be pregnant?

The electronic way of killing parasites is <u>safe if you use a frequency generator</u>. The frequencies of parasites and bacteria are <u>far away</u> from human frequencies. The treatment with each frequency is short. There are no side effects.

The zapper has not been tested and should not be used during pregnancy.

The herbal way of killing parasites has been used by pregnant women without bad effects but this is not enough safeguard. I recommend waiting until the baby is born if at all possible. The treatment is long and intense. The growing baby is exposed continuously to herbs. Perhaps this is preferable to the toxins produced by parasites. You must use your own judgment. Obviously it is wiser to take a chance on herbs than to take a chance on inheriting AIDS or "genetic" diseases.

Part two of regaining your reproductive freedom to have a child is removing pollutants. Gold, silver, copper and mercury can accumulate in the reproductive organs, wrecking the delicate hormone balance between estrogen and progesterone, or wrecking the motility of sperm. Research has not been done to search for dental metal in the uterus, ovaries and testicle of infertile couples. You can do this research yourself. Slides of ovary tissue cost less than $10.00 as do other parts of the reproductive system. Search for dental metal yourself. Remove <u>all</u> dental metal from your mouth, and replace it with metal-free composite. Extract teeth with root canals.

A Word Of Warning!

Be extra careful with contraception during the dental cleanup. You could get pregnant the very next day! **This is no joke**. It is a serious hazard to conceive a child while mercury is loose and rampant in your body from the removal process. It may be a <u>higher</u> risk than leaving it untouched. If you are pregnant no dentist will want to finish the job of mercury removal! **Don't try to get pregnant yet.**

You may have tried fertility pills, in vitro fertilization, and other methods for getting pregnant over a ten year time period, all to no avail. Then you start cleaning up your body and taking your mercury out and <u>suddenly you are pregnant before the job is complete!</u> It may seem unreasonable and illogical to have to be careful after ten years of no worries, but play it safe.

If you fail to observe this warning and do get pregnant too soon, you may pray for miscarriage. Otherwise, take vitamin C and thioctic acid and hope for the best. Men should add daily zinc and arginine (60 mg. and 450 mg, respectively) to their diets. Both men and women should add vitamin E (200 mg.), a prenatal multivitamin and multimineral tablet, eat freshly grown vegetables for folic acid, and add vitamin C (at least a gram daily, see *Sources*). **No other supplements!** Supplements polluted with heavy metals or solvents do more harm than good. If you are not sure of their purity, test one by eating it and searching for it in your immune system five minutes later. If it is there, it is harmful; eat no more.

Nausea

of pregnancy is the scourge of expectant parents. After waiting hard and long for the desired pregnancy, the mother-to-be feels rotten, salivates and gags at the thought of food, and wants no more sex. Maybe sex is ill-advised during pregnancy, no matter how reassuring the male or male-oriented obstetrician is! Maybe salivation is actually mercury excretion being attempted by the body. Maybe nausea is all about keeping toxins out of the body and away from the developing child. These are intriguing possibilities, worthy of your research expertise.

A few decades ago the treatment for nausea was a weekly B6 and B12 shot. Ask your obstetrician for this to see if it helps.

An older, herbal remedy was cinnamon tea: 2 tbs. cinnamon (bark or powder) in 2½ cups boiling water, steeped for 10 minutes. Strain and add honey to taste. Dose: ¼ cup three times a day before meals.

Nausea invites starch eating—pasta, potatoes, rice and bread. Starches can absorb. Perhaps they absorb the noxious substances causing nausea. Make sure you add vitamin C to grains. In any case you must still eat additional nutritious food to grow your baby. In spite of craving a pickles/chocolate pudding/carbonated beverage lifestyle, you must eat mainly good food. Craving can take strange turns. Search for the taste you crave in good food and in long forgotten childhood foods.

These are all the fertility cases I saw in a year's time. None were left out in order to hide failure. Assess the success rate yourself:

Domilita Renshaw and her husband had been trying for six years to get pregnant. Both had been tested and treated in assorted ways. Domilita's period was irregular, a sure sign that all is not well in

121

the area of reproduction. I gave them the usual warning about not risking pregnancy during their deparasitizing and depolluting procedures they both would be going through. Her hormone test showed slightly high (125 pg/ml) estrogen levels for day 22 (if it really was day 22!) and higher still if it was not yet day 22! Obviously, something was irritating the ovaries into overproduction of estrogen. She had oxalate and urate crystals and was put on the kidney herb recipe. She was switched to milk (3 glasses 2% a day) as her primary beverage besides water. She was toxic with nickel (dental metal) which would invite hordes of urinary tract bacteria, dangerously close to the ovaries. She made her dental appointment. She had sheep liver flukes and was started on the parasite program. She broke out in hives from a new hair spray polluted with praseodymium which got into her ovaries. She prepared to clean her liver for her frequent hives. Then she called to cancel her next appointment because she was pregnant (four months from first visit). Fortunately she had one visit with dentist completed. Nine months later she had a beautiful perfect baby.

Lindy Maloy and her husband had been trying for eight years to have their second child. They all had *Ascaris*, including, of course, their house dog. They wormed the dog monthly and did not want to part with it since they did not believe it mattered. They used the pet parasite program, but five months later she had higher *Ascaris* loads than ever. She also could not rid her uterus of intestinal fluke stages in spite of killing them with a frequency generator and using the parasite herbs. She remained full of solvents, bacteria and platinum from dentalware. Her endometriosis continued. They gave up.

Rosemary Peterson, age 33, had been trying to get pregnant for fourteen years. She had seven laparoscopies for endometriosis and very hard cramps with her period. She had intestinal flukes and sheep liver flukes in her uterus. There were sheep liver flukes and human liver flukes in her liver. There were intestinal fluke redia and cercaria in her saliva. The solvents in her uterus were methyl butyl ketone, acetone, carbon tetrachloride (from drinking store bought water), styrene (from drinking out of styrofoam cups), xylene (from carbonated beverages) and decane (from cholesterol-reduced foods). She also had a chronic yeast infection, treating it constantly with Nystatin™. She killed the flukes and yeast electronically before leaving the office and started herself on the parasite program and diet restriction. She got pregnant immediately, and did not return.

Elisabeth Tran, age 37, had tried to get pregnant for five years. She did get pregnant recently, on a special "gift" surgery program, but lost it. Her ovaries and uterus were toxic with mercury and thallium from polluted dental alloy. She also had barium and titanium in them, probably from lipstick. We did not see her again, we hope she solved these problems.

Christopher Gravely, a young man of 26 and Frederica, 22, promised faithfully not to get pregnant until their cleanup was complete. He was found by his doctor to have slow moving (low motility) sperm. He was robust and healthy looking but suffered a lot from low back pain—a clue to swarms of bacteria in the lower abdomen. An electronic search of his testicles and prostate (which had been infected once) revealed iridium, platinum and yttrium. This implicated tooth metal. He was also started on kidney herbs. Eight months later he had completed all his tasks, his low back and pain with urination had stopped, and this encouraged him to continue with his fertility program. We started him on thioctic acid two a day and zinc (60 mg.) two a day, switched him to an electric razor so he wouldn't have to use any chemicals on his face, and recommended that he ventilate his garage which was attached to the house, to reduce fumes in his home.

Meanwhile, Frederica, his wife, was also checked for toxic elements. She had antimony (from mascara) in her ovaries and breasts. She had sensitive painful breasts during her periods which were quite irregular. She also had indium and gallium, dental alloys in the ovaries and breasts. She, too, was started on the kidney herbs and instructed to get metal tooth fillings replaced. After two months they canceled their appointment. Frederica was pregnant! Not for long, though, and a wiser couple returned a few months later. Frederica finished her dental work. Both started the parasite program. Frederica's periods became regular. She was started on thioctic acid (one a day) plus zinc, (one a day), until her first missed period. Twelve months later they sent me their baby's picture: he was two months old.

Ginger Hart had been trying for three years to get pregnant. After an endometrial biopsy, a D&C,[11] and laparoscopy she was diagnosed with "inadequate corpus luteum." We found her ovaries toxic with nickel and europium from tooth fillings and strontium from toothpaste. She was delighted to understand her problem and set about correcting it.

Marjory Davis, age 28, had been on the "pill" (synthetic hormones) a long time but was off now and couldn't get pregnant. She actually got pregnant about one year ago but lost it at one month. A toxic element test showed her ovaries and uterus were full of beryllium (gasoline and coal oil), gadolinium and gallium. The metals are alloys of gold used in dentistry. She wore a lot of jewelry, just loved her chains, necklaces, rings, etc. But she agreed to go off all except two rings which did not have these alloys. To reduce fossil fuel fumes in the house she removed all gas cans and the lawn mower from the attached garage. They parked the cars outside. She was started on kidney herbs and promised to use contraception until she was done. She was to drink three glasses of 2% milk a day and take a magnesium tablet and stop drinking other beverages. Three weeks later her husband canceled her appointment because she was too embarrassed and delighted to call herself.

Prostate Problems

If urination is not complete, so you must soon go again, especially in the night, it is suggestive of pressure on the urethra from an enlarged prostate gland. Keeping a little urine from being voided is conducive to bladder and kidney infection, too, because bacteria soon find this "free food."

The prostate collects toxins as if it were a designated dump site, especially for nickel. Urinary tract bacteria quickly find "their" metal, nickel. Any supply of nickel will attract bacteria

---

[11]A surgical procedure, called *dilation and curettage*, meaning dilate the bladder with air and scrape away the inner lining.

as quickly as crumbs and cheese attract mice. Urinary tract bacteria are making use of your urea as their food. To digest it, they first break the urea molecule apart into two ammonia molecules. It is the ammonia smell of the urine that gives away their presence. The urine should have no ammonia smell. Our bodies do not make ammonia. Only bacteria can do this! Their digestive enzyme is called *urease*. In order to do its job, this enzyme requires the element nickel.

Nickel is plentiful in the soil which is undoubtedly where these bacteria belong, breaking up and utilizing the urine and droppings left there by animals. They perform an essential task in our environment, destroying animal excrement and thereby cleaning-up the soil around us. What folly it is to load ourselves up with nickel so that in one short hop from the earth they are residing in us! Bacteria are all around us doing their valuable jobs. We cannot stop associating with bacteria. We were not meant to feed them, however. If we did not supply them with nickel, as if we were just another patch of earth, they could not gain a foothold in our urinary tract and then to the prostate.

How can we rid our bodies of nickel? This is the challenge. Are we eating dirt? A small amount of dirt can't be avoided on our food. But we can stop sucking on nickel as if it were a lollipop. Our spoons, forks and knives are made of nickel! Stainless steel is 8% nickel! Does it really come off as you eat? When you stick a knife into the mayonnaise jar, it is stained in a few minutes. Try it. The mayonnaise has reacted with the metal loosening the nickel. When you smear the knife over your bread, this film comes off and you eat it. If you were to put the knife in your mouth, now, you could taste the metal. You will later wash the knife but not before you have eaten enough nickel to supply all the bacteria in your body with the daily allowance of their essential element, nickel. Nickel is not our essential mineral. Even plants keep their nickel levels very low. But due to pollution of animal feed with it, even a hen's egg now has 3 mcg/100 gm of nickel in it.[12] To produce a nickel-polluted egg, the chicken must be polluted.

Especially infants and children should <u>never</u> be given metal cups or cutlery. They need all their immune power to combat the barrage of new bacteria and viruses that is emerging in this age of AIDS. Nickel is part of dirt and belongs there, not in our pots and cutlery.

Another large source of nickel is metal dentalware. It is used to harden gold! If you suffer from prostate problems, remove metal from your dentalware. Nickel is used to make bridges, gold crowns, retainers, amalgams. Exchange it all for plastic ware and composite buildups (see *Sources* for more dental information). Stop eating and cooking with metal utensils; use old fashioned wooden or sturdy plastic cutlery instead. Always use a plastic knife for butter or mayonnaise. Never buy foil-wrapped butter.

Nickel is fat soluble and is stored in your skin fat temporarily when a surge of it enters the body. Your skin oils may be loaded with nickel causing "allergies" in the skin. Male pattern baldness is such an allergy. The sweat tries to excrete it for you. Always wash off your scalp sweat to help with this excretion. The skin oils dissolve nickel from metal jewelry (sometimes leaving your skin with a greenish black color) and transport it into your body. Don't wear metal jewelry. Earring posts should be plastic. Metal watches and metal rimmed glasses should be replaced with all plastic types. Metal rings should be replaced. After lowering your total body nickel levels and your prostate disease is only a memory, you might notice scalp hair returning to sparse areas. Search around the edge of the hair line for the first returnees.

Bacteria cannot live in the prostate without nickel being present. You can cure your prostate problems with the simple tactic

---

[12]Food Values by Pennington and Church, 1985

of stopping nickel pollution of your body. Notice that you get a fresh attack after accidentally using metal cutlery in a restaurant or eating mayonnaise-style salad with a metal spoon stuck in it. It might be wise to take a **histidine** capsule (about 500 mg., one a day for three weeks, see *Sources*) when this happens. Histidine is a nickel chelator. Taking **zinc** is helpful too (60 mg. two times a day for a month). Possibly, the nickel was poisoning zinc enzymes. Read about the benefits of **flaxseed**, too, but remember to test every product for pollutants before accepting it as a supplement.

Prostate problems of all kinds clear up when bacteria are zapped, the Kidney Cleanse is done, dental cleanup is done, and the Bowel Program is followed.

Richard Traylor, age 71, had suffered from prostate and urinary tract disease for three years. Scar tissue had to be removed occasionally from prior treatments of them. He was started on the kidney herbs and in two weeks (13 days) he had a considerable improvement in urine flow. At his follow-up visit we searched for toxins. He had radon, chromate, yttrium and strontium in his genital and urinary tract. He got rid of his water softener (such salts are polluted with chromate), toothpaste (strontium source) and opened the crawl space vents (source of radon). This cured these problems in less than two months. It also cured his stomach ulcers for which he had to take medicine. He was so pleased he decided to install a crawl space fan and pursue a parasite program and dental health just to see what extra health improvements he might get.

Omer Whitney, age 45, had always been a strong, healthy, hard worker. He could now barely walk, due to weakness and pains of several kinds; his prostate problems began several years ago. Our tests showed 4 kinds of kidney stones. He was started on only half a dose of the herbal recipe to give them a chance to dissolve more slowly. One month later he still had some stones although his leg cramps were already gone. At this time we found *Ascaris* (both kinds) which he killed with a frequency generator. We also found carbon tetrachloride and pentane (in decaf beverages) built up in him; also gasoline and TCE. He was considerably improved five weeks later and was quite eager to improve further. A toxic element test showed he was full of copper, antimony (from mineral ice massages), cobalt (aftershave), zirconium (deodorant), thulium (vitamin C fortified orange drink) and mercury (very high, from tooth fillings). He planned on cleaning all of it <u>out</u> of his body and regaining his lost strength.

Harvey Van Til, age 35, came in for his prostate and testicle swelling which began shortly after a vasectomy. He ached over the front right side of his abdomen. He was started on the kidney herbs and in four weeks he had eliminated his oxalate crystals and felt considerably better. We next found the adult intestinal flukes and human liver flukes in his prostate gland! After killing them immediately with a frequency generator and getting instant relief of pain, he got his own device and did not need to return.

Clayton Gamino, 26, had pain during urination which he interpreted as a left-over from a prostate infection he once had. He got all the metal out of his mouth, and did a kidney cleanse. A half year later he had no remaining pains and was able to father his first child.

Side Pain

Pain on the right side can come from problems at the ileocaecal valve or the appendix or the large intestine itself. It can also come from the liver which is higher up but is sending its pain message to your side. Pursue it as an intestinal problem first, killing parasites and bacteria and normalizing bowel movements with the Bowel Program. If the pain persists, especially if it reaches up the side to the

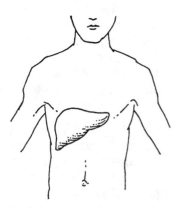

Fig. 22 The liver has a large lobe on your right side with the gallbladder tucked inside. The left lobe is smaller.

middle of the waist, it is probably due to the liver.

The liver is a large organ, mostly on the right side of the body, but with a smaller lobe on the left side. It is the chemical manufacturing plant for the body. It pulls in the food from the intestine (that you ate hours ago) and makes your body's chemicals from them. Toxic items are changed chemically into non-toxic items that the kidney is able to excrete into the bladder. Fatty things must be made water soluble for them to leave with the urine. The liver also makes bile and sends toxic items along with it to the intestine through the bile ducts. The bile enables calcium and fat to be absorbed. If the liver isn't getting much bile to the intestine , fat is left in the bowel contents and the feces will float in the toilet bowl. That is your clue to bile duct blockage.

Bile is bright green. Mixed with intestinal contents it turns the bowel movement dark brown. If the bile is <u>not</u> arriving in the intestine the bowel movement will stay light colored, even yellow or orange. This is another clue to bile duct blockage. Over a quart of bile should exit the body each day. Since bile is loaded with cholesterol this daily excretion of bile is a major method of keeping cholesterol levels low. If the bile ducts are choked with debris so only half as much (often only a cup instead of a quart!) bile is produced and excreted you can expect cholesterol levels to rise, and digestion to be bad. When food isn't promptly digested and absorbed the ever present, ever-ready bacteria will grab it for themselves.

Taking cholesterol-lowering drugs should be reserved for cases where natural excretion cannot be regained.

E. coli and other intestinal bacteria, which do no harm in moderate numbers, can overgrow in a few hours to give you bloating, gas and pain. <u>Your body produces no gas</u>. Only bacteria can produce gas. If your side pain is accompanied by bloating and gas, you <u>know</u> you have a digestive problem. And that this digestive problem stems from a congested liver if the pain is directly under it or over it, or if the feces are light colored or your cholesterol levels are high. Not everybody has all the symptoms.

To clear the clogged passages of the bile ducts, you simply do the liver cleanse (page 552) over and over until the problem is gone. There is one catch. If there are living parasites in the bile ducts, they will not <u>let</u> the bile ducts clear themselves. They are stuck fast to your ducts as a tick can be to your skin. They must be killed before they will let go. Zap them all, or you may use the herbal parasite program, staying on a twice a week maintenance program. Only <u>after</u> parasites are dead (after day 20 if using the herbal program) will you get a lot of "green stuff" and be able to clear "stones" out of your bile ducts. Only one large duct at a time will clean itself. We have hundreds of larger ducts and thousands of tiny ducts feeding into the larger ones! Stay on a schedule of cleansing the liver every two weeks (unless you are ill) until your side pain is gone, your digestion is normal, and you are bouncing with energy. You may also lose some weight, but only if you are overweight.

Remember that a clogged liver does not <u>necessarily</u> give you pain by itself. It is more likely the bacteria in the gall bladder and bile ducts, causing inflammation there and in your intestine, that cause pain. Don't wait till pain occurs over the liver. Use whatever clues you can to diagnose your clogged condition. Or just assume it is clogged. Do the cleanse, and see if you get any stones out. It can never hurt and can help a lot.

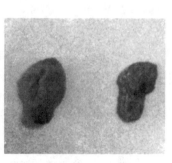

Fig. 23 Gallstones.

Bruce Hearn, 40ish, had severe side pain for several weeks and was rather gassy. He had seen a clinical doctor who found him in good health. But we found sheep liver flukes in the intestine and in the thymus! The thymus is an immunity-giving gland, so anything in the thymus is a very serious matter. He also had benzene in his thymus (inviting AIDS). He quickly switched from drinking soda to drinking milk. He went off everything in the benzene list. He killed the flukes electronically and started on the parasite program. Three weeks later the benzene was gone, his side was very much better and he could begin a kidney cleanse for his low back pain. He hadn't cleansed his liver yet! His improvement was probably due to improving his immunity which then controlled the bacteria.

Midabdomen Pain, Stomach Pain

The colon crosses over from your right side to the left side at the midabdomen. This is also the location for the bile duct to join your small intestine. Most midabdomen pain comes from either the colon or the bile duct connections. Kill parasites and bacteria by zapping or with the herbal recipe. Improve your digestion with diet clean up (off moldy food, boil dairy products). Sometimes the midabdomen pain stems from the stomach itself. The valves at the top and bottom of the stomach are meant to keep the food in. The valve at the top where the stomach joins the esophagus is a favorite location for bacteria.

You seldom feel them here though. This is just under your breastbone. They do their work quietly. Eventually, the tissue there is so weakened, the valve can't shut tightly and food is allowed to go back up the esophagus. This is called *reflux* and you may be told to sleep with your head elevated and to eat small meals, especially at bedtime. You may be given Reglan,™ a drug to help empty the stomach faster. Digestive enzymes will help empty the stomach, too, but may harbor molds. The real solution is to kill the bacteria in this area and keep them from reinvading it. Start by killing the *Salmonellas* and *Campylobacters* (zap them).

Within a day or so, however, the area can be re-invaded. Some bacteria are coming from your teeth! Some come from the liver! Often both sources are supplying bacteria to the stomach. The stomach allows a little bile to enter at the end of each meal, this is normal. But if the bile

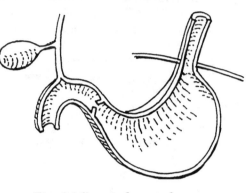

Fig. 24 Stomach, esophagus, diaphragm, gallbladder.

is full of live parasite stages and bacteria they may try to colonize the stomach, too. If there is insufficient stomach acid to kill them or if there is an accumulation of toxin in the stomach, they will get a foothold. Then they can burrow down deep to escape acid. Eventually, an ulcer can develop.

Stomach Ulcer

Often, such an ulcer is painless.

You are, therefore, not alerted to the parasites' presence until they have established themselves in good hiding places. Taking antacids, of course, works <u>in their favor</u>. The solution for both stomach pain and stomach ulcers is to kill parasites and bacteria, followed by dental and liver clean ups. One very common toxin that accumulates in the stomach is the pesticide **arsenic**. You inhale it right along with the flies and roaches you may be trying to kill with arsenic-laced pesticides.

Other inhaled toxins are fiberglass, asbestos, formaldehyde and freon. Your nose and mouth mucous traps a lot of these whereupon you swallow them and they glide into the stomach. Tooth bacteria and tooth metal get into the stomach the same way. You simply swallow them.

Clean up your air, don't use any pesticides (see other methods in *Recipes*). Your dentalware may be cleaned up in a few dental visits but the liver cleanses must go on for a year or two before it is reasonably clean. You may get pain relief in a few weeks but this should not derail your intention to revitalize yourself completely with a cleaned liver and stomach.

Hiatal Hernia

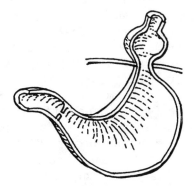

When bacteria have spread to the diaphragm and weakened it, along with the upper-stomach valve, food is allowed to get pushed up right through the diaphragm. Pressure in the abdomen from overeating or sitting in an easy

Fig. 25 Hiatal hernia.

chair pushes it up. Walk after eating. Empty the stomach before going to bed. Don't sit in recliners. Very many of us, about 25%, have a small hiatal hernia. It only hurts if it is inflamed. Work at clearing the inflammation first, to get pain relief. In time, the area will strengthen and the hernia itself may get smaller.

Jeffy, 3½ months, had been screaming a lot ever since birth. He was very gassy. He could not be put down without starting to cry. He was congested and had colds. He was on mother's milk exclusively so his chronic *Salmonella* infection must have come from someone who was a carrier, possibly his mother, although she

133

had no symptoms. The mother had platinum and tellurium in her milk (*Salmonella* can be transmitted in milk but this was not checked). The solution was to clean up the mother's milk by getting the dental metal out of her mouth, and washing hands before nursing. Jeffy's father had an *Ascaris* and intestinal fluke infestation. It is quite possible the baby had these also, giving him a nasty tummy ache in addition to the gas pains. The baby's older sister had screamed and cried the first nine months, too, so the parents were told it was a "familial thing." She also had ear infections, colds and a flaky patch of skin occasionally. She, too, had *Ascaris*. They were very pleased to be able to clear up the whole family's problems by killing parasites and removing toxins.

Ruby Adair, age 14, filled a page with her symptoms. She was also chronically fatigued and had consumed enough antibiotic "to fill a room." She had shooting pains from under her feet up her legs. A quick check revealed mercury and thallium in her immune system. Instead of being dismayed, this news filled her with hope for recovery. She arranged for dental metal replacement. Then she related her stomach "story". While at a wedding, a year ago, she began vomiting with diarrhea. She thought it was the stomach "flu" but she didn't recover for six months and had to miss school. The psychologist thought it was emotional. She was still only attending school one hour a day. We found *Fasciolopsis*, the intestinal fluke, in her stomach wall as well as in her intestine. She started the parasite program and in three weeks her appetite was back, insomnia was gone, fatigue was better and a significant improvement was evident.

Respiratory Illness

Asthma

is a very old disease described in the ancient literature. The only progress we have made to date with this disease is to give drugs to soothe the symptoms.

Asthma is associated in **all** (100%) cases with tiny *Ascaris* larvae. As soon as eggs hatch (in the stomach, immediately after swallowing filth) the microscopic larvae travel to the lungs, not the intestines. Imagine the distress of lungs full of tiny worms! One tries to cough them up, of course, but in our misguided effort to be polite we teach children to <u>swallow</u> anything they cough up! Some swallowing is inevitable and the young worms are back in the stomach, this time to set up their housekeeping in the intestine. Some never leave the stomach, causing children stomach aches and, of course, a large entourage of bacteria which, in turn, have their viruses.

Most cases of *Ascaris* infestation also show *Bacteroides fragilis* bacteria which, in turn, carry the *Coxsackie* viruses (brain viruses). Whether or not these bacteria or viruses will thrive in <u>you</u> depends on whether you make a good home for them, namely have low immunity in some organ. The preferred organs for *Bacteroides* are liver and brain (brain tumors always show *Bacteroides*). The preferred organs for *Coxsackie* viruses appear to be tooth abscesses and brain.

Not everybody with *Ascaris* develops asthma, even though they always go through a lung stage. Does it depend on the age of the person when the infection develops? Or how many *Ascaris* are present? Or the time of year when lung infection is present?

That innocent cough of early childhood should not be neglected, as simply "croup." At the first sign of a cough, use a frequency generator set to 408 KHz, the frequency for *Ascaris*, or use a zapper. Pay extra attention to washing hands before meals. Pay extra attention to the animals nearby. Kill their *Ascaris* with a zapper and keep it up daily or put parasite killing herbs in their food.

Asthma sufferers become **allergic** to many air pollutants such as pollen, animal dander, smoke. The production of histamine in the lungs and the vast interconnectedness of histamine to allergies has been well studied scientifically. Although invasion by worms is known to result in <u>both</u> histamine production and high eosinophil counts (over 3), and **asthma clients typically have both**, they are not routinely checked for worms clinically! They are simply given drugs to enable better breathing. More and better (though toxic) drugs have been developed.

But you can put an end to your asthma by terminating your *Ascaris* infection. Then wash your hands and fingernails with grain alcohol, and let no more filth past your lips. Wear plastic gloves for a week to break a nail biting or finger sucking habit. For children wash hands before eating anything, even between meals; keep fingernails short.

Dogs, cats, pigs and horses all get *Ascaris*. Never, never let a child clean up any vomit or mess left by an animal. This could lead to massive infection, the kind that could result not only in asthma but **seizures**. Kill the worms in animal messes before you clean them up too. Never use your dustpan or broom. Use cardboard, newspaper or anything that you can afford to throw away with the mess. Squirt povidone iodine (available at drug stores) on the mess–even if it's outside–and cover with salt before cleaning up. Discard it in outside trash. Wash your hands with grain alcohol, paying special attention to fingernails. If you are a food preparer, you could infect the whole family if you don't wash carefully.

If there is an asthmatic in your family, the whole family should be treated for *Ascaris* with a zapper or with the herbal parasiticides. Even after everybody including the pets have been treated, pets should not be allowed in the bedroom of the asthmatic person. Asthma is more than parasitism. It is also an allergic reaction, to the pet and to other inhaled bits of matter.

Clean the air. Smoke of any kind, fragrance and chemicals of any kind, all household cleaners, polishes, and so forth should be removed. Store essentials in the garage, not the basement, since basement air rises. Clean up the whole house. Persons who must use hair spray or nail polish should do so outside in the summer and in their own rooms with the doors closed in winter. Use a chlorine filter for the water, especially at the shower. Install central air conditioning if possible, with maximum filtering (but never with chemicals added to the filter and never with a fiberglass filter) at the furnace. A room air filter (not fiberglass) is next best. Use it for an hour in the bedroom ahead of bedtime so the air currents can cease. Just moving dust around is worse than leaving it there. Never do dusting when an asthmatic is in the house. Lungs heal quickly when the air is clean and there is no reinfection. The best place to recover is outdoors away from trees and bushes or indoors with total pollution-free air conditioning (free of asbestos, formaldehyde, arsenic, fiberglass, pet dander).

As your asthma lessens, reduce your inhalers, but always keep them on hand. When you suddenly need them, try to identify your source of reinfection or allergens. Use this experience wisely. Try to understand the recurrence of your asthma. Keep notes. It may take half a year with a dozen recurrences to finally learn and conquer! It will feel great to breathe without spraying yourself and taking medicine. If it comes back a year later, figure out what is happening that's seasonal. A pine tree near the house, a flowering bush, the first mown grass? Stay away from these until you are completely healed.

There are traditional herbs for helping lungs. Grow your own **comfrey** and **garlic**. Make **mullein** tea from the dried herb (see *Sources*). Read herb books for more help. Dry some for winter use, being careful to do it right and not let it mold.

Suzanne Carlyle, 45, had asthma from infancy. She was currently on Albutesol™ spray and tablets daily. Now she was beginning to have arthritis too. She was given arginine to replace caffeine. She had two species of *Ascaris* and was allergic to cats and other animals. She was started on the herbal parasite program after killing *Ascaris*, *Bacteroides* and *Coxsackie* viruses with a frequency generator. Her lungs showed kerosene, carbon tetrachloride, mineral oil, benzalkonium (from udder wash, she was also milk sensitive), aluminum from her cookware, and aluminum silicate from her salt. She had two extra lung parasites: *Paragonimus*, a lung fluke, and *Pneumocystis*. She was immediately improved after cleaning up these sources and canceled her future appointment.

Cay Wenkert, 63, had asthma for many years for which she took Proventil™, but this gave her such bad side effects she had to stay home now and not venture out. Her lungs were full of benzalkonium (toothpaste), arsenic (ant poison under kitchen sink), zirconium (deodorant), and nickel from tooth metal. She had dog heartworm in her lungs(!), in addition to her heart where she sometimes felt pain. She had *Ascaris* and *Naegleria*, *mycoplasma*, *Endolimax* and the intestinal fluke in her lungs! She coughed up blood, after her doctor had diagnosed *bronchiestasis* recently, meaning her lungs were not capable of sweeping out the daily refuse we all breathe in. In spite of killing these and cleaning up her environment she got no improvement. She repeatedly got parasitized. She had four or five root canal teeth which she was unwilling to have pulled. Hopefully, the tradeoff between teeth and health will soon begin to look poor.

Amy Newberry, 41, had recently begun to have asthma attacks. She had been on cortisone but now was on inhalers through the day (two puffs Ventillin™ 3x/day, plus three puffs Intel™ 3x/day plus four puffs Asthmacort™ 3x/day). She was often hospitalized for attacks. She also had stomach trouble and sinus problems (had pneumonia recently). She had *Ascaris* larvae, *Endolimax*, *Naegleria*, and *Acanthocephala* in her lungs! She also had arsenic and palladium (tooth metal). Going onto homeopathic medicine for stuffiness helped her avoid some hospital visits. It took several months (5 visits) to track her arsenic source to the bedroom carpets (stain resistance!). After steam cleaning it herself and doing a liver cleanse (after first killing parasites) she was amazed at her improvement. She had not been to the hospital in a month and was only using inhalers preventively. She planned to get dental work done. She got all her former health back.

Laura Brewster, 25, lived in a very old house. The slightest exertion would give her an asthma attack. She frequently got pneumonia, too. Her lungs had beryllium (coal oil) and asbestos, and two parasites, *Paragonimus* (lung fluke) and *Ascaris*. She got rid of all the old fashioned lamps and candles in the house, but could not find the source of asbestos. She got rid of the attacks but her cough and pneumonia bouts will continue until she moves from that house.

Brett Wilsey, 70, was congested most of the time, had chronic sinus problems, was getting allergy shots for dust and mold, and was on several inhalers for his asthma plus emphysema. He had asthma for eight years. He had oxalate, urate, and all three phosphate variety crystals in his kidneys. He was started on kidney herbs. His blood test showed high "total carbon dioxide" or "carbonate" showing that his air exchange was not good. His potassium was low, showing that his adrenals couldn't keep his electrolytes (sodium, potassium and chloride) regulated, in turn, giving him muscle weakness. His LDH was very high, showing that his heart muscle) was in distress, too. Fortunately, his RBC was slightly elevated, to help with oxygen delivery. (See Anemia page 285). His eosinophil count was high, as is the rule for asthmatics since they all have *Ascaris* worms. Besides *Ascaris*, he had pancreatic and intestinal flukes in his lungs(!) plus *Heterakis* (a chicken roundworm), human hookworm, and *Prosthogonimus*, another fluke. He was started on the parasite herbs. Two weeks later he felt a lot better although he still had some *Ascaris*. He was toxic with barium and hafnium (which were traced to his dentures) nickel, tin, rhenium. He stopped using commercial "denture-soak." His wife stopped using hair spray and they started leaving the car out of the garage and walked around to the front door, instead of using the attached garage. He also started drinking homemade comfrey tea. This made him feel still better.

When he removed his watch he got rid of his nickel source. Nickel has an affinity for lungs (as well as prostate and skin). He was now down to one puff of inhaler instead of two, only four times a day instead of hourly. He could breathe deeper than before. Then the lead in his water was found and traced to a single "sweated" joint in the pipes. He was started on food grade hydrogen peroxide, working up a drop at a time; now his cough became "productive", he was coughing up a lot.

He got the plumbing fixed and did a liver cleanse after which his fatigue lifted. He couldn't stop laughing and joking about the "emphysema" he was so worried over earlier.

139

Bea Karnes, 49, had asthma from childhood when she also had eczema. She was presently on several medicines plus allergy shots and antibiotics for it. She was toxic with antimony although she used no eye makeup and europium, tantalum, and gadolinium from dental metal. She also had hand swelling in the morning and was started on kidney herbs. She killed her intestinal flukes (in the intestine) and *Ascaris* in her lungs and was not seen for half a year. When we eventually saw her, she said her asthma had been "wonderful." She was faithfully controlling parasites with the maintenance program and occasionally drinking kidney herb tea.

Cynthia Prout's whole family (mentioned previously) had asthma. She was told it was inherited. The three young children and herself were on inhalers, nose sprays, cough syrups and antibiotics. Nola, age 10, also had ear infections and numerous allergies. Lewis, age 8, was a slight, nervous boy; he had been off wheat and milk for many years due to intolerance. Irwin, age 5, seldom went with the family due to his frequent stomach aches and the fact he could vomit without notice. The mother and two children who were with her (Irwin stayed home) had *Ascaris* infection and Lewis also had pancreatic flukes. Their home was toxic with vanadium, namely, a gas leak. The parasites were quickly killed and gas leak repaired. The whole family got well and canceled their next appointment. Some inherited disease!

Asthma is just one of our common respiratory problems. The causes are always a combination of *Ascaris* and other parasites with pollutants (allergies).

Bronchitis, Croup, Chronic Cough

- In **bronchitis** the bronchioles are the site of the problem.
- In **croup** it's further down.
- In cases of **chronic little hacky coughs** it may be heartworm!

Bud Portillo, 62, worked on earth moving machines. He frequently had a "bronchial virus" or "bronchial infection." He was always coughing. He had *Ascaris* infestation and arsenic pollution in his home. He also had palladium toxicity from tooth fillings. As soon as they removed the mouse bait from their home, tore down the hallway wallpaper (arsenic source) and changed wells (the well water had arsenic in it from seepage!)and killed parasites, his cough was gone. He also finished his dental work. All this took six months.

Gene Mizell, age 4, was constantly clearing his throat. His parents wondered if it was a "nervous habit." He had two species of *Ascaris* living inside his small body. He was started on a small dose of parasite herbs immediately, stirred into a daily dose of VMF syrup (see *Sources*). He also had PCBs, aluminum silicate, lutetium from recent painting in the house and xylene and toluene solvents. He was switched off soda pop and onto milk. We saw him five weeks later. He had gone through three treatments with vermifuge syrup. His throat clearing was gone, as well as his hacky cough and the blue circles around his eyes. He still had PCBs, which they later cleared by switching off detergent.

Carmen Castro, 30ish, had a chronic cough without being ill. She also had some heart irregularity. She had *Dirofilària* (dog heartworm) and *Loa loa*. There were no indoor pets. After killing the parasites with a frequency generator and starting on the parasite herbs she was still coughing a bit but her pulse was down to 80 (from 120). She still had toluene, TC Ethylene solvents and mercury, platinum and lead in her body. Then a gas leak developed in their home. She used moth balls and painted a room. After this she had to be on antibiotics for her extreme cough. This time she had *mycoplasma*, *Haemophilus* and influenza. She killed these electronically and her coughing stopped. Until she gets the dental work done she will continue to pick up new infections.

Hope Feldman, 57, had been coughing for half a year. She had seen many doctors including a reflexologist. She had *mycoplasma* and *alpha strep* at tooth #17 (lower left wisdom tooth). As soon as these were killed with a frequency generator her cough stopped. She was advised to wear turtleneck sweaters for extra warmth over her bronchii and get a cavitation cleaned at tooth #17.

Teresa White, 37, had bronchitis several times each winter and was put on antibiotic for the whole season to keep it from breaking out. Her lungs were loaded with tantalum from dental metal, cobalt from detergent and thulium from her vitamin C. She had taken herself off milk, thinking it might be a factor, and used an air cleaner but without results. As soon as she had the tooth metal replaced with plastic (in less than a month) she could go off antibiotics and also was rid of a chronic sinus condition, but still had a bronchitis bout. She had *Ascaris* larvae in her lungs and phosphate and oxalate crystals in her kidneys. Her diet was changed to include milk and fish, magnesium, lysine (500 mg one a day), vitamin B_6, and a vitamin A+D capsule. She started on the kidney cleansing herbs and then the parasite program. In another month the whole problem was gone. Wisely, she got ready to cleanse her liver.

Craig Stewart, 2, had a history of respiratory problems. He had been on Ceclor™ and Ventilin™ for a long time; he had pneumonia the previous year. He had whip worm (*Trichuris*) infesting his intestine which was promptly killed with parasite herbs (as much as his parents could get down him was effective). He was toxic with asbestos. When the clothes dryer belt was changed to a U.S. variety (imported belts contain asbestos which flies into the air when the dryer is used), Craig's health turned around.

Doris Gumb, 26, was on Isoniazid™, Tussionex™ and Rifodin™ for tuberculosis. It started with coughing. She was down to 98 lb. in weight. Her lungs were toxic with beryllium (coal oil fuel), mercury, uranium, and tellurium. She began by clearing all toxic items from her house and basement and then bringing an air sample for testing. She also had *Ascaris* larvae in her lungs and pancreatic fluke in her pancreas. In three weeks she was coughing less and producing less with each cough. The "clean" air sample still had uranium, tellurium, mercury and beryllium. She had no metal tooth fillings, though. In the next three weeks she found a hole in the floor to the crawl space. It was letting up uranium dust and radon. The mercury was traced to the carpet in a child's bedroom. After throwing it out, her sputum cleared up and she was on the way to recovery, although we never found the source of tellurium.

Breast Pain

Although lumps and cancer in the breast produce no pain, they sometimes do give you little warning twinges. These twinges cross into the breast from the armpit or from any direction. It is gone in a second, leading one to believe it couldn't be serious. If the breast has any unusual sensations, painful or not, investigate immediately.

Test yourself for cancer. (You may use a specimen of mother's milk as a cancer test since this has mitotic stimulants in it—see Curing Cancer page 331). If you have purchased a slide of breast tissue (mammary gland) you can search your breast for cancer. If not, but you find "mother's milk" in your white blood cells, assume it is cancer and clear it up immediately.

If you don't have cancer, search for the pollutants giving you these twinges of pain. Search for your deodorant, cosmetics, and soap in your white blood cells. Search for dental metal. The breasts are often full of nickel. Nickel is quite soluble in fat and the breast is mainly fat. Nickel is one of the top carcinogens listed by researchers. It could even explain the high incidence of breast cancer. But titanium and barium from cosmetics, as well as asbestos and fiberglass are also quickly accumulated in the breast. Clean up your dentalware and body products. Check for exposed fiberglass. Change your dryer belt. Buy a new non-CFC refrigerator. Never try to get rid of these pains with pain killers; let the pains show you whether the clean up has been complete.

Breast Sensitivity

Breast sensitivity can be quite uncomfortable to the point of not being able to wear a bra, especially near period time. It may be due to high estrogen levels; this is also conducive to breast lumps and breast cancer. Most of your estrogen is produced by the ovaries before menopause and later by the adrenal glands. Too high estrogen levels plague the modern woman. Certain food molds, particularly **zearalenone**, causes over-estrogenization. It affects men too. I have found it in popcorn and corn chips! And brown rice. Stop eating these. Eat white rice. If you make cooked cereals be sure to add vitamin C to them before cooking (1/8 tsp. per cup), to detoxify food molds. I do not know whether taking vitamin C <u>with</u> your popcorn would detoxify zearalenone. Don't risk it. The excess estrogen compounds must be detoxified by the liver. Yet, the liver may be incapable of this because you ate yet another food mold! See the section on moldy food (page 381).

Over-estrogenized women are over-emotional, seemingly on a roller coaster of enthusiasm and despondence. They can develop a high pitched voice, that almost sounds squeaky. High enough estrogen levels are important for fertility but too high levels can cause infertility. Your body is eager to set the level just right, if only you will clean up the ovaries of parasites and pollution. Don't stop your clean up until the breast feels normal again throughout your cycle and you don't feel over-emotional, even just before your period.

Breast Lumps

Breast lumps may or may not be painful. If you feel one, don't wait to be more certain, don't wait to analyze it with tests, don't wait for a doctor's diagnosis or a mammogram. Obtain a frequency generator or zapper and zap yourself immediately. Also do the herbal parasite program immediately (page 338).

Your body often turns the breast into a collecting station for toxic wastes that have been drawn downward from the top of your body. From your head where shampoo and hair spray and cosmetics leave their daily deposits, from your dentalware with its constant supply of heavy metals, from neck and armpits where cologne, deodorant and soap leave their toxic residues. The lymph nodes under the armpit and the region above the breast, collect it all and let it slip into the breast where it is bundled up in a cyst. Perhaps the kidneys are clogged so toxins are forced to go to a designated dump site instead of out through the bladder. Do a kidney cleanse. Don't rest until all your breast lumps are gone. They will begin to shrink in three weeks if you are removing the correct toxins. Even radon and asbestos go to the breast, so be meticulous with your cleanup.

When the platelet count (in a blood test) is very high (over 400) there is quite a tendency to form cysts or lumps since platelets make your blood clot. The platelet count goes up when parasites are present. Maybe your blood is attempting to clot them! These clots make "nests" for fluke stages which may be why breast lumps often become cancerous. If yours is over 300, (it should be 250,000/cu mm) start patrolling parasites regularly. Stopping the use of caffeine and taking vitamin E (400 u. a day) are helpful in recovery but don't rely on these minor measures. Breast lumps definitely invite breast cancer.

Leslie Yeager, age 37, had breast soreness and "fibrocystic lumps". She had cerium and nickel accumulated in her breasts. They cleared up in weeks after her dental metal was gone (she simply took out her retainer). Later she replaced it with a partial made of plastic.

Kari Pfeifer, age 36, had numerous cysts in both breasts and uterus. Her estrogen level was too high (187 pg/ml on day 22 of her cycle; the day of testing is important since it varies through the cycle). Her breasts were full of beryllium (coal oil from hurricane lamps) and radon. After these toxins were removed, all her breast lumps got smaller. After she did the kidney and Liver Cleanse, the lumps got softer and breasts were no longer painful. She had several root canals which filled her breasts with numerous bacteria, mainly *Histoplasma cap* (root canals develop infection around themselves). After starting her dental cleanup and killing bacteria with a frequency generator, all her breast lumps disappeared.

Claudia Davis, age 41, had breast soreness ever since a mammogram two years earlier. She had numerous other pains and indigestion. She had intestinal flukes in her intestine and fluke eggs in her blood: a dangerous situation. They might land in the breasts and start developing there. This is how cancer begins. But she did not have cancer yet. She had a buildup of niobium from polluted pain killer drugs and thulium from her vitamin C. She had *Salmonella* and several other bacteria in her white blood cells, which accounted for digestive problems. In eight weeks she had cleaned kidneys, killed parasites and gotten rid of her heavy metals. Her breast pain was better and a lump on her eyelid had also disappeared.

Stephanie Nakamura, 68, had six surgeries to remove breast lumps, going back to youth. Her recent mammogram was O.K. Her breasts were toxic with cadmium, lead, gold, radon, uranium, gallium, silver. Our tests showed she had kidney crystals and she was started on the kidney cleanse. She was given vitamin E, (400 units daily), sodium selenite (150 mcg daily) and vitamin C (1 or more grams daily). Her triglycerides were also very high showing again that she had kidney problems. She was given magnesium (300 mg daily), vitamin B_6 (250 mg daily) and lysine (500 mg daily). She killed parasites and cleaned up everything except gallium, silver, mercury, gold, cadmium. These must have come from her gold crowns. Her dentist advised against removing these and proclaimed they had nothing to do with her developing glaucoma, arthritis and stomach ulcers. It was a tough decision for her and she made the wrong choice. Perhaps if she had been up for the next breast surgery she would have gotten those "gold" crowns replaced with composite too.

Heart Pain

Pain over the heart region is usually quite real, even though an EKG does not find any abnormality. The most common cause is *Dirofilaria*, heartworm of dogs. It often begins as a pain just above the heart but spreads itself over the whole heart region. Kill it with your zapper. Parasite herbs can also be effective. If you did kill them, the pain often <u>intensifies</u> for a day before it leaves. Then the pain should be completely gone.

Heartworm is very easy to pick up again. If you have had heartworm, you should no longer keep a dog for a pet. Give it away.

Another heart parasite, *Loa loa*, is also a filarial worm and may be the causative factor. Both *Dirofilaria* and *Loa loa* can be obtained as slide specimens to use for testing yourself. Heart muscle can also be obtained as a slide specimen, but a chicken heart from the grocery store or snippets of beef heart (make sure to sample all 4 chambers) will do.

Follow up on your heart, even when no pain remains. These tiny heart parasites have stages that you may not be able to purchase in slide form and therefore can't test for. These stages, if not killed, will become adults so a maintenance parasite killing program, herbal or electronic, is essential. Virtually all dogs have *Dirofilaria* in spite of monthly medicine to kill it. They pick it up immediately after their last treatment for it and can give it to you again. The only way to live safely with pets is to give them parasite killing herbs daily in the feed.

Other heart problems such as irregular beat and mitral valve prolapse can clear up along with the pain. Or they may be due to bacteria (see Heart Disease, page 318).

Meredith Zackman, age 53, came for her diagnosed cardiomyopathy (heart disease). She owned a beautiful, old, very big dog, and of course she would never part from him. We knew she would lose her battle against heart disease. She had both *Dirofilaria* and *Loa loa* which we killed instantly with a frequency generator. She was on Lanoxin™, Furosemide™, Captopril™ and Metoprolol.™ We found she also had *Cytomegalovirus*, *Staphylococcus aureus*, *Streptococcus pneumonia* in her heart. The *Staph* bugs were also in tooth #17. She had copper in her heart (from tooth fillings) and cobalt and PCB from her detergent. There was zirconium from her deodorant and fiberglass from somewhere. Her pulse was typically in the 90's. Eight days later, after her dental work to replace metal was done her pulse was normal (low 70's), both worms were gone and she felt much better. But she still carried four bacteria, five viruses and two tapeworm stages: *Taenia solium* scolex in the spleen (she had chronic pain there) and *Taenia pisiformis* in the liver. She was started on Rascal (an herbal combination) for these. Six days later she had all of her problems back including *Loa loa*. She repeated everything, then she had to go off her heart medications because they lowered her blood pressure and pulse too much. She started the dog on the parasite program but continued to be heavily laden with parasites and bacteria that always found their way to her heart. She purchased her own frequency generator and was quite faithful with dog treatments. She may outlive her dog and then regain her health, finally.

Bruce Walby, age 42, had chest pain for three years. We found he had *Dirofilaria* and *Loa loa* in all four chambers of his heart. When he zapped them, the pain left a day or so later.

D'Ann Fonties, age 22, had a lot of chest pain but was told by her doctor it was simply "gas bubbles". She also had a serious digestion problem. She had *Dirofilaria*, high levels of styrene (from styrofoam drinking cups) and benzene. This information delighted her and she planned to change her habits.

Sheila Osborn, age 27, had chest pain when she lifted objects. Her pulse was slightly elevated (81) and slightly irregular. She had *Dirofilaria*. Five weeks after starting the parasite program she was feeling much better but still had the chest pain. This time she had *Loa loa* (but not *Dirofilaria*).

Wendy Lewellen, age 28, had a chronic cough and chest pain at midsternum (the sternum is the bone attached to the ribs and runs up the middle of the chest). She had *Dirofilaria* in one chamber of her heart (right auricle). She had xylene and toluene solvents which came from her daily beverage, Mountain Dew.™ She was also full of asbestos from her trips to do laundry nearby (this could not be proved, but when she switched laundromats, the asbestos went away). Two months later, after killing parasites, she was free of heartworm and her cough and chest pain were almost gone. She was probably healing very slowly due to the asbestos which was still present.

Lupita Cline, a young mother, had a chronic hacky cough and irregular heart beat. She had *Dirofilaria* in all chambers of her heart and *Loa loa* in her blood but not in her heart. She had carbon tetrachloride, propyl alcohol, hexanedione, toluene, and TC Ethylene buildup from drinking Pepsi™ and Mountain Dew.™ Her pulse was slightly elevated at 80. There were no pets in the house. She was started on the parasite program and two months later was rid of her heartworm but now had *Loa loa* in her heart and was still coughing a bit. She was full of platinum, mercury and palladium from tooth metal as well as vanadium from a gas leak in her home and paradichlorobenzene from using moth balls. She was on antibiotics for a "bronchial infection" and was happy to learn about a better solution.

Slow Pulse/Syncope (Passing Out)

Mason Heckler, 30s, was a mechanic by trade and could not afford to pass out on the job. Yet, it had been happening off and on for 10 years. He had acquired high blood pressure in his teens! This was soon followed by an extremely slow pulse (50 beats/min). No medicine worked (he had been tried on many) so he was on none. Then he got high blood pressure, it was 160/80 currently. He also had constant chest pain around the left nipple. He had heartworm and was started on the herbal parasite program. He never had a dog. In five weeks his pulse was 72; the parasite was gone. I presume his syncopes were due to sudden blood pressure changes or missing a few heart beats in a row. He began the kidney cleanse next to lower his blood pressure.

Chest Pain

When there is a tightness or just a little pain at the middle of the chest, especially under the breastbone, you may be merely having an allergic reaction. You might be feeling little spasms coming from the esophagus, and reaching up toward the throat from gallstones. You might also have HIV/AIDS disease which has a similar symptom over the sternum. So it is very important to pay attention to even a minor symptom in the chest.

Ruling out HIV disease ranks first in importance. Search for its emission at 365 KHz, or purchase a microscope slide with the dead virus on it as a test specimen (see *Sources*). Or purchase a set of slides representing all the stages of *Fasciolopsis buskii*. Without this parasite you can't get the HIV virus. Purchase a slide of the thymus gland or make your own specimen of throat sweetbreads. Check yourself for benzene buildup in the thymus. (See Using The Syncrometer page 462.)

If you have neither the benzene nor the parasite stages, you have no risk. Your chest distress is due to something else. Improve your air quality so that your lungs are not in distress. This includes radon, chlorine (from the bleach bottle under the sink), colognes, room fresheners as well as the usual pollutants (asbestos, arsenic, formaldehyde, fiberglass, freon).

If you feel waves of pain reaching up to your throat, you probably have a gallstone stuck in a bile duct. Epsom salts can relax that bile duct in 20 minutes. Take a tablespoon in ¾ cup water <u>but only on an empty stomach</u> or you may feel quite ill. Taking a large dose of valerian herb (6 to 8 capsules) may also buy you a little time by relaxing the duct. If you do get relief, you can be <u>sure</u> it was a spasm of some kind. The magnesium in Epsom salts relaxes spasms. I would recommend cleaning the liver (page 552) a number of times to try to dislodge the sticking gallstone. The instructions for liver cleansing advise you to kill parasites and cleanse the kidneys first. But if your throat pain is severe enough, you might just zap and go ahead with it at once.

Upper Back Pain

The main pain may be a dull ache over a shoulder blade, or between the shoulder blades or running right through you from the front to the back of the chest. These are all gallstone pains coming from the liver! Get yourself ready to clean them out. Clean the kidneys first, kill all the parasites that might be residing in the bile ducts and blocking them (flukes, pinworms and roundworms) and get onto a maintenance parasite program. Then mark your calendar for your first liver cleanse. Even if your first cleanse gives you only a dozen bits of green "stuff" you have done well; you have accessed the bile ducts. The pains will probably be "magically" gone the next day, but they might start to return in two days. The bile ducts are having spasms again due to the remaining stones.

After you have cleaned out 1,000 or more, you will get permanent relief. Repeat every two weeks, unless ill, until the upper back pains are gone, permanently. If chest pain or upper back pain is severe, try going off your favorite high fat food (ice cream, butter, cheese). Also try taking 6 valerian capsules, 4 times a day including bedtime to relieve the spasms.

Shoulder Pain

Some shoulder pain is called *bursitis* and some is called *arthritis*. But it always derives from stuck gallstones in the bile ducts of the liver! You can prove this by taking a tablespoon of Epsom salts in ¾ cup water at 6 p.m. instead of supper <u>and on an empty stomach</u> (or you may feel quite ill). If some of the pain subsides then you have evidence as to its true cause, because Epsom salts relax the bile duct valves.

Get started cleaning the liver (page 552). By the time you have chronic or acute shoulder pain you have about 3,000 stones! Count them roughly, as they float in the toilet after the liver cleanse so you know how much progress you have made toward the final goal. Don't start cleaning the liver until you have killed parasites and spent three weeks cleaning the kidneys though. This improves elimination of liquid toxins so a liver cleanse is promptly cleaned up for you.

151

What emerges from the liver is the most contaminated mess imaginable, full of bacteria and viruses and parasite eggs and stages (all dead we hope) of every kind. It needs prompt clearing from your body. The diarrhea sees to the bowel elimination. But some toxins can only pass through the kidneys. Kidneys should be clean and capable of doing the job. Remember it is unwise to clean the liver before all parasites are dead, especially flukes, because they produce a substance that <u>inhibits</u> any action of the bile ducts!

You are only one day away from freedom of shoulder motion and sleeping on your side again. Permanent improvement, though, depends on progress with your total stone count. Your bursitis can return in a few days or a few weeks. Be patient. You may only cleanse once in two weeks, and not if you are ill. After six cleanses you can be quite sure of being relatively pain free.

Between cleanses use valerian capsules to stop the spasms. It takes 6 capsules 4 times a day to be effective.

Typically only some bile ducts are spasming, and typically those ducts have a single fatty food trigger. Stop eating the high fat food you consume the most (it's probably your favorite). If that hasn't helped in two days choose a different high fat food to omit. The most common culprits are ice cream, potato chips, salad dressings, cheese, butter, cream, and milk.

Perhaps the pain is actually caused by bacteria living in the blocked bile ducts and invading the shoulder. This point has not been clarified. Using your zapper or frequency generator does no good for this pain. Only liver cleaning brings your shoulders back to their youthful mobility.

Upper Arm Pain

Excruciating pain in the upper arm soft tissues can keep your arm hanging straight down for fear of worsening it with motion.

Magnets of high strength (2x5000 gauss) taped to your arm, under your sleeve, can get you through the day. Also try valerian capsules (6 capsules four times a day). Go off all fat in the diet to let the spasm subside. Then start your liver cleanse at 6 p.m. If you used pain killer drugs during the day, the cleanse may not yield anything but it's worth a try anyway. You might be lucky and pop out the chief culprit stone. If not, you should wait several days before trying again; this time avoid pain killers the day of the cleanse. Be sure to zap parasites the day before or earlier.

Peggy Patton, age 60, had shoulder pain and painful feet in addition to aching all over. The aching was due to *Trichinella* which both she and her husband had. It took six months on the parasite program before it stayed away. She had clay colored stools, evidence of bile duct blockage. Then two liver cleanses cured her shoulder pain, nausea and remaining pains. She started gardening again and immediately picked up hookworms and *Trichinella* again. But she learned to sanitize her hands with grain alcohol after washing away dirt and this kept her parasites in check.

Jessica Atkinson, a middle age school teacher, developed a pain in the right cheek quite suddenly. She also had pain over the right mid abdomen and right side at the waist but X-rays and scans showed nothing (she had been X-rayed three times). She struggled for seven years to stay employed. She was having severe pain attacks over the liver and described her stool as almost white after these attacks. She cleaned her liver at least 30 times before she related, one day, that her joy in living had returned. Her gallstones were exceptionally large (½ x ¾ inch). Eventually the abscesses in her upper teeth were found, clearing up her cheek pain and protecting the liver from recurrent infections from these bacteria. Only then did she get permanent and complete pain relief.

Lisa Mattie, 72, had her right arm hanging limply by her side. It was so painful she bent forward to let it hang straight down. But in seven months she had done 6 liver cleanses, getting over 3,000 stones out. All pain was gone although some numbness in that arm persisted. She could also stop using Tums™, stop coughing, and no longer was bothered by her hiatal hernia.

Elbow Pain

One variety of elbow pain is due to an inflamed tendon there; it is sometimes called "tennis elbow." It is not due to playing tennis or any other arm use. The inflammation is caused by a liver full of stones and parasites, especially flukes which manufacture a chemical that affects tendons. Kill all flukes and cleanse the liver for quick relief. Using your elbows while they are inflamed is traumatic to them, like working with a sore thumb. Don't play tennis or do other arm exercises until they are pain free.

Parasites consume large amounts of your vitamins and minerals. Give yourself vitamin A (25,000 u daily), zinc (60 mg. daily), and B_6 (250 mg twice a day) until the pain is gone.

Wrist Pain

Tendons passing through the wrist can become inflamed from the unnatural chemicals produced by fluke parasites in the liver. Using the wrists to work further traumatizes them (injures them) making it harder for them to heal. A small hole between the tendons lets the nerve and blood vessels through into the hand. Fluke parasites also make chemicals that thicken tendons. When tendons at the wrist thicken, they can squeeze down on the nerves and blood vessels until the hand or fingers feel numb. If you have pain at the wrist or numbness in your hands, killing parasites and cleaning the liver may give you the permanent cure. Wearing a wrist bandage or support can help reduce trauma damage to the wrist while it is healing.

Numbness of hands, without wrist pain, is more often due to a brain problem with parasites and pollutants. Lead, mercury, fluke parasites are the usual culprits.

Thumb Pain and Hand Pain

can be due to liver parasites. Get yourself ready for a liver cleanse. If the pain goes away beforehand, while you are on the kidney cleanse, it shows you had deposits in your joints. You were headed for arthritis in your hands. Read the information on arthritis (page 78) to protect yourself.

Finger Pain

This is pain in a joint, often accompanied by some enlargement or knobbyness of the joint. It is not hard to recognize these as deposits of the same kind as we saw in the toes. You can test yourself to identify the variety. **Uric acid** and **phosphates** are the commonest types. Read the section on toe pain (page 55) for detailed instructions. You can greatly reduce your finger joint deposits and the size of the knobs. In six weeks after starting the kidney cleanse and changing your diet, the knobs may already be shrinking. A large magnet (5000 gauss—used only as directed) may bring pain relief but only dental cleanup and environmental cleanup will give you lasting improvement.

Back Of Neck Pain

The back sides of the neck seem to be highways that run between the teeth and liver. Both contribute to pain at the back of the neck. Pulling an infected tooth or cleaning a cavitation can bring complete relief, only to return the next time a tooth is extracted. Extractions should be followed by cleaning out the cavity created so an infection can't start here. Cleaning the liver can also bring immediate relief, only to find pain and stiffness to return months later. You must cleanse many times for permanent relief.

An allergic reaction to potatoes and tomatoes can express itself in neck pain too. When the liver can no longer detoxify the chemicals (solanine, etc.) in this food family they are free to roam the body with the circulation. Perhaps they prefer to attach themselves at a particular neck site and cause inflammation here. Perhaps an injury was already there, beforehand. Whiplash is often blamed for back-neck pain and indeed chiropractic adjustments can bring total relief. Perhaps the trauma of whiplash first invited all of these contributors. Merely killing bacteria with a zapper is not long lasting. But dental cleanup plus liver cleansing is.

Front Neck Pain

Lymph nodes under the jaw strain your body fluids of the head, removing bacteria and toxins. They are sometimes called "neck glands." If the stream of bacteria is endless such as when they are coming from a hidden tooth infection, the lymph nodes will enlarge to do a better job. They will also try to remove toxic metals, mouthwash, and toothpaste for you.

To see what is affecting your lymph nodes, purchase a slide of lymph nodes. Since we have lymph nodes in many locations in the body, you can't single out the neck nodes for study. So you will get to see all the toxins affecting lymph nodes everywhere: PCBs in your underwear being removed by groin lymph nodes, lead in your intestinal lymph nodes

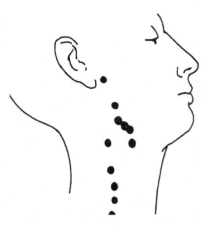

Fig. 26 Lymph node neck glands

from the water you are drinking, mercury in your neck lymph nodes from amalgam fillings. Eliminate all these. Don't rest as long as any of your glands are enlarged.

Roland Sanford, 23, had minor pain and a lot of stiffness along the sides of his neck. His arms had some numbness. He only had one metal tooth filling but his whole body was toxic with samarium, beryllium, indium, copper, cesium, and mercury. When it was replaced, his neck pain and numbness got better.

Audrey Doyle had severe neck pains she attributed to sitting all day and sleeping in her wheelchair. She had to take pain killers to get to sleep at night because they were so bad. She knew eating cream and butter made it worse but she had no will power, she said. After a liver cleanse, getting "thousands" of tiny stones, she was free of it...for one day! But it was enough to convince her and she was determined to be off pain killers.

Temporal Mandibular Joint (TMJ) Problems

Pain at the angle of your jaw is not due to a poorly fitting joint. It fits perfectly but the muscles nearby are pulling it out of joint with their frequent spasms. There is <u>always</u> a hidden tooth infection present. Ask the dentist to search for hidden tooth infections and to clean your cavitations (you will need to find an alternative dentist, and read Dental Cleanup, page 409). Begin immediately to heal these bone lesions with vitamin D (40,000 to 50,000 units once a day for 3 weeks, followed by 2 such doses per week forever), milk-consumption for calcium, and a magnesium oxide tablet. (See bone healing, page 87).

Kill pinworms with a zapper or frequency generator in yourself and family members twice a week and keep everyone's fingernails short for extra hygiene in the family for a month to prevent reinfection. Pinworms can cause tooth grinding and contribute to TMJ dysfunction. For extra muscle relaxation, take two magnesium tablets at bedtime and valerian capsules.

Tooth Ache

Before the pain becomes acute and excruciating, kill bacteria of the mouth, including "tooth decay" and "tooth plaque" frequencies (see frequency list, page 561). Make your dental appointment immediately. If zapping bacteria several times in a few hours relieves pain enough to get you through the night or past the weekend, do not delay a single day. Zapping does not reach into the middle of an abscess—it circles around, so some bacteria are left to repopulate.

Try to understand the problem. If there are teeth with root canals near the location of pain, extract them. The toxic materials of the root canal jeopardize your total body health. Removing them <u>always</u> helps and may let the jaw heal normally where they were extracted. Since the pain is caused by a bulging infection pressing on a jaw nerve, and because each tooth has a related organ(s) it is especially important to clear up all infections to protect these organs.

defenses and regularly invade the eye if they get into the body somewhere.

We get *Toxoplasma* from cats; the infectious stage is in cat feces.

Toxoplasma infection could be the beginning of a lifetime of eye disease due to weakening of the eyes at an early age. *Toxoplasma* also invades the brain, frequently causing a dull ache or pressure at the back of the head. *Trichinella* is another common eye parasite, invading the eye muscles, so that a muscle is weakened and doesn't allow perfect alignment of the two eyes. Dogs and cats are the source of these.

**There should never be a cat box in the house.
Never let a child near a cat box.**

By killing all the large parasites plus a few bacteria (*Staphylococci, Chlamydias, Neisserias*) the eye can become pain free in a few days. If pain returns, you missed something or reinfected yourself. Everyone in the family including pets needs to be treated for all the parasites. No indoor pets should be kept by a person of low immunity, since infecting yourself daily and then killing parasites daily is not a solution.

Herpes of the eye is not a single actor. The true host of this virus is a larger parasite, possibly a tapeworm stage. Tapeworm stages should be killed with an herbal preparation, Rascal, or with a zapper. (Not with a frequency generator. Only a zapper can kill all the segments and eggs at once, leaving nothing alive to wander about and find a new tissue to invade.)

Mary Rauch, age 60, filled a page with different pains and problems. Even her eyes had a dull ache around and behind them, sometimes reaching to the back of the head. Her teeth hurt when she ate and she had been getting B$_{12}$ shots once a week for 36 years for pernicious anemia. She was full of *Ascaris*, amoebas and pin-worms which kept her legs twitching and jerking in bed at night, even waking her up. She was so much better after the kidney cleanse and parasite program she was eager to cleanse her liver. Before two months had passed her eye pain was gone.

Jessie Healy, middle aged and in good health otherwise, had carried the anxiety of having inherited *retinitis pigmentosa* for forty years. Now her drivers' license was in jeopardy due to fast progression of her disease. Numerous heavy metals had accumulated in her retina, including cerium from dental floss, arsenic from pesticide, tin from health food brand deodorant, PCB from skin salve, cobalt from dish detergent and indium from tooth metal. She had eight parasites in the retina including *Toxoplasma* from association with cats years ago. Removal of dental metal alone arrested the disease process. Two years later she was slightly improved and still driving her car.

Macular Degeneration

Dolores Bollapragada, 50ish, had suffered from clinical ergot poisoning in the past which put her in a coma for several weeks. Ergot is a grain (especially rye) fungus, very toxic to the liver. Its byproducts are used in migraine medicine. She had overdosed, somehow. Perhaps her liver never recovered. It no longer detoxified solvents for her, allowing them to accumulate in her retina. There she had propyl alcohol, benzene, carbon tetrachloride, acetone, butyl nitrite, styrene, gasoline, wood alcohol, paradichlorobenzene (moth balls), pentane, methylene chloride and decane. She stopped snacking on cold cereal through the day. She had many habits and products to change. But she was determined to salvage her sight. She did.

Headache and Migraines

Headaches can take the joy out of living. They can lower your motivation level so low that you don't even want to do anything about them! People with daily headache deserve our deepest sympathy since they must carry on with life's daily duties in spite of it. Often, no medicine helps. Although there are common headaches, sinus headaches, migraines, and others, the causes of all overlap a great deal.

> Tooth infection, urinary tract infection, bowel problems, and a wormlet, *Strongyloides* are the common causes.

There are also allergic connections which include milk, eggs, citrus and salty foods. But the allergy-approach is difficult to put into practice. It is almost impossible to stay off these foods for long time periods. Eliminating bacteria and *Strongyloides* leads to a permanent solution.

Possibly the parasite wormlet comes first, since even young children can suffer with migraines. *Strongyloides* is a microscopically small threadworm that horses are plagued with, but humans and our pets pick it up easily. Every migraine sufferer (100%) has high levels of this tiny worm. Perhaps it is really the special bacteria it brings with it that cause the blood vessels to seep or to spasm in the brain, causing pain. Zap it immediately.

Bacteria hidden under a tooth filling or root canal or in a space where once a tooth was pulled can be the cause. *Staphylococcus aureus* is a favorite, but various *Clostridia*, *Streps* and others are often seen, too. You don't feel pain from this small abscess because the pressure isn't building up inside it. It has found a way into your body–namely, your brain!–so no pressure builds up to alert you. Find an alternative dentist with experience cleaning cavitations and finding small hidden abscesses. If you get immediate relief from dental work, only to lose ground again later, the abscess may have formed again (they are notorious for forming again). Go back to the dentist. Irrigate the dental wound site with white iodine (potassium iodide, 12 drops) or Lugol's (6 drops) to ¼ cup water using a curved-tip syringe.

Do not use iodine if you know you are allergic to it.

The colon is always a thriving mass of bacteria. It should be emptied at least twice a day to keep their levels down. Use the simple herb, *Cascara sagrada,* senna tea, or magnesium oxide tablets (2 to 3 a day) to help you eliminate frequently if your own regularity is lacking.

Gallstones in the liver and a congested liver are sources of bacteria, too. Do several liver cleanses and note the effect.

Is it the toxins made by bacteria or the inflammation from the bacteria or wormlets themselves that produces the headache? Certainly, one can <u>eat</u> the toxins by themselves in foods like yogurt, cheese, wine, sour cream and develop "royal" headaches. Stay away from these **tyramine** containing foods. Boil all your dairy foods to prevent *Salmonellas* and *Shigellas* from swimming into your beleaguered brain. Don't eat dairy foods that can't be boiled for ten seconds.

Begin by killing all *Strongyloides* and other parasites, bacteria and viruses with a zapper. Hopefully, this will only leave a few stragglers behind in abscesses, gallstones and the colon contents. If the colon bacterium, *E. coli,* is your headache cause, start the Bowel Program. Search for the source of your *E coli* in food or polluted water. Stop reusing water bottles. Most people get their *Strongyloides* back in a few days from pets, other family members, and themselves! Zap every day for three weeks. Try to "clean up" family members and pets. Never let a horse or pet salivate on you. Never put your fingers in your mouth. Always sanitize your hands with grain alcohol after using the bathroom.

To summarize the steps to cure migraine headaches:

1. Kill *Strongyloides* and bacteria by zapping.
2. Do the herbal kidney cleanse.
3. Clean up dentalware.
4. Do the Bowel Program.

5. Boil all dairy foods.
6. Do liver cleanses.

This has never failed to substantially reduce migraine intensity and frequency.

Headaches are also caused by toxins in your environment; especially things you breathe in. Household gas is the most common offender. You don't smell it after you get used to it! Gas pipes are notoriously leaky. Conducting gases through pipes with joints in them, where gases could escape, must be the most ludicrous of all modern "conveniences". Would you try to conduct water through pipes with holes in them? You would soon see the water on your kitchen or bathroom floor. But gas doesn't land on the floor, it doesn't make a puddle, so you, the consumer, are left helplessly believing you don't have leaks. Every gas pipe that has a seam should have a clear plastic boot around it containing indicator compound to let it be known when gas is escaping. Other methods could be invented to make the gas utility safe. As you will see from the case histories, very many persons are living in a cloud of poisonous gas.

The telltale element is **vanadium**. When your vanadium test is positive, you have a gas leak that your body found, even though the gas company may not. Many gas companies use outmoded equipment to search for it. Four out of five gas companies miss the gas leak. Health Departments and building contractors use modern equipment that detects even the tiniest leak; call them.

If you are a headache sufferer, fixing the pipes is not good enough. Switch from fossil fuels to electric. There will be many dividends. (Remember not to use candles as part of your lifestyle, nor to be a smoker.) Your air needs to be clean: clean of perfumes and colognes, clean of potpourri and air fresheners, clean of air sprays, pesticides, formaldehyde, freon, carpet and car odor, fireplace lighter, and of wood smoke.

Janette Donovan, age 52, had migraines every day but could not tolerate <u>any</u> medication for it. She walked about "like a zombie" most of the time. She frequently had vomiting with them. She was gassy, had pain in her right groin for many years and chronic bladder leakage. Our kidney stone test showed urate crystals. Her urinalysis also showed urate crystals and a slight amount of blood, obviously chronic urinary tract infection. The parasite test showed *Strongyloides*, *Trichuris* and *Fasciolopsis buskii* in the intestines. Her heavy metal test showed beryllium. This was tracked down to hurricane lamps that once held coal-oil in them— it filled her house air unbeknownst to her. Thirty five days later she had done an herbal parasite killing program, done the kidney cleanse, cleared out the hurricane lamps and all fuel containers. Her headaches were "more like pressure" now than pain. She still had *Strongyloides*. Four months later she had some headaches still but not migraines. They were down to once a week. Three months after that she had done a liver cleanse and gotten abut 3,000 stones out! She was still getting some headaches. She tested positive to *Histoplasma* and *Coxsackie virus #4* (a common brain virus) probably stemming from dentalware. She had many root canals and couldn't decide what to do. Keep her teeth and risk return of migraines; or get partial dentures. After eight months of indecisiveness she was back up to ten headaches per month, although not migraines.

Patsy Olsen, age 30, had migraines daily, frequently with vomiting. She had *Strongyloides* as well as *Ascaris*, and other bowel parasites as did her husband and two children. She couldn't tolerate any medication and had to give herself an enema daily for constipation. The whole family was put on parasite killing herbs. A gas leak was found and fixed and the baby's diapers were changed to non fragrant. Ten months later, the whole family still had *Strongyloides*. By one year she was experiencing a couple of good days a month although she still had *Ascaris*, *Coxsackie* viruses, and various tooth-related bacteria. Her two and a half year old had swollen neck glands, was toxic with bismuth from disposable diapers but did not have *Strongyloides*. The eight year old was also toxic with the lotions and fragrance of baby-stuff in the home; she was constantly congested and coughing but became free of *Strongyloides* in six months. After another ten months (the baby had been potty-trained meanwhile) the mother began to have headache-free days.

Donald Schaible, age 14, had migraines, learning disabilities and severe acne. The parasite test showed *Strongyloides*, *hookworm* and *Ascaris*. In spite of being on the parasite program two weeks and zapping, he still had *Strongyloides*.

Kenneth Jones had migraines for thirty five years and had tried all the new medications. They worked for a while, then stopped helping, but he continued taking them anyway. He usually went to the emergency room for the really bad ones, once a week but lived with the constant daily variety. There were two house dogs. They and the whole family had *Strongyloides*. After cleaning up an asbestos problem, killing parasites for five months and clearing kidneys of urate stones, he was down to two to three mere headaches a week. Two months later, he was getting migraines again; they all had *Strongyloides* again. With renewed efforts, one month later his bad headaches were down to one a month, although his low level chronic headache persisted: they had the dogs on a strict schedule of parasite killing herbs as well as themselves. He had not been to the emergency room for a month.

Angelina Gander, age 46, had daily headaches, not migraines. She also had persistent urinary tract infection and sinus infection. She was put on the herbal parasite program and four weeks later was much better. She also lost her chest pain due to heartworm and regained her milk tolerance.

Gracie Arlington had a boy age 6 who wet the bed, a girl age 8 with a behavior problem at school. She was stressed by an unfaithful spouse and thought she should go back to school for a Nursing degree so she could support the family. But she was getting two or three migraines a week in addition to colitis attacks which she feared would make her unable to study. The two cats, a dog, the children and herself all had *Strongyloides*, *Ascaris*, and a variety of other intestinal parasites. The humans were promptly zapped for parasites and the boy was dry that night for the first time in his life. A few nights later he was wet again. This time the animals were zapped and put on the pet parasite program and the children's toileting was carefully supervised. When she dropped her extreme vigilance over all, they all relapsed. After a year of trying, they gave away their beloved dog, put the cat box in the porch

167

and the mother did the cleaning herself but nothing prevented relapses. A half year later, her six year old son asked if he could launder his own sheets and blankets. This request broke her heart and she planned to give away one cat. Even with only one cat, the girl's behavior and grades fluctuated extremely, the mother had a migraine a week and the boy wet. During a vacation the mother loaned the last cat, (her cat) to which she was very endeared, to a friend, to see if it made a difference. The boy never wet again, the girl made straight A's, and the mother's headaches became sinus headaches. Some intensive dental work cleared these up. She brought her Nursing diploma to our office two years after beginning. She should have had another diploma for **Intelligent Parenting.**

Earache

Earache is particularly common in children. Bacteria, mainly *Streptococcus pneumoniae*, have built up to a high level. Zap them. They were probably introduced by some larger parasite. But why did they multiply and thrive in your child's ear? There must have been food for them and protection from the immune system. Probably the Eustachian tubes are full of mucous, providing habitat. The mucous is present because some air toxin is irritating the sensitive linings. Clean up the air: not just asbestos, fiberglass, formaldehyde, freon, and arsenic, but perfumes, fragrant school supplies, potpourri.

Being housebound, as in winter, makes the air-toxin problem worse. Use summer time to strengthen your child for the winter—spend summer outdoors. Always wash hands a lot. Stay away from moldy food. Give small doses of niacin (25 mg., niacin thins mucous so it can run away) along with vitamin C (250 mg.) at bedtime.

Putting in "tubes" is a short term solution that is better than perpetually staying on antibiotics, but neither should be necessary.

To hasten healing, as soon as earache is suspected put room temperature olive oil in both ears, tug the earlobe to let bubbles out, and stopper them with cotton wool salvaged from vitamin bottles (other types are polluted with mercury). Put on a light hat that covers the ears.

When adults get earache, the *Strep*s are hiding under tooth fillings and in gallstones. Clean up these two sources and zap.

Drinking non sterile milk adds *Salmonellas* and *Shigellas* to the *Strep* ear infection! Small wonder milk is thought to make people mucousy. The ears must now battle them, too. Even a few bacteria consumed in milk can start a whole colony if bowel bacteria have been disturbed by antibiotics. If your child has become "allergic" to milk or gets mucousy, remove cheese and ice cream–not milk–from the diet. Even cheese can be eaten if baked as in pizza or casseroles. Milk must be boiled. Try to reduce the child's *Salmonella* sensitivity by avoiding unnecessary antibiotics. Keep immunity high by avoiding moldy food!

Ear Noises And Ringing

This is also called *tinnitus*. A hissing or buzzing sound is heard in one or both ears. It can be continuous or pulsing off and on. It can be as loud as roaring.

Tinnitus is caused by three things acting in partnership: toxic elements, an allergy to *salicylates* (the aspirin family) and a bacterium *Streptococcus pneumoniae* (the pneumonia bug). This "bug" can be carried in the chronic state after a bout of pneumonia or what seems to be a head-cold. It is always present in earache. It is easily activated by exposure to cold wind or drafts and certain toxic substances. For this reason I recommend keeping the ears warm in winter by keeping them covered or wearing a cotton plug or ear-muffs. The *Strep* bug can also cause *Meniere's syndrome*, congestion, loss of balance and chronic sinus problems. Often an antibiotic of the penicillin family helps immediately, then loses its effectiveness. This shows you that bacteria are involved but cannot be truly vanquished with antibiotics.

Streptococcus pneumoniae often hides in pockets under infected teeth and in holes left where teeth have been pulled—especially wisdom teeth. These can be found by alternative dentists who clean these cavitations. *Strep* also resides in the liver; clean them out with liver flushes.

Certain foods and many medicines, especially cough medicine and lozenges contain salicylate.

To cure the tinnitus we must stop using aspirin or any high level source of salicylates. We must also stop the exposure to certain toxic elements—lead, beryllium, zirconium, benzalkonium. They are present in the air at gas stations and in many of our body lotions, soaps and salves. Switch to safe varieties. Niacin tablets, such as 100 mg, taken three times daily is another treatment, intended to increase the blood supply to the inner ear. Taking a thyroid tablet, by prescription, often helps too.

These methods never fail to improve tinnitus but a complete cure is seldom possible.

William Thall, 47, had a headache daily and was on pain medicine for it daily. He had tinnitus, a loud humming noise in the right ear. He had *Shigella* (producing nerve toxins) and *Borellia* (Lyme disease virus). He had *Gaffkya*, a respiratory bacterium under two wisdom teeth (right side). He also had *Campylobacter* and *Anaplasma* growing on him somewhere. He had *Strongyloides* too. He was toxic with vanadium (gas leak) and asbestos. After ten weeks he had two cavitations on the right side of his jaw cleaned, he had been on the parasite program and his tinnitus was gone, (he still had occasional headaches indicating he still had some *Strongyloides*).

Billie Scott, 26, had a history of ear problems, and lots of headaches. She was started on the kidney cleanse. Then she added the parasite program including their two dogs. She had a cyst in her left buttock, due to PCBs traced to the well water. She stopped using this well and switched off detergents for laundry and dishes. She switched off soda pop, onto milk. In 3½ months her tinnitus was gone and the cyst was shrinking.

Larry Pelegrini, 59, had tinnitus in both ears but was otherwise a strong, tall, intelligent person, who cared for sick people, whether family or not. As soon as he saw how simple it was to kill invaders with a frequency generator, he bought one. Preventing their recurrence was his big challenge since he had neither the means nor insurance to do dental work. He was toxic with aluminum, copper and PCBs. After switching to borax for all washing purposes, he got rid of aluminum and could feel his memory improve. The kidney herbs cleared him of uric acid and oxalate and he felt more supple. He had to go off his favorite beverage to get rid of pentane and methyl ethyl ketone. Twice a week he killed two dozen parasites and bacteria, that just seemed to pop up from nowhere, in order to feel better and reduce his tinnitus. But he lived alone, had to cook, garden, take care of animals and his sick friends which gave him a lot of parasite exposure. Sometimes he would be toxic with arsenic (a new pesticide he tried out) or vanadium (gas leak) but mainly it was tooth filling metal. If only this wonderful man could afford his dental work: what a blessing to society he could be for a long time to come.

Scalp Pain

Infection anywhere in the head can cause sensitive scalp and scalp pain. Even a common cold can cause bouts of scalp pain. Clean up your dentalware and environment.

Lumps on the scalp are often called *sebaceous cysts,* actually this is where your body has sequestered PCBs (polychlorinated biphenyls, extremely hazardous, now banned in the U.S., but often a pollutant in detergents.) Get rid of them by switching off detergents for all purposes. See *Recipes* for dishwasher liquid, dishwasher detergent, and laundry detergent replacements.

171

Non-Painful Diseases

Explanations for many of these "mysterious" diseases become rather obvious when you see a **common parasite, or pollutant, or both** consistently show up in case after case.

Diabetes

All diabetics have a common fluke parasite, *Eurytrema pancreaticum*, the pancreatic fluke of cattle, in their own pancreas. It seems likely that we get it from cattle, repeatedly, by eating their meat or dairy products in a raw state. It is not hard to kill with a zapper but because of its infective stages in our food supply we can immediately be reinfected.

Eurytrema will not settle and multiply in our pancreas without the presence of **wood alcohol** (methanol). Methanol pollution pervades our food supply—it is found in processed food including bottled water, artificial sweetener, soda pop, baby formula and powdered drinks of all kinds including health food varieties. I presume wood alcohol is used to wash equipment used in manufacturing. If your child has diabetes, **use nothing out of a can, package or bottle** except regular milk, and **no** processed foods.

By killing this parasite and removing wood alcohol from the diet, the need for insulin can be cut in half in three weeks (or sooner!).

Be vigilant with your blood sugar checks. The pancreas with its tiny islets that produce insulin recovers very quickly. Even if 90% of them were destroyed, requiring daily insulin shots, half of them can recover or regenerate so insulin is no longer necessary. The insulin shot itself may be polluted with wood alcohol (this is an especially cruel irony—the treatment itself is worsening the condition). Test it yourself, using the wood alcohol in automotive fluids (windshield washer) or from a paint store, as a test substance. Try different brands of insulin until you find one that is free of methanol.

Artificial sweeteners are polluted with wood alcohol! Instead of helping you cope with diabetes, they are actually promoting it! Do not use them.

Drugs that stimulate your pancreas to make more insulin may also carry solvent pollution; test them for wood alcohol and switch brands and bottles until you find a pure one. You may not need them much longer, so the extra expense now may soon reward you.

Many persons can detoxify the amount of wood alcohol that pollutes our foods. They do not have a food mold, **Kojic acid**, built up in their bodies as diabetics do. I have found Kojic acid in coffee, and potatoes with gray areas inside. Do not eat discolored potatoes or peels, even if cooked or baked. Being able to detoxify a poisonous substance like wood alcohol should not give us the justification for consuming it. All poisons are bad for us. Do not consume them.

All diabetic persons also carry a virus, *HA virus* in the pancreas. This virus grows in the skin as a wart but is spread quite widely in the body such as in the spleen or liver besides pancreas. It is not necessary to kill this virus since it disappears when the pancreatic fluke is gone. The HA virus undoubtedly belongs to the pancreatic fluke. The question can be asked: Does the fluke or its virus cause diabetes? There might even be a bacterium, so far missed in our observations, that is the real perpetrator.

While recovering from diabetes, it is very important to check your blood sugar every day. Improvement is so rapid, you may suddenly be over-insulinized by your next shot. Cut down your dose to suit your actual need.

There are additional aspects to diabetes that have been studied by alternative physicians. For instance, allergy to wheat and other grains containing gluten is common. Perhaps the pancreas and its islets would heal much faster if grains were out of the diet for a while. Perhaps the 50% improvement that is consistently possible just by killing parasites and stopping wood alcohol consumption could be improved further by a month of grain-free diet. Eating **fenugreek seeds** has been reported to greatly benefit (actually cure) diabetes cases. Are they a specific fluke killer, virus killer, or neither? It seems like a good idea to add this to your diet if you are a diabetic. Wood alcohol also accumulates in the eyes, and there is a connection between diabetes and eye disease. **Bilberry leaves** are an herbal treatment for both diabetes and weak eyes. Do they help by counteracting wood alcohol or detoxifying Kojic acid? Make a tea for yourself, using ¼ cup leaves to three cups water. Drink ½ cup a day. **Chromium** is another must for diabetics (200 mcg three times a day). It helps insulin enter your cells.

Gold is attracted to the pancreas. Heavy metals should be removed from dentalware including all gold crowns and no metal should be worn next to the skin as jewelry, including all gold items.

Blythe Jenkins was on Micronase™ (5 mg) daily for her diabetes but she still had a morning blood sugar of 183. She had pancreatic flukes and sheep liver flukes in her pancreas, vanadium (a gas leak) in her home and cadmium in her water (old pipes). After killing parasites and cleaning kidneys her morning blood sugar was down to 148. She also got rid of her hot flushes, groin and leg pain. This encouraged her so much she did the rest of her body cleanup and could go off her medicine completely.

Robert Greene, age 65, had been on insulin five years already, getting two shots a day (25 u each), and even this was not controlling his blood sugar which was 288 in the morning. He was raised to 30 units without much improvement. His legs and feet were too painful to walk without a walker to lean on. He had *Loa loa* in his pancreas. (This is another example of a parasite going to the "wrong" location, this time the pancreas instead of the heart. I believe the solvent makes this possible.) Also *mumps virus, HA wart virus, mycoplasma, flu virus, chicken pox virus, Adenovirus* and *Shigella*, all making their home in his pancreas! This was possible because he had wood alcohol accumulated there, from drinking various beverages and using artificial sweetener. As soon as he stopped this practice and killed everything with a frequency generator his blood sugar fell below 100 in the morning and he had to reduce his insulin to 20 units. He was also on chromium 200 mcg (2 three times a day). Meanwhile, he cleared 2,000 stones out of his liver. He could now walk well again and decided to take a part time job. The whole process took one year.

Ralph Dixon, age 72, had been switched to 30 units of insulin, once a day, after six years on pills for his diabetes. He still had a fasting blood sugar of 242. He had the pancreatic fluke and a host of bacteria and viruses in his pancreas. He had a poodle. After killing the pathogens and cleaning his kidneys, his blood sugar dropped so he cut his insulin to 25 units (blood sugar was at 111). Soon he had to cut it to 20 units. He was also on chromium 200 mcg (2 three times a day), manganese 50 mg. (one a day), fenugreek capsules (2 a day), and bilberry leaves, each supplement by itself. He also lost his angina and fatigue with all this body-cleaning. But if he went off the maintenance parasite program he would promptly get a spike in his blood sugar, showing how easy it was for him to reinfect and how new parasites would immediately find his pancreas.

Melissa Bird, 54, had major illnesses including heart disease (2 angioplasties), numerous other surgeries and diabetes. She took 15-18 units of insulin once a day. Besides pancreatic flukes in her pancreas, she also had intestinal flukes there(!), plus widespread *Ascaris*. She also had warts and candidiasis. Fortunately there were no pets. Her parasites were instantly eliminated with a frequency generator and she was started on kidney herbs for her other problems. Seven weeks later she stated she had to cut down her insulin because her morning blood sugar had dropped to 90. Then she eliminated the decafs and artificial sweetener that were giving her wood alcohol, started the parasite herbs and did a liver cleanse. The day after the liver cleanse her blood sugar went up to 164 but was completely normal after that (under 100) and she did not dare take any more insulin or pills. We advised her to keep monitoring her blood sugar and be very, very vigilant and to please stop smoking.

John Angert, 65, was not on any medicine in spite of his diabetes. He was too embarrassed to tell us his blood sugar. He had a long list of other health problems, too. He was toxic with thulium (vitamin C) and palladium (from tooth fillings). He had a variety of parasites. After doing some dental work and parasite killing his fasting blood sugar dropped to a normal 98. But his leg cramps kept returning in spite of doing a kidney cleanse. Only after changing his diet to include milk did the phosphate crystals stay away and eliminate his cramps.

Cornelius Edens, age 33, came for his diabetes, although he also had fatigue, digestion problems, and headaches. He had numerous other minor symptoms like chest pain over the heart, soreness in testicles, etc. His diabetes was only diagnosed one year ago. he was on insulin (Humulin™ 20 long acting plus 6 regular units) in the morning. He often omitted the evening dose which should be 14 long plus 6 regular. This brought his fasting blood sugar down to 166 in the morning.

He had pancreatic flukes in his testicles besides in his pancreas. His aflatoxin level was very high; he was told to stop eating grocery store bread, eat bakery bread only. He had silver, nickel and very high levels of gold–probably all three coming from his gold crowns–he was to have them all replaced with composite. He had fiberglass in his pancreas. Wood alcohol was present in large amounts in his pancreas as expected. He was to stop drinking all store bought beverages, whether frozen, powdered, or ready to drink. He did not test positive to benzene, propyl alcohol, Salmonellas, Shigellas, or E. coli. But he had Staph aureus growing at high levels in his pancreas. The usual source for this is in teeth, so he was told to ask his dentist to search for cavitations and clean up hidden tooth infections while replacing the gold crowns. He was to find the exposed fiberglass and seal it off. He was to zap parasites every other day for 1 month. His supplements were vitamin C (1 tsp. with each meal for constipation; then 1 tsp. daily), vitamin B-50 complex (2 per day), thioctic acid (2 per day). He was to start the Kidney Cleanse recipe for his testicle problem, and after 6 weeks do a Liver Cleanse. He was to follow up with us in 3 weeks, after dental work was completed. He never returned. Four months later we received a phone call he was too embarrassed to make himself. He needed no insulin and was doing fine. Another 3 months later he was still doing well, and off insulin.

Prediabetic

Alyce Dold, 64, came because she was worried about her blood sugar and chest pain. Indeed, a blood test showed her fasting blood sugar to be 136, just beginning to show insufficient insulin production by her pancreas. She had pancreatic flukes and wood alcohol there. Also mumps virus and HA virus. She had six more solvents accumulated due to eating raisin bran and other cold cereals each day. She was glad to be forced off this routine: she switched to 2 eggs every other day with biscuits or bread (not toast) and cooked cereal in between. Her chest pain was due to dog heartworm and *Staphylococcus aureus* bacteria that originated at teeth #16, 17, 1, 32. The worms and *Staph* were killed with a frequency generator. She was referred to a dentist for cavitations and started on kidney herbs. Two weeks later, there was still a little residual heart pain due to *Staph*; dental work was not yet done. She was given chromium (600 mcg per day) to help her insulin regulate sugar. Her LDH (See tests) was still high from the recent heart stress, no doubt. But she had accomplished a lot and planned to get it all done.

Diabetes Of Childhood

The problem is the same for diabetes of childhood as for diabetes of later onset, but much easier to clear up, underline provided underline the whole family cooperates.

Wesley Evanco, age 6, had his onset at age 11 months. Prior to that he had chicken pox and his baby shots. He had pancreatic flukes and their reproductive stages in his pancreas as well as wood alcohol. He had no other solvents accumulated. The problem was clearly due to these two enemies of his small body. Wesley's father did not have pancreatic flukes but his mother had very high levels, along with wood alcohol. She had to clear hers up before Wesley could recover. She chose not to. She couldn't believe the connection. Our most persuasive efforts were not successful. We hope Wesley can forgive us all in due time.

Herpes

The *Herpes* family of viruses includes *Herpes Simplex Virus* (HSV) 1 and 2, *Epstein Barre Virus* (EBV), shingles or Chicken Pox (*Varicella zoster*), *Cytomegalovirus* (CMV) and some newly discovered ones.

Herpes simplex virus 1 is the virus that breaks out around or inside the mouth. We call it a cold sore because it often follows a cold in childhood. As children, we may get HSV 1 once or twice each winter. When they come more often the child's immunity is low. Adults who get repeated attacks also have low immunity (this is obvious from a blood test where the white blood cell count is less than 5,000 per cu mm).

Herpes simplex virus 2 breaks out in the genital area. It is often blamed on promiscuous sex but I believe it has quite different origins.

I believe the virus is introduced to our bodies by another large parasite. Perhaps it is pinworms, or *Ascaris*. Perhaps it is a tapeworm stage, picked up from dust and dirt.

I have some evidence that it is released from dog tapeworm stages when these are being killed by your immune system. It is probably the same tapeworm stage as releases the *Adenovirus* (cold virus) which would explain why children frequently get "cold sores" during or after a cold. (See Curing The Common Cold, page 357.)

Nevertheless, you would not get sick from these viral releases unless your immunity was lowered.

Herpes lives in your nerve centers (*ganglia*) and it is from here that you can be attacked after the initial infection. Evidently your immune system can destroy them as quickly as they emerge. But a meal of **aflatoxin** or other **moldy food** suddenly "gags" your white blood cells and lets a viral attack happen.

The viruses can also be "triggered" which lets them out of hibernation (latency) to multiply and travel along the nerve fiber to the skin. Triggers are things that put these nerve centers to work: sudden cold and heat, trauma from chafing and friction. Never drink water with ice cubes in it. Never eat hot soup with a metal spoon. Don't tweeze hairs.

Begin your prevention program by raising the immunity of your skin; this means removing all toxins from the skin. Use only natural lotions, softeners, cleansers on your skin made from recipes in this book. Health food brands are not superior. This will get rid of nickel, chromate, titanium, zirconium, aluminum, and benzalkonium from your skin and probably your whole body! Do laundry with borax and washing soda, only, to eliminate commercial detergent as a source, too.

As soon as you feel that warning tingle or sensation of *Herpes*, zap or use a frequency generator at 293 and 345 KHz (HSV 1) or 360 and 355 KHz (for HSV 2). Immediately take a **cayenne** capsule and 8 **lysine** tablets (500 mg each). The cayenne slows down travel of the virus along the nerve.

Attacks probably occur when the triggers act at the same time as an immune drop occurs. Immune drops happen frequently due to eating moldy food. Of course, mercury in amalgam tooth fillings keeps immunity chronically lowered. Many persons report they stopped breaking out with *Herpes 1* after replacing their amalgams. Stopping wearing tight synthetic underpants helps reduce *Herpes 2* out breaks.

When you get an outbreak, mop up a droplet of the blister fluid and prepare it as a specimen for yourself. If you search for it in your white blood cells when your attack is over, it will not be found because it is in hiding inside your nerve cells. Zapping does not reach them inside your own cells. Nevertheless, you can totally eliminate them by repeated zapping provided you kill them at their earliest warning. Evidently, they haven't multiplied yet, so gradually their numbers go down.

Even after you have been *Herpes* free for a long time, stick to your preventive principles. Avoid the trigger foods, peanuts, and chocolate, or be ready to zap. Avoid cold wind or direct sunlight on your face. Don't eat abrasive or acid foods like popcorn, nuts, toast, crackers, candy, citrus. Although you may stop the virus in its tracks by zapping, healing the lesion takes time. Keep the skin softened with a cornstarch or sodium alginate recipe (see *Recipes*).

A lysine mush helps too: crush a lysine table with a large wooden spoon, add a pinch of vitamin C powder and a pinch of zinc oxide. Save part of this mixture for later use. Wet a small bit of it with a few drops of water to make a paste. Apply to lesions.

Bazezew Hailey, 38, started breaking out in the genital area after a period of antibiotic use. She was started on lysine (500 mg, 8 a day), cayenne caps (one with each meal). She was to fill her prescription for Zovirax™ from her doctor, though. By the time she had it filled, the next day, her lesion had stopped enlarging, and she could reduce her supplements. Her skin was full of mercury, lead, strontium, aluminum. Her white blood cell count was low, showing low immunity. Her ratio of segmental to lymphocyte white blood cells was low, evidence for a chronic viral condition. Her bone marrow contained lead and radon. She stopped using toothpaste (strontium), salt, deodorant, detergents (aluminum). She got the metal out of her mouth and eliminated her radon problem by opening crawl space vents. The lead source was never found, but

181

after she moved to a new house it went away. *Herpes 2* stayed away. A year later she still hadn't opened the Zovirax™ bottle.

Fatigue

Fatigue, whether minor or extreme, is always associated with blood sugar disturbances. The more disturbance, the more fatigue. We have three organs that do most of the sugar regulating: our **adrenals**, the **liver**, and the **islets in the pancreas**. In severe fatigue, that keeps you partly bedridden, all three organs are heavily parasitized. *Epstein Barre Virus* (EBV) is running amok in your body, as a rule, even when clinical culture techniques cannot find it. With your frequency generator and Syncrometer you can find it emitting at 380 KHz. Killing the viruses is not as important as killing the larger parasites and getting your organs functioning for you again. The viruses will go away by themselves.

The liver's role in blood sugar regulation is to get it out of storage when needed. When sheep liver flukes have taken up residence they're spewing their chemicals as well as their own bacteria and viruses into your circulation; it is surprising that the liver has any sugar in reserve and can function at all. Sheep liver flukes are commonly seen in fatigue syndrome cases.

The adrenals (the outer layer called the cortex) help to regulate the blood sugar in a complex way. Some adrenal factors influence the thyroid which is another energy-related organ. Both adrenals and thyroid have toxic buildups in fatigue cases! Their work is hampered.

The heart of sugar regulation is in your pancreas in the tiny islands of cells that secrete insulin, called the *islets of Langerhans*. Here we always find the pancreatic fluke in residence. It actually breeds there when wood alcohol accumulates in it. Wood alcohol is a common pollutant of food, even in artificial sugar which is often recommended to replace real sugar and spare the pancreas. There is wood alcohol in store-bought drinking water, fruit juice, powders meant to be stirred into beverages, even if they are health food varieties. It's probably being used to clean tubes and hoses in the manufacturing plant. The only beverage you can safely buy (not safe unless you sterilize it, though) at a grocery store is milk. Make your own beverages using recipes in this book.

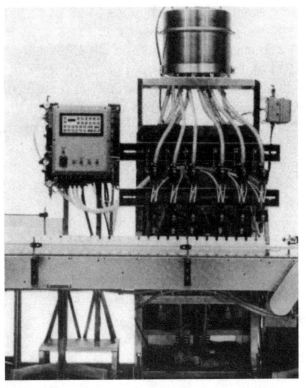

Fig. 28 Bottling equipment should be rinsed with ethyl (grain) alcohol, not propyl alcohol or wood alcohol.

Your first step toward curing your fatigue syndrome is to kill the pancreatic fluke and all other living invaders of the pancreas, liver, adrenals and thyroid. Use a zapper. Drink milk or buttermilk for several days afterward to provide lactic acid for the "good" bacteria to feed and recover on.

Your second step is removing metal from your mouth, particularly gold. Gold from teeth and jewelry readily goes to the pancreas! Do everything in the *Easy Lifestyle Improvements* chapter.

Your energy can bounce back in a few weeks by attending your liver, adrenals and pancreas. Help these organs heal and grow strong again. Avoid food molds (read Moldy Food, page 381). The most powerful assistance to the liver is a cleanse. This will eliminate liver viruses such as EBV and *Cytomegalovirus* (CMV). Be patient. Do it on a schedule until you have over 2,000 stones out. Take **vitamin C** at least 3 gm/day, to help both liver and adrenals. Take B_2 **and** B_6 to help adrenals and kidneys. Take glucose tolerance factor, **chromium** (two 200 mcg tablets 3x/day). See *Sources* for all of these. Take these supplements for three weeks, then cut the dose in half, and take on alternate days only, as a hedge against possible pollution in these.

Although your energy may be normal in three weeks, you are at higher risk for fatigue than the average person. Reinfection with anything will put the new parasites right back where the old ones were. Other bacteria, solvents and toxins will head for the pancreas, liver and adrenals again because these are weakened organs. It could take two years to build your health to its previous level, but is well worth it to have youth, initiative, and a beautiful appearance again. Going back to school is a good use of your time when your initiative has returned but your physical strength is still not up to housework or a job. When your energy comes back to you, it is tempting to overwork: to clean the whole house or to get into some gardening.

> ## It is better to be moderate today than in bed tomorrow.
>
> Anyone who has suffered from Chronic Fatigue Syndrome (CFS) or recurrent EBV has learned that lesson well.

June Timony, age 38, was diagnosed with Chronic Fatigue Syndrome), EBV and *Candida* around 1½ years ago by her family doctor. She also had a thyroid problem and a high estrogen level (165 pg/ml). She had severe depression at times. Our test showed her body was full of bismuth (fragrance) and silver (tooth fillings) especially in the ovaries. She cleansed her kidneys and killed parasites but could not make up her mind to do the expensive dental work.

Janice Brown, age 21, had EBV with chronic fatigue and depression along with a dozen more symptoms. Her skin, kidneys, breasts, brain, ovaries and pancreas were all loaded with mercury, platinum and other metals. She was full of radon and bus exhaust and the plumbing was shedding cadmium. Rather than do all this she and her husband decided to move. Before the moving date arrived she had cleansed kidneys, killed parasites and done dental work and was feeling noticeably better. Then they moved. She immediately was very fatigued again and worried that the move had been in vain. This time she had a liver full of *Salmonella* and a return of phosphate crystals in her kidneys. But it was easy to clear up and it was a very useful lesson to her to avoid unsterilized dairy products. She was much more careful after this.

Dee Safian, age 36, came especially for her low energy. She had EBV once. It left her extremely nervous. We advised going off caffeine but not substituting for it by drinking decafs. Her tissues were full of arsenic from pesticide; her urinalysis showed kidney crystals and her eosinophil count was high 5.5% (parasites). She had sheep liver flukes and stages in her pancreas due to a buildup of wood alcohol there. In four months after killing parasites and doing a kidney cleanse she was much improved.

185

Josefina Linzer, age 32, came for her fatigue and depression. Her tissues were full of arsenic, PCBs, chromate (eye makeup), mercury, yttrium, radon and terbium. She needed tooth metal replacement but could not schedule it immediately. She had *Ascaris* and pancreatic flukes in her pancreas and reacted to sugar in her diet quite strongly, so avoided it. She also had *Strongyloides* and *Trichinella*. She killed all these with a frequency generator and started on the kidney herbs. Her wood alcohol buildup was coming from carbonated beverages. She went off. In 6 weeks she had done everything except the mercury removal and was feeling much better.

Brigette Dawn, age 21, had Chronic Fatigue Syndrome with EBV, along with other problems. She cleaned her home and cleansed kidneys, killed parasites, and did two liver cleanses. Still the fatigue would return two days later. Meanwhile, though, her infertility problem got solved (she got pregnant) and this encouraged her to continue the battle against fatigue after the baby was born.

Hector Garcia, age 14, was getting gamma globulin injections every three weeks for his chronic fatigue syndrome. He had pancreatic flukes in his pancreas, sheep and human liver flukes in his liver and intestinal fluke in his intestine. He had a buildup of benzene, propanol, and carbon tetrachloride, as well as aflatoxin from his granola breakfasts. He also had *Candida* and measles in his white blood cells. He killed parasites with a frequency generator and went off the solvent polluted items in the propyl alcohol and benzene lists. He immediately (in 20 days) felt much better.

Dana Levi, age 16, had chronic fatigue syndrome and dizziness; he was not in school. He had pancreatic fluke in his pancreas, sheep, human and intestinal flukes in his liver! Both benzene and propyl alcohol were present in his immune system. As soon as the parasites were killed (with a frequency generator) and he changed a lot of his products, he felt better but soon lost his improvement. At the next visit, our tests showed a buildup of vanadium (from burning candles in his bedroom). When he stopped this, he was better again for a while only to relapse again. His propyl alcohol level was up as was aflatoxin. But getting a taste of normal energy gave him the determination to get himself well! He embarked on a liver cleanse program and still more careful food selection.

Dennis Dillard, age 16, was beginning to do poorly at school due to fatigue. He had to stop athletics although his regular doctor pronounced him well. He was also getting chronic sinus infections. His lungs and trachea had accumulated seven heavy metals: vanadium, palladium, cerium, barium, tin, europium, beryllium. His fasting blood sugar was low (73 mg/DL) and LDH very low (90 u/L; it should have been 160). The body makes LDH in response to lactic acid levels. When the muscles aren't making much lactic acid from their normal metabolism, LDH levels will fall too. Was he developing a muscle disease? The gas leak was fixed (vanadium), the garage was sealed off from the house to eliminate barium and beryllium but the other toxic elements came from his dental retainer. As soon as his retainer came out, and they stopped using flea powder on their dog, his energy became normal and sinuses cleared up. A year later he still had not been ill.

Evelina Rojas, age 12, was having extreme fatigue with mood problems and sudden fevers. She killed *Ascaris* and sheep liver flukes with the parasite program but promptly got them back due to a benzene buildup I believe due to using products containing an herbal oil. Her high levels of *Streptococcus pneumoniae* (cause of fevers), *Staphylococcus aureus* and *Nocardia* could not be eliminated until her three baby teeth (with root canals) were pulled. After that, she was well.

Elaine Perkins, 48, came specifically for her low energy and nervousness. She was toxic with arsenic, a substance that replaces energy with nervous excitement and exhaustion. She also had a backlog of antimony (using baby oil), aluminum, rhenium (hair spray), benzalkonium (toothpaste) and radon. In four months, she had the arsenic and three other toxins eliminated and already had more energy.

Neil Youngblood, 53, was so fatigued, he had to brace himself even while sitting. A blood thyroxin level (T_4) of 1.0 instead of the normal 7.5 mcg/DL explained his fatigue. He had a mouthful of assorted dental metals which were accumulating in the thyroid, inviting viruses, particularly CMV, into it. He had to be on four grains of thyroid to feel near normal. After he had all his tooth metal removed, he only needed one grain to feel O.K. This encouraged him to clean up more of his body.

187

Scott Pennington, 50ish, was on thyroid medicine for his hyperthyroidism. He had been on iodine-radium earlier. He had the *miracidia* of the intestinal fluke, sheep liver fluke, and pancreatic fluke in his thyroid! Adult human liver flukes were also there! His thyroid was toxic with iridium, nickel, tellurium and mercury (metal tooth fillings) and decane, TC Ethylene and pentane solvents. He had been drinking a great deal of regular tea, which let oxalate crystals deposit in his kidney and slow down the excretion of toxins. The parasites were killed with a frequency generator, he changed his diet to get rid of solvents. In two weeks he was feeling better, had more energy and better sleep. This encouraged him to do the dental work.

Skin Problems

Sebaceous Cysts

Your body, in its wisdom, keeps toxins together and out of harm's way by making a cyst out of it. All the *sebaceous cysts* I have seen are filled with *polychlorinated biphenyls* (PCBs).

Get rid of PCB sources in order to clear PCBs from your body. This can take 6 to 12 months. Change <u>all</u> detergents (for dishes, laundry, and body use) to borax and/or washing soda.

Commercial detergents are wonderful cleaners...

but are unquestionably toxic. <u>Whether you have cysts or not</u>, it is always a good idea to use borax and washing soda instead.

If you have a particularly visible cyst, try to poultice it to the surface. Washing away some of it would be a great help to your body. Read herb books on poultices or just take whatever wild leaves you can gather; make a mush out of them with a blender, mix with honey or homemade skin softener to make it spread like peanut butter and cover the cyst with it night and day, covered with a piece of plastic. The wetness has drawing power. The plant juices have other benefits. If you can't poultice and must rely on kidney excretion, be sure to take kidney herbs at the same time.

Skin Rash

Rashes can be caused by many things. To find the cause, follow a logical pattern. It may be due to:
- HIV
- Yeast and Fungus
- Allergy
- Childhood Diseases (rubella, etc.)

HIV is the most alarming possibility. Eliminate it first by testing for it. It's often too early for a clinical test to be positive for HIV, so use the Syncrometer (page 457). I often see the rash disappear within days of eliminating the virus.

Probably the most common cause of rash is **yeast**. *Candida* has a resonant frequency of 384-388 KHz. If you test positive for it, stop all commercial soap and detergent for all possible uses. Zapping *Candida* may drive it away for a few days. The fungus is hosted by another parasite but finds your skin quite satisfactory for a home, at least while your skin immunity is low. It may be low from wearing metal jewelry, having metal tooth fillings, aluminum (from lotions and soaps), cobalt (from shaving supplies), and zirconium (from deodorant.). When all these are removed, the skin will dry up quickly in open air or under a heat lamp.

In babies' skin, immunity is low from diaper chemicals (mercury and thallium), wipes, and soap and detergent chemicals. Tight fitting, mercury treated diapers are a modern atrocity. Always line them with a tissue and keep them loose fitting.

The skin that has rash or fungus should be dried with paper towels, unfragranced and uncolored, in order not to contaminate the cloth towels, and thereby transport the tiny infectious spores to other skin locations. You may use skin healers.

Only the skin healers given in *Recipes* are safe to use. Keep them refrigerated when not in daily use. Commercial lotions, including health varieties, all contain toxic ingredients.

Many adult rashes are due to **allergies**. Allergy to nickel is common, the reaction is easiest to see under rings or watches. The metal is pulled into the body for elimination. Since nickel is used by so many bacteria, especially urinary tract bacteria, it doesn't get eliminated, it gets taken up by bacteria. It also piles up in

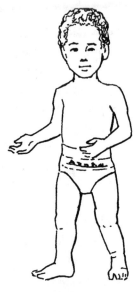

Fig. 29 Tight diapers are a modern atrocity, forcing mercury and thallium into the baby's sponge-like skin.

kidneys, adrenals, bladder and prostate where bacteria thrive on it. Strangely, it also accumulates in the male scalp (and in women's scalps who have male pattern baldness).

Allergy to strawberries, perfume, deodorant or chlorinated water, however different they are, can all be expressed the same way, in a rash. The liver has refused (been unable) to detoxify the chemicals in these items and allows them to circulate in the body. Not for long, though, since great damage could be done to brain and other tissues. Mercifully, the skin grabs these chemicals into itself. Ultimately, it must still be removed. The allergic reaction and your immune system come to your skin's rescue, although bringing you discomfort.

Why didn't the liver detoxify the chemicals given to it? The answer is based on a simple experiment. Try cleaning your liver (page 552) several times or until 1,000 bits of refuse have been washed out of the bile ducts. This relieves the back pressure on that part of the liver, and allows it to do its work again. The physiological details are not understood. Fortunately, the results are instantaneous. The day before the liver cleanse you would never eat a strawberry or peanut for fear of a reaction. A few days after the cleanse, your body "knows" which food it might tolerate and as you try a bit, you notice <u>no reaction, no rash</u> This simple experiment suggests that the liver couldn't detoxify these foods <u>because of the refuse in its ducts.</u>

Each liver cleanse "cures" a different set of allergies suggesting that the liver is compartmentalized—different parts having different duties. It follows that by getting <u>all</u> the stones out <u>all</u> your allergies will disappear. Experience shows this to be true, although it can take two years to carry out such a program.

Meanwhile, avoiding the offensive food or product is very important. It is quite destructive to bathe the brain in strawberry chemicals or your toes in maple syrup chemicals. Stay off allergy-producing foods and products even if you can tolerate a little or can be "desensitized" to them with shots or homeopathic methods. Use these methods for <u>relief,</u> not <u>license</u> to continue using items that tax your body.

Certain **childhood diseases** produce a rash and this can be diagnosed by testing for the suspected disease with a slide or culture of it. Then use a zapper to kill both the bug and any larger parasites that may have brought it in.

Hives

Sometimes your body will break out in hives instead of a rash. Again, gallstones in the liver and gallbladder are responsible. Do the Liver Cleanse.

Acne

The more severe cases of acne cover parts of the body as well as face and can pit the face so badly there is hardly any clear skin left.

In ten days you can reverse this, so most of the skin is beautifully clear. There are bacteria involved and skin oils of youth feed these bacteria. Acne has been extensively studied by scientists. Perhaps the true culprit was too big to be seen with a microscope or too small (antigen) to be recognized or just too unimaginable. I inevitably find *Trichinella*, one of the four common roundworms that infect humans.

Test yourself to *Trichinella* with the slide called "larvae in tissue." Search for it in your skin. It is generally believed to reside in muscles, especially the diaphragm, but in acne cases it is in the skin.

If you only have a frequency generator, set it at 404.5 KHz and at neighboring numbers, extending 5 KHz on each side, to be sure to include all eggs and other molt stages. Or zap.

Psoriasis, Eczema

Psoriasis and eczema are both caused by *Ascaris*. Their molting chemicals are quite allergenic; perhaps it is these that are affecting the skin. Since pets pick these worms up daily, there is chronic reinfection in families with pets. Keep zapping.

Bernadette McNutt, 34, had acne on her back, chest and face. She had been treated since teen age with ultraviolet light, Retin A, and antibiotics. She already had a history of shingles and fungus, two more skin conditions. Her skin was toxic with strontium and her kidneys had cadmium, silver and beryllium deposits inhibiting excretion. She had only one parasite, extremely high levels of *Trichinella*. Her children were also infected as was the cat. In spite of using parasite herbs for months she got no improvement until the baby was out of diapers. Then she cleared up.

Royce Hamilton, 17, had acne so dense on his face there was no good spot the size of a dime anywhere. He had it about one year. His urinalysis showed "amorphous" crystals (stones of all kinds) and a trace of protein. He had *Trichinella* worms throughout his organs. He was very fatigued. He was started on kidney herbs so there would be good excretion after killing the *Trichinella*. His thyroid and kidneys were full of zirconium and titanium from all the lotions he used for his skin. He didn't need deodorant. Evidently even his armpit bacteria had been affected. It took four months to clear his *Trichinella* although there were no young children or pets in the house. His face was beginning to heal, but three months later he had a recurrence, although his parent was not a carrier. After this, he cleared it up again and his face looked as beautiful as a child's.

Evan Knight, 36, had psoriasis at elbows and knees from age 9 but now it was spreading to his fingers and scalp. He occasionally had bronchitis and puffy eyelids, indicative of *Ascaris* but at the time of his visit he had *Trichinella*, fluke stages and *Echinostomum* in his skin. He was started on the parasite program and in three weeks it was clearing instead of advancing. He switched to milk for his beverage to raise his immunity and removed the arsenic, formaldehyde and thulium (from his vitamin C) by doing the necessary cleanups.

Gerry Chastain, 41, had a red nose, erupted along the sides. He had been on sulfa drugs and Emycin.™ He had *Leishmania tropica*. He killed it in the office with a frequency generator and got immediate improvement but four weeks later it was back. He had four solvents built up in his body: benzene, TCE, TC Ethylene and hexanedione. This situation would make recovery impossible since he was no doubt reinfecting himself. He also had titanium, platinum and silver accumulated in his tissues and needed to replace his dentalware before expecting a permanent cure.

Floyd Oldham, 50s, was getting pimples on his nose. His whole face was red and flushed looking. His bowels were loose and he had some urinary urgency. He harbored two kinds of *Leishmania* (*braziliensis* and *tropica*). He killed the *Leishmanias* with a frequency generator and started himself on the kidney herb program. Five weeks later the pimples were gone but general redness had reappeared. The *Leishmanias* were still gone but this time he was toxic with cobalt.

Cobalt is known to promote skin cancers and also heart disease. This was discovered decades ago when an outbreak of heart disease occurred in England. It was traced to a pub (where they all partook) where cobalt was added to the beer to make the foam rise higher! In fact, the foam will just stay in place like a hairdo, if you add cobalt. It was made an illegal additive. Gradually, it has crept back into consumer's products: first toilet cake (blue), then window washer (blue), then dishwasher detergent, and now even mouthwash. If you see a blue colored product, **stay away from it.** It accumulates in the heart and skin. People with skin cancers often have cobalt build up.

Floyd stopped using all these products and cleared up again.

Grethe Driscoll, middle aged, wore tons of make up, so skillfully applied that scars from a face lift could never be detected. When she had minor breakouts, which usually occurred while away on a trip, it seemed like a catastrophe. She tried everything available but could not get to her parasite herbs until she was back home several weeks later. After one week on them (5 day high dose plus maintenance) her complexion was perfect again.

Crofton Thornton, 15, had an embarrassing case of acne. He had *Ascaris*, hookworm and *Strongyloides* (he also had migraines) all reacting in the skin. He stopped drinking commercial beverages that gave him solvents. He killed parasites electronically and with herbs and got a considerable improvement. But he still had *Strongyloides* one month later. Nevertheless, he had seen the connection and he knew it was just a matter of persistence to a clear complexion. Note, he should have had *Trichinella*—did I miss testing for it?

Warts

Could we get warts from playing with toads in childhood? We don't play with toads anymore. Yet we get warts. We don't know how we get them. But after learning how to get rid of them, you will probably know how you got them. Not all warts are the same. In fact, they might all be different: each one is made up of 5 or 6 different viruses, not just one as we had believed.

Peel a tiny fragment off one of your warts. Prepare it for testing by placing it in a small bottle. Add a few tsp. filtered water and a ¼ tsp. grain alcohol. Label it with the location you got it from: like "left middle finger knuckle. " First, search your body for other locations of this wart (organs that test positive to your sample). You can easily find them in your skin, of course. But also search electronically in your liver, spleen, muscles, stomach, heart, pancreas. **Notice how often they are present in the pancreas**. The pancreas seems to be a wart-virus heaven. Are they in the islets or the rest of the pancreas?

Without a zapper, you will need to find the frequency of each virus to completely destroy it. Attach your frequency generator and search between 400 and 290 KHz. When you find its resonant frequency, kill it by treating yourself for three minutes at 10 volts from a frequency generator. Will your warts fall off?

In a few days one or two of your warts will begin to shred. After a week you may lose one or two completely, and find that several more have become smaller. The remainder are unchanged. Continue to identify and kill them. Notice that they are not necessarily gone from the pancreas or other organs at the same time as they are gone from the skin. Perhaps warts are not the benign entities we have believed them to be. They may, in fact, ride into the body on some common bacteria, like *Salmonella*, or common parasite like pinworms or tapeworm stages.

Zapping doesn't reach all the viruses in a wart either. It takes repeated zappings to start the shredding and gradual killing of warts.

Guy Laird, age 11, had warts on his lips besides fingers. His job was feeding the three outdoor dogs. He was full of *Ascaris*. He had *Taenia pisiformis* and *Taenia solium* bladder cysts in his liver. These were shedding viruses into Guy. He was started on Rascal for six weeks (this was before the zapper was invented). Maybe his benzene buildup was responsible for letting so many parasites (and their viruses) survive and multiply in his body. He stopped using toothpaste, killed *Ascaris* (408 KHz) and some flukes (434 to 421 KHz) and improved his diet. All except one wart came off (without bleeding). He was given different chores, too, to reduce his contact with animals and their parasites.

Georgianna Mills, a middle age music teacher, broke out with warts all over her hands, at least 30 in total. A few months later she was diagnosed with bone cancer; she always wondered if there was a connection. She cleared up her cancer and killed her viruses and bacteria with a frequency generator. Nearly all her warts disappeared. But her indoor pet brought new parasites daily, especially *Moniezia* tapeworm stages. With each *Moniezia* infection (about once a month) she got new warts. She was never able to clear them completely.

I concluded that each wart is actually composed of 3 to 6 viruses and these viruses are distributed throughout our bodies! How satisfying to be able to rid our bodies of them, once and for all even in internal organs. There is a catch. Small remnants of some warts do not disappear in spite of killing most of them. More accurately, they disappear and then reappear in our internal organs. Could this suggest to us their true origin? Could it be a tapeworm stage?

Tapeworm Stages

Our bodies harbor numerous stages of tapeworms. But not the tapeworm itself, which may belong to a dog, cow, or pigeon. Tapeworms lead complicated lives, much like insects with their caterpillars, larvae, larval molts, pupae and eventual adults. Tapeworms shed eggs with the bowel movement of the animal host. The eggs blow in the dust and reside in the earth. A vegetarian animal nibbling vegetation near this filth, or licking dirt and dust off its coat, swallows the eggs. Humans, too, eat plenty of filth by licking their fingers. As children we all eat dirt simply by eating with unwashed hands.

The Jewish society discovered the great importance of washing hands before eating, thousands of years ago. But many of us choose to ignore truths that seem old fashioned. In our own relatively short life times we cannot see the whole picture as well as the prophets and seers of ancient cultures could. We eat plenty of dirt and along with it, the eggs of tapeworms. Dog and cat tapeworms are most prevalent, but sheep, cow, pig, and seagull tapeworms are also common.

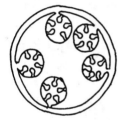

There is hardly a predator species in existence that doesn't have its own characteristic tapeworm. Whatever animal species you live near, or once lived near, you probably swallowed some of its filth and some tape eggs. The **eggs** hatch in your stomach and the tiny **larvae** burrow into a neighboring organ without any consideration that this is your stomach wall or spleen or muscle. The larva's plan is not to grow into a long worm—that can wait. The larva must simply

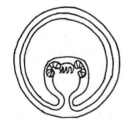

Fig. 30 Some cysticercus varieties (types) have multiple heads.

survive until you can be conveniently eaten! A wolf or a tiger will surely come along! In bygone days it did.

The larva is about ¼ inch long, surrounded by a "sac of waters," like a tiny water balloon. Looking very closely at this sac, called a **cysticercus**, we see a head (scolex), complete with hooks and suckers, turned inside out, inside a bladder.

As the tiger's teeth bite down on the cysticercus, the pressure pops it out. The head is now right side out with hooks and suckers ready for action. Now it grows in the tiger!

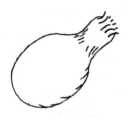

It quickly hooks into a loop of intestinal wall so it can't be swept away and begins its growth into a regular long **adult** tapeworm. The tiger is the true or **primary host**. We were merely the sec-

Fig. 31 Emerged cysticercus.

ondary or **intermediate host**. Why does the adult tapeworm prefer the tiger instead of us? Only Mother Nature knows. But the best way to get to a carnivore is through its prey.

You can find these larval cysts in your organs using slides of the *cysticercus* stage of various common tapeworms. Search in your muscles, liver, stomach, pancreas, spleen, intestine and even brain. **You will not find even little bits of them in your white blood cells.** My explanation for this curious finding is that the tapeworm leaves no debris to be cleaned up by your white blood cells. Evidently your body builds a cyst wall around the larva to tightly encase it and <u>prevent</u> toxins and debris from entering your body. Thus your white blood cells are not alerted in any way. Of course, the larva is much too big to be devoured by tiny white blood cells anyway. Yet, it seems that if a pack of white blood cells had attacked the larva just as soon as it hatched from the egg they would have been able to devour it. Perhaps it enlarges too rapidly. Perhaps our white blood cells are preoccupied. In any case, we begin to load up on tapeworm stages from infancy and by the time we are middle aged we have dozens tucked away in our organs.

Some do die in the course of time. Perhaps their true secondary host is a rabbit or a mouse instead of a human. The short life span of these other hosts might mean that the life span of the *cysticercus* is also quite short, not 40 years! When they die, the white blood cells do clean them up and we can see them in our white blood cells at this time. It can take several weeks for the *cysticercus* to be completely gone by this natural method. During this time, we become ill! Numerous bacteria and viruses spring up, as if from nowhere, in our organs.

Don't be surprised if you are testing yourself during illness to find a tapeworm or two in your white blood cells! It is well worth searching for at such a time. Help your body dispatch the tapeworm stages all together with your zapper. A frequency generator is bound to miss some. Some cysticercus varieties consist of many heads, and each head has even more heads inside it! These might have different resonant frequencies. Only killing them together has the desired effect. Remember bacteria and viruses are released by killing tapeworms, so always follow with a second zapping in 20 minutes, and a third zapping 20 minutes after that. Only then can your tapeworm-related illness disappear.

If you do nothing, your body will be kept busy killing bacteria and viruses as the tape cysticercus wears down and eventually dies. You may not wish to identify all of them (but at least search for *Adenovirus*, the common cold) and just note where you are being attacked: your nose, throat, ears, lungs, bronchi. Internal organs are attacked too. It seldom takes more than three weeks, though, for your body to clean up a tape stage even without any help from a zapper. The attendant illness will be gone by then, too.

Watching these events in your body gives you insight into the very powerful forces at work, called immunity or body defense. The body "knows" a great deal more than we have surmised. There is yet so much to discover.

What initiated the death or dying process of the tapeworm stage in the first place? Has your body been trying all along and finally succeeded? Has the *cysticercus* reached the end of its life span naturally? Have its (the tapeworm's) own viruses and bacteria gotten the upper hand and killed it? Did it accidentally absorb something that killed it?

By taking a herbal combination, Rascal, you can soon find a tapeworm stage in your white blood cells where you could not find it earlier. It is now dead or dying. This proves the effectiveness of Rascal, even though it is slow.

Since we all eat dirt and inhale dust that is laden with dog feces or other animal excrement, we all harbor tapeworm stages, although none may be present in our white blood cells. **Are they harming us?** Perhaps they are living out their lives as quietly as they can in our organs, the way mice or ants try to live in our dwellings. Yet, when tapeworm stages are being killed, either spontaneously by your body or with a zapping device, we see an assortment of bacteria and viruses spread through the body, including the common cold.

Getting rid of the tapeworm stages in your organs seems a very worthwhile goal. Since each of us has been associated with dozens of animal species in our past, we probably have dozens of varieties of tapeworm stages in us. I cannot identify more than a handful due to lack of prepared slides. You can find them without identifying first, though, by listening to their emission frequencies. Their emissions are often extremely weak, possibly due to being encased in a cyst. Search between 510 KHz and 410 KHz. You may wish to "track" them for a while before killing them. You may wish to search for identical frequencies in your pet's saliva. Or you may wish to dispatch them as rapidly as possible. Use the zapper, not a frequency generator. Remember to "mop up" after your tapeworm killing by zapping again to kill bacteria and viruses that have been released from the tapeworm.

You may be disappointed not to feel any different after ridding yourself of numerous tapeworms and their pathogens. Evidently, the tapeworm stage itself doesn't make you sick; it is simply there like a wart is there, without making you sick. Its viruses <u>can</u> make you sick. Depending on which virus it is, it can make you very sick or not sick at all. Different viruses invade different organs. And some of these turn into warts!

The Flu

Influenza is a virus that can cause "the flu." Does it belong to us as humans or to a larger parasite we are hosting? It is easily transmitted from person to person and in less than a year can spread across the planet. Some flu examples are Influenza A, B, C and Swine flu.

However, much that is called "flu" is actually caused by a bacterium, either *Salmonella* or *Shigella*. If someone in your family is "catching" a flu, test their saliva for the presence of dairy products, implicating the *Salmonellas* and *Shigellas*. Also test for influenza A, B, and C. Children's "flus", especially when there is a fever, are usually due to *Salmonellas*. Even after zapping it can take an hour for the symptoms and fever to go away.

Go straight to the refrigerator and throw away all dairy products. Throw away all milk, cheesecakes, buttermilk, cream, butter, yogurt and cottage cheese, deli food and leftovers. You may wish to identify the food source of your family's bacteria first, and save the uncontaminated food. Use the sick person as a subject, searching for foods that appear in her white blood cells (or search their saliva sample for the food offender). If the flu is "going around" your neighborhood, you might wish to tell

201

some of your neighbors which foods you found were contaminated. They may have purchased the same food! Obviously, when a contaminated shipment of dairy products arrives in your grocery stores, quite a few people will be consuming it, setting the stage for a "bad flu" that "goes around".

Why can some people eat contaminated food without getting sick? Maybe their *Salmonellas* don't multiply rapidly. Maybe their stomach acid is strong enough to kill most of them. Maybe their bowel movements are frequent enough to expel them quickly. Maybe they haven't been on frequent treatments with anti-strep antibiotics. The answer is not known yet. After a serious bout with *Salmonellas* or *Shigellas* the body does not completely clear itself of them. They stay in hiding somewhere. When a new batch of bacteria arrives, even though very sparse, as in 1 tbs. of milk, the two subtypes can hybridize and produce a much more vigorous offspring. This is called *virulence*. You are made much sicker by more virulent subtypes of bacteria. You may have diarrhea, vomiting, illness. Especially if you believe you have "lactose intolerance," pay attention to *Salmonella* and *Shigella*.

If your flu is due to an influenza virus, kill it with your zapper. Some family members may prefer to take a homeopathic flu "remedy" such as Oscillococcinum™ or Flusolution.™ Others may take herbs. These probably act by prying the viruses out of your cells' gateways and channels so the white blood cells can easily devour them.

But flu due to *Salmonella* is not easily zapped away. Remember, the zapper current does not penetrate the bowel contents, which is exactly where *Salmonella* lives! Besides zapping to clear them from your tissues, you must eliminate them from the bowel by using the Bowel Program (page 546).

Lugol's iodine solution (see Recipes) can quite quickly get rid of Salmonella throughout the body. Use 6 drops (small drops from an eyedropper) in ½ glass of water four times a day. If no more *Salmonella* is consumed, it will be vanquished in a day or two.

If your flu brings you a fever, use Lugol's.

Fever

Fevers are there to help your body fight the invaders...up to a point. Don't use a fever medication unless the body temperature goes over 102°F, and then only enough to bring the fever down a bit.

Most fevers, especially **"fevers of unknown origin"** are due to *Salmonellas* and *Shigellas*. Your body may be young and strong enough to kill them but not strong enough to kill an everlasting supply of them coming from dairy foods you eat on a daily basis. Stop eating salads at restaurants immediately. Stop eating food made by others' hands unless it is sterilized. Stop eating dairy foods until you have cooked them. Stop eating those that can't be cooked.

Sam Ellis, age 7, had two episodes of severe abdominal pain with fever lasting two weeks. He got hyperactive with milk products, had a frequent cough and stuffy nose. (Here the picture is quite clear. The milk products were bringing him *Salmonellas*, *Shigellas* and other bacteria which grew in his intestine to produce pain. But why only Sam and not his brothers?) Sam had a buildup of benzene from using bathroom soap containing a special herbal oil. Sam also had hookworms, intestinal fluke, and rabbit fluke, probably due to his lowered immunity from the benzene. Then his mother boiled Sam's milk, removed the polluted soap (she planned to use it herself!) and killed his parasites with the parasite herbs. His fever went away and stayed away. He said he enjoyed all this because now he "could play after school" without a stomach ache and he wasn't being sent to the nurse's office because of a fever. Notice the bacteria causing the temperature went away by themselves, probably due to the return of his normally strong immune system.

203

Jalene McCormick, 46, had been passing lots of kidney stones (hundreds) for years and had a temperature most of the time for which she was on antibiotics. It took her six months on our kidney herb recipe to dissolve and pass so many they no longer showed up on X-ray, and to stop making them. Then her fever left, not to return.

Kristen Jane Johnson, a young mother, had recurrent fevers and fatigue but, besides EBV, her doctors found no cause. We found HIV virus and a lot of bacteria and parasites. The fever-causing bacterium was *Salmonella*. To stop her *Salmonella* attacks she had to raise her immunity besides boiling all dairy products. Moldy foods (pasta) and lunch meats (benzopyrenes) were the source of liver toxicity. Each new *Salmonella* attack immediately invaded the liver so a vicious cycle was set up. When she stayed meticulously on the parasite program, meticulously off unsterilized dairy products, and meticulously off benzene-polluted items, she cured herself of fevers and night sweats and the HIV infection. Perhaps in two years the liver will have recovered enough to kill *Salmonella* that enter it, but she is not taking any chances till then.

Although Kristen was eating food polluted with both *Salmonellas* and *Shigellas* she only "picked up" *Salmonella*, never *Shigella*! Why is that? In contrast, people with multiple sclerosis "pick up" *Shigellas*, not *Salmonellas*.

Multiple Sclerosis & Amyotropic Lateral Sclerosis

Multiple sclerosis (MS) is a disease of the brain and spinal cord. It is called *lateral sclerosis* if the disease is mainly in the spinal cord.

It is caused by fluke parasites reaching the brain or spinal cord and attempting to multiply there. Any of the four common flukes may be responsible. Kill them immediately with your zapper or a frequency generator (434 KHz to 421 KHz). They cannot return unless you reinfect yourself. Stop eating meats, except fish and seafood. All meats are a source of fluke parasite stages unless canned or very well cooked. Pets and family members are undoubtedly carriers of the same flukes, although they do not show the same symptoms. Give away your house pets. Don't kiss your loved ones on the mouth. Make sure your sex partner has also been freed of fluke parasites.

The most important question you must be able to answer is why did these parasites enter your brain and spinal cord? When the brain contains solvents, it allows flukes to multiply there. The solvents, **xylene** and **toluene** are common brain solvents always seen in MS cases. Evidently these solvents accumulate first in the motor and sensory regions of the brain, inviting the parasites to these locations.

Xylene and toluene are industrial solvents used in paint and thinners. It is also a pollutant of certain carbonated beverages (I found it in 7-Up,™ ginger ale and others that I tested). Stop drinking them.

All MS cases I have seen also harbor *Shigella* bacteria in the brain and spinal cord. These come from dairy products. They are manure bacteria. Be absolutely meticulous about sterilizing dairy products. Even one tsp. unsterilized milk added to scrambled eggs could reinfect you. Not even heavy whipping cream or butter is safe without boiling. Kill bacteria every day with a zapper. *Shigellas* produce chemicals that are toxic to the brain and spinal cord. Eliminating *Shigellas* brings immediate improvement.

All large parasites like flukes have their own entourage of bacteria and viruses. Perhaps it is these that initiate the brain's reaction, which is inflammation and scar tissue formation in the outer covering of brain cells and nerve fibers. Perhaps it is the fluke stages themselves. Your brain is trying desperately to heal these lesions, only to be assailed by a fresh batch of solvent and *Shigellas* and another generation of parasites and pathogens.

The other pollutant associated with MS is **mercury** from dental metal. The mercury that is constantly released in the mouth does not all get excreted by the kidneys or eliminated by the bowels. Some of it travels up to the brain and gets into the spinal cord as well. You will be able to eliminate and excrete more mercury by doing a kidney and liver cleanse. The mercury may itself be polluted with **thallium** which is even more toxic. For this reason mercury removal should be done extra thoroughly to be sure no thallium has been left behind.

If you are concerned about MS-like symptoms, purchase slides of the brain regions, cerebrum, and cerebellum. Or purchase pork brains at the grocery store and snip out a portion of the sensory lobe and cerebellum. Prepare these as test substances (sterilize your hands afterward). Test your daily foods and body products for their presence in these brain areas. Also test for parasites, bacteria (especially *Nocardia* and *Shigella*) and other pollutants such as arsenic and pesticides. If the disease (tremor and lack of sensation) has not progressed too far, you can cure it. In all cases you can stop it from progressing further by cleaning up dentalware, the environment and diet.

Brandi Rainey, age 34, of Amish religious culture, was diagnosed with MS four months earlier after an MRI confirmed it although she had symptoms for many years. She was told she had inherited a gene for it and that Amish folk are particularly susceptible to MS for reasons of inbreeding. She had a constant pain running down the side of her neck, and headache. Her legs were getting too heavy to get up stairs. Our tests showed her brain was full of scandium (tooth metal alloy) and fluoride (toothpaste). Her vision was getting worse; her eyes were full of wood alcohol. She lost no time in getting dentures: there were no teeth that could be saved. She had several bacteria growing in her jaw bone: *Strep G* (sore throat bacteria), *Staphylococcus aureus* (this was raising her pulse to over 100), *Clostridium tetani* (causes great stiffness), and *Shigella* (produces nerve toxins). She killed these with a frequency generator. Five weeks later the pain and stiffness in her neck were gone, her pulse was down to 100, her periods were free of pain and her hands seemed to shake less. She was put on the parasite program plus thioctic acid (2 a day) and histidine (500 mg, one a day to keep nickel levels down)and advised to cook and eat with non metal. Four weeks later her pulse was down to 80, her legs were much better. She zapped four remaining bacteria. Two months later the numbness and tremor had left; her legs still felt tired and her hands sometimes shook but she was quite reassured that MS would not claim her life. Nor had a gene betrayed her. A half year later she was walking and working normally, doing liver cleanses and keeping up her vigilance against parasites and pollutants.

Kendra Welch, 56, was diagnosed with MS a year ago, by MRI. She went to a chelating doctor and this cleared up her temporary ischemic attacks (T.I.A's) which were occurring daily. But she had lost her balance, eyesight was getting worse, her feet and hands stung. Her sister also had MS but nobody else in the family did which baffled her doctor. Her brain tissue was full of barium, europium, gadolinium, and platinum. These are dental alloys, although barium could come from bus exhaust (she wore no lipstick). She was advised to have all metal removed from her mouth immediately. Two days afterward she came into the office without any neurological symptoms. She stated she was afraid to stop her new health program, though, and this was good policy.

Lynne Ceretto, age 15, was diagnosed with an "MS-like syndrome" by MRI. She had intestinal flukes and stages, human liver flukes and *Trichinella* in the brain. She had no tooth fillings. But there was benzene in her thymus keeping her immunity low. She also had propane and asbestos in her brain from leaky pipes and a worn washing machine belt. She, too, was told she had a "bad" gene. She was barely able to walk with help. It took several months to track down the source of benzene—the drinking water. Sometimes it was polluted; sometimes it was not! When the pump was oiled, some of it dripped onto the cement platform. Rain washed it to the center and down the pipe in the well. They eagerly removed the platform, found the oil on the water surface, cleaned everything up carefully, until no benzene could be found which put her on the road to recovery. A year later she had recovered further.

Norma Luellen, a young mother, had tingling, numbness and weakness on the entire left side of her body. She was in process of clinical tests for MS. Her body was full of pentane, possibly from her workplace since 12 other persons working there also had MS (such a situation should make our government eager to jump at investigations)! She had intestinal flukes and their stages, not in the intestine or liver or thymus, but in her brain! We found her home air toxic with bismuth too, probably from cosmetics. In spite of staying on the parasite program she got reinfected with sheep liver fluke, probably from eating hamburgers. She was not able to stop her carbonated beverage habit and frequently showed xylene, acetone, methylene chloride in addition to pentane in her white blood cells.

Shannon Synder, age 44, had been getting more numb over her whole body for several years and was presently considered by her doctor to have MS. Her muscles twitched all night, making sleep impossible, and her hands shook. She had intestinal flukes in the brain (cerebrum and cerebellum) but none in the intestine ! The brain also had wood alcohol from drinking Diet Coke.™ She also had bismuth (cosmetics), palladium, copper, samarium, and tellurium (tooth alloys) in her brain. She began to improve enough to be off Prednisone by her 10th day of the parasite program.

Erica Blake, age 41, was diagnosed with MS two years earlier although her symptoms went back 13 years. She was on Prednisone™ but her balance was getting so bad she had to be in a wheelchair. Chelation treatments kept her from deteriorating further. Her brain was full of gasoline; she used to work at a gas station and now was getting it from the attached garage. Her hands and feet were completely numb. She had 5 root canals extracted and a few days later was able to stand. She could now walk with a cane. She had human liver flukes, sheep liver fluke and Trichinellas and dog tapeworm stages in her cerebellum (motor control center). After killing parasites and starting to take thioctic acid (4 a day) and cleaning up her environment she improved enough to drive a car again, walk without a cane in her home. She regained enough feeling in her hands and legs to do her housework, too.

Kurt Nielsen, age 43, was told he had peripheral neuropathy. His feet were so numb he had to look at the clutch to drive. Also both hands were numb. He was full of kerosene and benzene possibly from fuel oil that he pumped for a living. There were fluke stages in his brain and a dozen bacteria and viruses. He also had mercury and thallium in his immune system which came from tooth fillings. However, he had all his metal fillings replaced two years earlier! He thought there was no mercury left in his mouth! Actually, he had little bits (called tattoos) left somewhere. And they were giving him the classical symptoms: numbness of hands and feet and gradual destruction of his nervous system. His peripheral neuropathy was due to thallium poisoning. The dentist couldn't find tattoos, and he was left in his predicament. (This was before I found mercury and thallium sources in many personal products.)

Duncan Wood, a middle age father of 5 young children, could still slowly shuffle along when he arrived. He could not raise his arms to eat. He had uncontrolled inappropriate laughter every minute. He was diagnosed with MS two years earlier and told he had a "bad" gene. The fact that one child was beginning to show similar symptoms strengthened their belief in the gene theory. Ten days later his inappropriate laughter stopped; he could get his right hand to his face, he walked twice as fast and had very little tremor remaining. Strong chelating treatments obtained at a Mexican clinic had drawn much of the mercury and thallium out of his brain. He killed the flukes and *Shigella* bacteria electronically and stopped consuming unboiled milk. The brain solvents, xylene and toluene were removed quickly, too, as well as asbestos. His fast improvement showed them how important it was to remove the source of these pollutants in his home.

Two days later he regressed considerably which made him feel quite depressed, since his chelating treatments had not stopped. Was there still an unknown factor? It was a return of *Shigella* bacteria! He had inadvertently eaten a non-sterile dairy food: milk added to soup when it was already done cooking! This was a valuable lesson. Nothing else had returned. He was away from the asbestos and xylene from the workshop at home. He zapped the bacteria again and applied greater vigilance to eating only sterilized dairy foods. He recouped his losses in one day.

Then they scheduled their dental work, which had already been done once two years ago! He had leftover mercury and thallium. Now, selecting a dentist with experience in finding tattoos and cleaning cavitations made much more sense to him than it had before. He also planned to do a kidney and liver cleanse after re-

209

turning home. And to stay out of the workshop until the asbestos-containing belt had been replaced and the furniture painting had been moved to a different building.

Shigella also causes irritability and depression, a frequent problem for MS cases.

High Blood Pressure

High blood pressure is one of the easiest problems to correct without resorting to drugs.

The most important change to make is to stop using caffeine as in coffee, tea, or carbonated beverages. Don't use decaffeinated coffee or tea either because of the solvent pollution in them. Switch to hot milk or hot water if a hot beverage is desired, or any of the beverages given in the recipe section. If being without caffeine leaves you fatigued, take an arginine tablet in the morning (500 mg).

Blood pressure is mainly controlled by the adrenal glands which sit like little caps on top of the kidneys. Whatever is affecting the kidneys is probably affecting the adrenals, too, since they're so close to each other. You must find out what it is.

You could do your search in the kidneys since kidney tissue is available in grocery stores. Adrenal tissue is available on microscope slides. What will you find? Probably **cadmium**.

Search for the cadmium source in your drinking water! Cadmium comes from the metal pipes. In fact, you could scrape a galvanized pipe to get a cadmium test substance. Conducting or storing drinking water in containers of metal is as foolish a practice as eating food off the floor. Water picks up everything it touches <u>simply because it is wet</u>! You may not <u>see</u> what it picked up any more than you can <u>see</u> if it has picked up sugar or salt. The cadmium and other metal is <u>dissolved</u> in the water. The older the pipes the softer, more corroded they are, and the more metal is picked up as the water rushes by. If you find cadmium in your hot or cold water, you will <u>never</u> be able to filter it out. Nor should you switch to bottled water. The amount of cadmium in your clothing from doing laundry with this water is already too much for your adrenals and kidneys.

Change your galvanized pipes to PVC plastic. If you believe you already have plastic pipes or all copper (which leads to leukemia, schizophrenia and fertility problems) you will need to search every inch of plumbing for a very short piece of galvanized pipe left in the system! A piece as short as a 2 inch T or Y can be causing all the trouble.

The toxicity of cadmium, in fact, the high blood pressure connection, has been known a long time. After finding the cadmium start on the kidney cleanse. You might miss the cadmium problem if you don't attend to it first. Also remove all metal from your mouth.

All (100%) cases of high blood pressure I have seen could be easily cured by eliminating cadmium and other pollutants, followed by cleansing the kidneys.

To test whether you still need your blood pressure medicine, wait until your pressure is down to 140/90 or better. Then cut the dose in half. Check it again next day. If it has climbed back up you are not ready; go back to ¾ or a full dose of medicine. Try again a few days later. If your blood pressure stays down, cut your medicine in half again (you are now down to ¼ the regular dose) and see if your blood pressure stays improved.

When you are down to 130/80 go off completely. But stay on the kidney herb recipe. At 120/80 try yourself on a few shakes of sea salt. The amount of salt eaten, once the pressure is down, has little influence. In fact increasing salt intake <u>improves</u> energy without raising blood pressure. Take no more than one teaspoon a day (2,000 mg sodium), total, including cooking. Better yet, make a salt that is a mixture of sodium and potassium chlorides (see *Sources*). Mix it for yourself in a 1 to 1 ratio or whatever your taste can accept. The sodium portion could be sterilized sea salt (test and make sure it has no aluminum silicate in it first).

Mold toxins have specific kidney effects! Especially **T-2 toxin**, found mostly in dried peas, beans and lentils. Rinse these thoroughly first, throw away shriveled ones, and add vitamin C to the cooking water. All cases of serious kidney disease show a build up of T-2 toxin. Be extra careful to avoid moldy food (read Moldy Food, page 381).

Bala Cuzmin, age 72, had high blood pressure for ten years but the upper (systolic) pressure remained high in spite of various medicines that were tried. She had three kinds of kidney stones and only one functional kidney. She stopped using caffeine, switching to arginine tablets to get over the let-down. Her diet was changed to reduce phosphate and add calcium, and she took magnesium and Vitamin B_6 to assist the kidneys. She was very anemic and her mean cell volume (MCV) was high due to *Ascaris* infestation. She killed parasites, cleansed kidneys but saw no drop in blood pressure which stayed at 150 to 170 systolic. Her adrenal glands were choked with copper and platinum. She had all the metal in her mouth replaced and promptly saw a blood pressure drop to 145-150. Three months later it was at 128 to 133 on half her medicine. She had not been tested for T-2 toxin yet, nor changed her copper water pipes.

Sabrina Patton, 66, had a long list of health problems, including high blood pressure for six years. She was on Corgard™ and diazide drugs which kept it down to 140-160/74-80. She had phosphate crystals in her kidneys and was started on kidney herbs and a diet change to include milk and exclude soda pop. She had high levels of mercury and copper in her immune system. She was feeling so much better after the kidney cleanse that she decided to remove her last fillings and replace her bridge, too, since it was shedding ruthenium. On her way home from the dentist, her ears stopped ringing and soon her blood pressure was down to 126/68. She was still on half a dose of drugs because she was too afraid to go off entirely. But when her pressure stayed down she found the courage to go off completely. This gave her the energy she wanted to play basketball with the grandchildren again.

Rolf Ehrhart, 61, had 80% blockage of heart arteries and high blood pressure for which he was on a Hydropres™ patch, Tenormin™, and Logol™ (diuretic). He had phosphate and uric acid crystals in his kidneys. He was started on kidney herbs followed by the parasite herbs. His *Ascaris* and flukes were zapped. He stopped using store-bought beverages. Then he could cut back on his medicines, measuring his blood pressure daily to guide him. After seven weeks it was down to 140/85, so he decided to do without medicine, a bit early. He was also getting chelation therapy and was now able to walk 2-4 miles a day. His next chore, which he approached gladly, was removal of all metal from his mouth.

Len Gerald, 45, was on Vasotec™ for high blood pressure. He was constantly sleepy; his blood test showed a low thyroid level in spite of being on Euthyroid.™ He was started on kidney herbs followed by parasite herbs. In two weeks, barely into his program, his blood pressure dropped. He had to go off his blood pressure medicine. It stayed at 126/80. He still had some *Ascaris* and other health problems but was highly motivated to clean them up, too.

Glaucoma

In glaucoma the pressure in the eyeball gets too high, putting pressure on fragile retina cells that do your seeing. The first question to ask is: "Is my blood pressure too high?," because there is a link between high blood pressure and elevated eyeball pressure.

Your blood pressure should be 120/80. Your doctor may say 140/85 is "not high." He or she is kindly refraining from giving you drugs until this level of pressure is reached. It is your tip-off, though, that something is not right and you should correct it now, when it is easy, and before other damage is done. Read the section on high blood pressure (page 210) to learn how to reduce it by going off caffeine, checking for cadmium poisoning from your water pipes, and cleansing the kidneys (page 549). Even though your doctor has explained how the tiny tube draining your eyeball is too narrow, you should ask: was it not too narrow <u>before</u> high blood pressure struck? Simply getting your blood pressure to normal is sufficient help for beginning glaucoma.

Antonia Guerrero, age 51, had glaucoma for five years and was deteriorating rapidly. She cleansed her kidneys, killed parasites and changed her diet to the anti-arthritic one since she also suffered from arthritis in her hands for ten years with painful enlarged knuckles. She didn't get relief from taking aspirin. She got rid of her asbestos toxins by bringing her own hair blower with her to the hairdresser. After seven months she had pain relief for her arthritis (without aspirin) and her glaucoma was pronounced stable by her ophthalmologist.

Tooth Decay

The strongest part of our body structure is our bones. The strongest bones are our teeth. How can they decay? We must look at the **enamel**, **dentine** and **root** of the tooth as well as the bone they rest in for some answers.

Scientists have already searched very hard and long for answers. But their work is hampered by commercial interests that try to shape the results. Since commerce determines which research can be done (that is, paid for) sacred territory can be ignored. For example, the effects of sugar-eating, gum-chewing, tooth brushing, fluoridation, tooth filling materials and diet can be ignored if it interferes with product sales. Trivial studies such as comparing shapes of toothbrushes, studying the chemical composition of plaque, and studies of bacterial structure and genes are done instead. Studies "at the molecular level" do not threaten existing industries.

Important research has lapsed since the 40's and 50's. Perspective on tooth health was sound and clear in the mind of Dr. Weston Price in the 1930's. His scientific studies stand as a beacon even today because truths, once found, do not change. He traveled the world over in search of good teeth. Anywhere and anytime he found them, he described the people who had them. This is excellent science. It lets you draw the conclusions. He described what he saw in a book, titled Nutrition and Physical Degeneration.[13] They came to these conclusions from the following observable facts:

1. Skulls of primitive peoples who lived along coastlines, such as Peruvians, Scandinavians and various islanders, and whose staple foods included fish daily, showed perfect teeth; not a single cavity in a lifetime. They had strong bones that didn't break even once in a lifetime of 45 years. Skeletal structure was fully developed, meaning the jaw bone was not undershot or cheek bones squeezed together, forcing the teeth to grow into a smaller than ideal space. Consequently, there was room for the wisdom teeth, and no need to crowd the remainder. They saw no crooked teeth or unerupted wisdom teeth. The authors estimated a daily consumption of **4 to 5 grams of calcium** in their fish containing diet.

Our daily consumption of less than 1 gram calcium daily is small by comparison. Our wisdom teeth erupt poorly, our other teeth are often crooked. But today bad teeth go shamefully unheeded because we don't need to chew our food, we can lap it (ice cream) or suck it, or gum it (applesauce).

2. These primitive peoples got all the calcium, magnesium, phosphate, boron and other bone builders they needed simply from eating (fish) bones. Mexican peoples got 4 to 6 grams of calcium a day from **stone-grinding** of corn for their staple, tortillas, instead of from fish.

---

[13]It is still available from the Price-Pottenger Nutrition Foundation, a non-profit organization that seeks to keep his observations alive. Their address is PO Box 2614, La Mesa, California 91943, (800) 366-3748.

Where do we get our calcium? Milk is our only supply. One quart supplies one gram. There is little excuse for a carnivorous society like ours to regularly throw away the bones of its food animals in view of our dire shortage. It leaves us dependent on milk alone. Milk has so many disadvantages. It is impossible to milk a cow by machine and not get a few manure bacteria, *Salmonellas* and *Shigellas*, into the milk. These bacteria are not completely killed by pasteurization the way more susceptible bacteria are. It takes boiling temperature to kill all of them. Why isn't milk sterilized? Water was sterilized for human consumption in distant decades. Chlorination of water is not ideal but it did sterilize the water. Milk could be sterilized by boiling or flash-heating.

Milk has other disadvantages: dozens of antibiotics, both by feed and by shot, bovine growth hormone, chemicals added in milk processing, the bad effects of homogenization, and allergy to milk. Yet, in a choice between milk drinking and bone loss, one must choose the milk. This would not be necessary if bones were properly salvaged–ground to powder and added back to the meat where it belongs–to offset the acidifying effect of the phosphate in meat. One gram of calcium is not much bone (½ tsp.) but it requires a whole quart of milk. Bone powder added back to ground meat, soups, stews could greatly improve our tooth decay problem, bone density problem, and skeletal growth problems.

Softened teeth set the stage for decay; bacteria do the dirty work.

Zapping bacteria does not kill them all. The zapper current does not reach into abscesses under metal filled teeth or around root canals. *Staphylococcus aureus*, which we are constantly stuffing in our mouths as we lick our fingers, finds an immediate hiding place in a crevice where it can't be zapped. Many other bacteria hide here, too: those that cause ear ache, sore throats, bronchitis, stiff knees, joint disease. You can try zapping all the *Clostridia*, *Streps* and tooth decay or plaque bacteria. But the only way to successfully eliminate them is to pry them out of hiding and wash them away. This is a job for the dentist (see Dental Cleanup page 409).

Strep. mutans is considered to be the bacterium that causes tooth cavities. I have found it in milk, evidently another pasteurization escapee. All the more reason to sterilize dairy products.

Frannie LaSalle, 52, was getting compression fractures in her spine, but the weak bone condition was evident in her mouth (many teeth were loose—they could be jiggled!). Her gums were red and inflamed. A low thyroid condition (she needed 2½ grains a day of thyroid—in one day the normal body goes through 5 grains of thyroid products) contributed to this. Her blood phosphate level was high (4.7 mg/DL—should be below 4.0) and her alkaline phosphatase was 205, also high, showing she was dissolving her bones (including tooth sockets) at a rapid pace. Her whole system was too acid, as could be seen in elevated CO_2 levels (28, when 23-30 is normal).

Only the major minerals, sodium, potassium, calcium and magnesium can have an impact on this major disturbance. The dentist said she had to have all her teeth pulled and replaced with dentures. Her kidneys showed all three types of calcium phosphate crystals. She drank no milk. She had only three weeks before her oral surgery appointment. She was started on ½ cup 2% milk, 6 times a day plus 50,000 units of vitamin D (a prescription dose) to make sure she absorbed all the calcium. She also took magnesium oxide (300 mg. once a day) and vitamin B_6 500 mg (one a day).

She was started on the kidney cleanse to help activate the vitamin D and to help the adrenal glands make *estrogen*. Her estrogen level (5.2 pg/ml) was too low to get the calcium deposited back into her bones. She was also given licorice herb for their estrogen-like action to help with this and vitamin C, 1 gram (1,000 mg) 2 to 3 a day.

Her mouth care was to be as follows: potassium iodide (white iodine, made up by dissolving 88 gm potassium iodide in one liter/quart water). Purchase a new very soft toothbrush. Use no toothpaste or store bought floss. Use 2 lb. or 4 lb. (the 4 lb. is coarser) fish line (rinse first). Brush twice a day; floss only once at bedtime before brushing. Use 6 drops of food grade hydrogen peroxide for daytime brushing. Use 6 drops of potassium iodide for nighttime brushing. Use no mouthwash, chewing gum, candy. In three weeks her teeth could not be jiggled. Her dentist was astonished (but was not interested in how she achieved this). In six weeks her mouth looked normal and she could chew some foods. Her vitamin D was tapered as follows: Take 6 a week for the first week (miss one day). Take 5 a week for the second week (miss two days). Take 4 a week for the third week. Then 2 a week indefinitely. She never lost a tooth.

Muscle Diseases

There are a variety of muscle wasting diseases, thought to be genetic in their cause. Yet, what could be more easily inherited than a parasite? Persons living together share food, living habits, refrigerators, and parasites. Their shared genes indeed give them similar susceptibilities but if we take muscle parasites away, muscle diseases "magically" disappear.

Of course, there is no magic involved. It is actually hard work. Hard work to rid the whole family of parasites that are shared and possibly were present even at birth. Parasites that normally don't go to the muscles. For example liver flukes and intestinal flukes. They belong in the liver and intestine! Yet, in muscle disease they show up and reproduce themselves in the muscles. The reason for this becomes clearer when you see that certain solvents have accumulated there. Heavy metals, bacteria, and viruses have accumulated there, too. The host's muscles, instead of kidney and bowel, have taken on the duties of toxic dumping grounds. Could it be that the regular routes of elimination were overwhelmed? Or did the muscles, traumatized by these unusual parasites, invite the toxins? A tantalizing question.

But in seven minutes you can methodically kill everything and anything that is alive in your muscles and shouldn't be there. Zap until you are free of all parasite invaders. Your muscles will feel lighter afterward.

Muscular Dystrophy

In muscular dystrophy the solvents, **xylene** and **toluene** are seen to accumulate in muscles. These also accumulate in brain and nervous tissue! (See Alzheimer's page 269 and multiple sclerosis, page 204). Could it be that these solvents are actually present in the nerves of the muscles?

Fortunately these solvents will leave your body, by themselves, in five days after you stop consuming them! Stop drinking all store bought beverages, including water and powders that you mix, and including health food varieties. Water claims and health food powder claims sound as convincing and strong as a twelve inch plank to walk on. But if the plank leads out over the side of a ship, would you walk it?

Throw all your possible sources of solvents out. Flavored foods are the chief offenders (cold cereals, sweets and candy too). But of course, you should check in your basement or attached garage for cleaning solvents. Places where painting is done or automobiles are worked on should be off limits to you.

If you've been wondering whether you have muscular dystrophy, which I consider to be a fluke disease, search your muscles electronically. Use prepared slides of flukes along with a sample of hamburger meat to represent your muscles. If flukes have already taken up residence in them, you should diagnose

219

yourself as "Positive". If not, but other parasites and toxins are present, you have pre-muscular dystrophy.

Also, the likelihood of finding thallium is quite high, judging by the case histories.

Mel Rickling, age 18, had been seeing a specialist for bouts of muscular weakness for several years, but no diagnosis was given. His condition was not yet severe enough although it was difficult for him to raise an empty glass or get upstairs. It began at puberty, not too long after his first mercury tooth filling. He had asthma in childhood. The flukes attacking his muscles were liver fluke, intestinal fluke, and pancreatic fluke. Other parasites in his muscles were Leishmanias, several dog tapeworm cysts, and pinworm.

He also had assorted bacteria in his muscles. The solvents propyl alcohol, benzene, toluene, and xylene were accumulated there too. Ortho-phospho-tyrosine (cancer test) was already positive. His doctors had not searched for cancer in their biopsies. His drinking water contained lead and since he had lived in one house since birth he was probably drinking lead every day of his life. He also had high levels of mercury and some thallium accumulated in his muscles; these came from the tooth fillings in his mouth and could explain why his problems began after his first filling was put in.

His flukes and other large parasites were killed immediately with a frequency generator. He was started on the herbal parasite program to prevent reinfection. His diet and body products were changed to exclude solvent pollution. He could have no commercially prepared beverages except milk which needed to be boiled to kill bacteria. In twelve days his daily stomach pains were gone, so he was able to eat more and gain some much needed weight. The rash on his face was gone, the pain at his right side was gone, his muscle twitches were gone, his joints no longer ached and his mood was much better. The whole family was put on the parasite program and Mel was scheduled for dental cleanup. The plumbing repairs removed lead from the water and he was soon able to walk upstairs, in fact run upstairs.

A young man, seeing himself regain normalcy, wants nothing more than to "lead a normal life" which includes reckless behavior. But after several warnings from his muscles he stuck to his restrictions and gained the weight he wanted in order to participate in athletics.

Myasthenia Gravis

is probably a fluke disease. Some chemical, possibly coming from the fluke, may affect the acetylcholine receptors, thereby causing an allergic reaction so they become inefficient. This is most noticeable in the eyelids. They droop from lack of strength to lift them.

The thymus is often involved, too. The thymus is extremely sensitive to benzene and with so much benzene pollution in our products and foods (pollution from gasoline is negligible by comparison), you will probably find benzene accumulated there. Search the thymus and the muscles for parasites, bacteria and tooth metal as well as toxins in the foods eaten daily. Kill invaders twice a week with a zapper or stay on an herbal parasite program until all danger of recurrence is past (one to two years).

Clean up dentalware, diet and environment. Keep no indoor pets since any new parasite, however tiny, will surely find the niche left behind by the flukes and give you a new myasthenia gravis-like disease. The whole family must be parasite-free to protect the member with myasthenia gravis. But it is a task easily accomplished and desirable in its own right, so discuss your plan immediately with family members. Don't delay. The flukes don't waste a single minute. They go right on feeding and breeding.

Carmen Opsal, age 37, was told by her specialist she had her myasthenia from birth since she didn't have the strength to nurse. She had pancreatic fluke stages throughout her body. Her plan was to start on the parasite killing program, clean her kidneys, remove toxic elements, kill bacteria and clean her liver. Long before she accomplished this, in one month, she was feeling better and had return of her strength on some days. She still had the solvent, methylene chloride, from drinking "pure" orange juice and praseodymium from eating foil-packaged foods, also thulium from her

221

brand of vitamin C. She was full of auto exhaust and nickel from dental metal. There was hafnium from nail polish and hair spray and zirconium from deodorant. She planned to get rid of it all, and never need to return.

Universal Allergies

If minor allergies are due to a disabled liver, then extreme allergies must be due to an extremely disabled liver. This is the case for persons suffering from "universal" allergies, namely "everything", like the lacquer on floors, plastic chairs, the neighbor's flowers, and the grocery store.

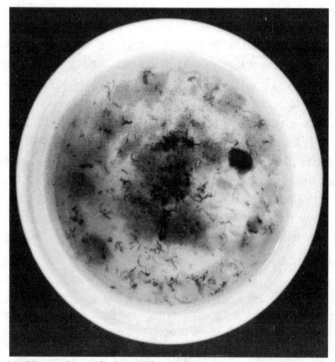

Fig. 32 Sheep liver flukes. Black threads in toilet are indicative of fluke remains.

They have more than merely clogged bile ducts. They have the sheep liver fluke living in the bile ducts! A tip-off to this situation is allergy to wool and wool fat (lanolin). A few flukes might not be noticed but a liver full of flukes that spill over into the intestine can give the worst case of allergy imaginable.

Sometimes the body manages to kill them with its own resources (maybe you ate something even too toxic for them!) They come through the bowel in a torrent. In the water of the toilet bowel they explode, spewing their infectious eggs all over in little black threads. Because these look like hairs, you may believe you passed "things with black hairy legs." These are actually burst flukes with black strings of highly infectious eggs. Why some people are literally taken over by these flukes is unclear. Amongst sheep, only certain sheep will be severely affected, being called "liver-rot." The disease in animals has been extensively studied.

Kill flukes with a frequency generator (434-421 KHz) or zapper. Come to the aid of the liver by avoiding food molds, removing dental metals, stopping chronic *Salmonella* infection and finally cleaning the kidneys and liver.

Environmental Illness

is another name for "universal" allergies. When more than a few flukes are present in the liver, they keep the liver from doing its major job: detoxifying all the food and chemicals that are taken into your body.

Different parts of the liver have different detoxifying jobs. One part detoxifies plastics and solvents, another part detoxifies perfumes and another newsprint ink, and so on. Foods have natural chemicals that need detoxification. By changing our food constantly we avoid overburdening any one of our detoxifying mechanisms. This is probably the basis for wanting differ-

ent food at each meal and different meals each day. We somehow "know" when we're ready for the same food again.

Less extreme forms of allergy can be due to other flukes in
the liver, such as human liver fluke (*Clonorchis*), or just plain
clogging with numerous cholesterol crystals.

Anything that is lodged in the bile ducts obstructs the flow
of bile. This causes back pressure in that part of the liver so it
produces less bile.

The bile duct system is a gigantic tree with lots of intercon-
necting branches. Remember how "stringy" liver can be when
you buy it in the grocery store. These strings are bile ducts.
When one is obstructed, others take over its job. But when a
whole section of the liver gets obstructed and it can't detoxify a
whole set of chemicals you dare not get those chemicals into
you again.

What if you do? These chemicals go coursing all over your
body! They are taken up by various organs. The brain has special protection, called the *blood brain barrier*. But this can get
broken by parasites that burrow. Now chemicals can roam
through the brain. Some attach themselves and cause an
"allergic reaction". Beryllium, from "coal oil," kerosene and
gasoline attaches itself to the brain easily. Then other things attach themselves to the beryllium!

The extreme form of allergies simply requires killing the
sheep liver fluke and other flukes inhabiting the liver. They tend
to overflow the liver and inhabit the intestine, too. In this case,
you might actually see some in the bowel movement after killing them. They won't let go of you as long as they are alive.

They have two attachments to hold onto you, yet, they are
not difficult to kill, even with herbs. Use the herbal parasite
recipe (page 338), zapper, or a frequency generator.

Sheep liver flukes might actually be breeding, that is, multiplying in the liver of the hyperallergic person. This is not normal. Sheep liver flukes "should" only spend their adulthood in

our bodies. When the baby stages are also found in our bodies, (instead of in minnows or snails) there is undoubtedly a specific solvent involved. Environmentally ill persons have quite a few solvents accumulated in their organ tissues. Which one enables the sheep liver fluke to go through <u>all</u> of its development in the human is not known yet.

Obviously, the extremely allergic person, should remove all solvents from their diet and environment. Begin with eliminating propyl alcohol and benzene. The <u>same</u> products have other solvents too. It is processing of foods that puts solvents into them. Go completely natural. Dairy products are free of solvents, except for some cheeses. Remember to boil them to get rid of bacteria. Salt, olive oil, butter, and honey are free of solvents. With electronic technology, you can find solvent free products. Otherwise, if it didn't grow or you didn't make it from scratch, you must assume it has solvents! Cook from scratch, make your own pasta, bread, fruit juices, beverages.

Often, <u>but not always</u>, persons with sheep liver fluke, have a specific allergy to lanolin, a sheep product. Since lanolin is widely used in other products, this becomes a very broad range allergy. Such persons "can get no fat" at mealtimes or wear no wool without a considerable reaction. The allergy to lanolin does not disappear the day the flukes are all dead. But cleaning the liver with several liver cleanses (page 552) after killing parasites will start the recovery process.

Which comes first, the flukes or the solvents? That can't be answered. But what happens next is easily seen. The more flukes, the less able the liver is to detoxify solvents. The more solvents the better able the fluke is to multiply. A vicious cycle is set up that accelerates the illness.

Perhaps neither of these came first. Perhaps something else poisoned the liver so both solvents and flukes are given a home in your liver! Such a powerful liver poison would be a food mold: *aflatoxin, cytochalasin B, sterigmatocystin, zearalenone, ochratoxin, sorghum mold, griseofulvin, citrinin, T-2 toxin, Kojic acid, ergot* and others. Avoid food molds—see Mold Free Diet, page 365. The diet must be quite limited at first, to allow the liver time to "regain" its detoxifying capability.

Of course, it is assumed that environmentally ill persons have had their dental metal replaced by metal free composite. This includes gold. Gold accumulates in the pancreas, another organ of digestion. This may mean choosing partial dentures. Read the section on healing the jaw and Bone Strengthening (page 87) to ensure this move brings you success.

The liver is a versatile organ. It can regenerate itself but it won't if food molds block regeneration. Given half a chance it will become like new. After killing parasites do the liver cleanse (page 552). If it has been a month or more since you killed parasites, then go on a high dose parasite herb treatment the week before, or zap. Don't use the herbs <u>the day</u> of the cleanse. With one major allergy gone after each cleanse and by timing liver cleanses two weeks apart, it takes only six months to have a reasonably normal life again. You can endure indoor air again, sit on plastic chairs, read newspapers, wear cotton clothing and leather shoes without reacting. You must still be patient and careful as you take back the world for you to live in.

Delores Flores, 53, was brought by her husband to the driveway in front of the office. There she put on her mask and advanced to the outdoor bench. She did not dare to come in. Without doing any testing her condition was obvious. She must start killing liver parasites. But it seemed too simple to be believable. And she knew she'd be allergic to the parasite killing herbs (this was before the zapper). She decided to do nothing.

Patricia Humphry arrived wearing an industrial painters' mask. It smelled rubbery. Her winter boots smelled moldy. And a faint scent of mothballs came from somewhere. Even her car had an engine problem, spewing exhaust fumes into the driveway. I suggested she begin with some basic reading material on allergies. She did not return either.

Arlene Kelly, 50ish, could eat no fat—not the tiniest snippet. But at Thanksgiving she allowed herself a little gravy. The consequences were swollen eyelids, swollen face, swollen throat: quite a dangerous situation. After killing *Ascaris* and the flukes, and cleansing the liver (all in time for Christmas) she dared a little pie—and got along quite well!

Alcoholism

When the portion of liver that detoxifies ethyl alcohol (the drinking kind) is hampered you are at risk for alcoholism. The other contributors to alcoholism are **beryllium** and **ergot**. Perhaps there are even more contributors.

Beryllium is plentiful in coal products such as "coal oil", and in gasoline to which kerosene or coal oil has been added. Fuel for "hurricane lamps" is a common offender, filling the air with beryllium. Liver blockage can force beryllium to circulate through the body; if it happens to attach itself to the addiction center of the brain, you're in a heap of trouble. Beryllium is very reactive. Any other allergen coursing by can react with it. If this happens to be alcohol–the drinking kind–you will be alcoholic unbeknownst to you.

When the liver is quite disabled, there may still be alcohol coursing through your body the day after you drank even a little bit! It is bound to find the beryllium stuck to the addiction center. Together, they turn the brain into a uncontrolled machine. Neurotransmitters are released that shouldn't be; others not released that should be. Mood is affected in a typically "alcoholic" way. Depression may be lifted—or caused!

Alcoholic persons should remove all fossil fuels from their environment, and <u>never</u> choose a career that exposes them to paint, cleaners, or automotive products. They should do liver cleanses until 2,000 stones or more are out.

Of course, they should never touch a drop of alcohol: not even the Black Walnut Hull Tincture in the herbal parasite program. The aqueous recipe should be made for them. Since alcohol is produced anyway, in the body, the liver should <u>never</u> be poisoned by molds, especially <u>ergot</u>: the very mold that is so abundant in alcoholic beverages! Alcohol and ergot interact to make each more toxic.

To help the brain recover its neurotransmitter status, take glutamine (500 mg.), a B-50 complex, and niacinamide (500 mg—to help detoxify ergot), with each meal.

To prevent alcoholism, protect your liver from food molds, especially ergot. Add vitamin C to nuts, pasta cereals, grains and even alcoholic beverages! Avoid fossil fuel pollution of your home by switching to all electric utilities.

Alcohol Addiction

There are many definitions of addiction. My definition is based on the special brain toxins, *beryllium* and *ergot*.

The brain has a region called the addiction center. If this center is stimulated it produces pleasure-chemicals. It is carefully controlled so that not too much pleasure or happiness can be experienced.

When a toxic substance, beryllium, is inhaled it circulates with the blood to the brain and may land at the addiction center. The more beryllium is inhaled the bigger the chance that it will occupy the addiction center. The brain cells in the addiction center have receptor sites for *glutamate* (the same glutamic acid that comes from the protein in our food). Normally, glutamate activates the addiction center. But when beryllium has "stolen" these seats, the glutamate is powerless to activate the joy and happiness center. The result is a low level chronic depression. The more beryllium there is to clog the receptors the worse the depression. Giving glutamic acid does not help but giving **glu-**

tamine does! Addicted or depressed persons should take glutamine, no less than 3 grams (3000 mg) a day. It comes in 500 mg. tablets. It is completely harmless.

When we drink alcohol or put it on the skin (as in mouthwash, tinctures, medicine) or produce it by fermentation in the intestines (*Candida* produces alcohol) a substance, *salsol*, is formed. Salsol reacts with beryllium. If the beryllium is in the pleasure center it reacts with it there. This reaction has the effect of activating the cells! Now a large amount of pleasure-chemical can be released. The amount is larger than normal because so many clogged cells are activated together. This explains the alcohol "high". In all the alcohol-addicted persons I studied, salsol was present, along with beryllium, on the receptor sites normally activated by glutamate (or NMDA or kainate). As we removed the beryllium we saw that the salsol also disappeared.

The solution to alcoholism is to avoid ergot contaminated food and avoid beryllium inhalation. We also remove the brain beryllium using **thioctic acid**. Stopping the use of alcohol may save a life or career but does not correct the problem. Even after 30 years of abstinence, I still see the beryllium present in the addiction center and the salsol, derived no doubt from endogenous sources, still attached to the beryllium. This is why the addiction is never gone even after years of abstinence.

If any member of the family is, or was, addicted to alcohol the house should be searched for beryllium sources. Hurricane lamps or antique lamps are the most common sources. Remove them permanently. Washing does not clean them. Remove all solvents, cleaners, lighters. Switch to a butane lighter. The air should be tested for beryllium. The garage door to the house should be permanently closed. and the car and lawnmower kept out of it. Addicted persons should not be painters! Nor walk into a dry-cleaning business. Soon you will see a more cheerful disposition in the addicted person and this will be rewarding for the whole family.

Miguel Alcorn's wife cleaned up the environment for Miguel, whose alcoholism was 30 years long. Even lighter fluid was removed. The garage was sealed off from the house. She added vitamin C to his meals so he didn't have to "take anything". She was very careful about moldy grains. He lost his preoccupation with drinking after killing parasites. She believes he is not sneaking any. Our hats are off to her.

Seizures

are <u>always</u> caused by tiny *Ascaris* larvae in the brain.

I suppose they find their way to the seizure center by accident. It is not normal for them to be in the brain, they typically travel between the stomach and lungs. *Ascaris* eggs are present everywhere in animal filth. Dogs, cats, horses and pigs all get *Ascaris*. Their excrement dries and flies about in the dust, but mostly it resides in the soil. Children playing in the dirt cannot help but pick up *Ascaris* eggs. The eggs hatch in the stomach and the tiny larvae, microscopic in size, travel first to the lungs. Here they go through a *molt*. This causes some coughing.

Whenever a child coughs for part of the day do not assume it is harmless. Use a frequency generator set to 408 KHz, or use a zapper. Children should be treated for *Ascaris* anyway, whether coughing or not, once a week. The tiny larvae are in the cough up. Children should <u>not</u> be taught to politely swallow this. They could be swallowing their own future seizures, asthma, or eczema. Teach children to use tissues for all spit up. The lungs are doing what they can to rid the body of these invaders. Your intelligence must cooperate with your lungs.

Ascaris do not come sweet and clean in themselves. They bring their own bacteria and viruses. One of these bacteria is *Bacteroides fragilis*. *Bacteroides* <u>needs</u> a host like *Ascaris* so it can be oxygen-free. Such a requirement is termed *obligatory anaerobic* meaning "must have absence of air."

Being transported to the brain inside *Ascaris* larvae is probably the means by which *Bacteroides* gets into the brain. Brain abscesses and brain tumors usually have *Bacteroides fragilis* growing there. Brain tumors will not shrink unless all the parasites, bacteria and viruses are dead. *Bacteroides*, in turn, are big enough to house thousands of viruses. Two common viruses seen with *Ascaris* are *Coxsackie B$_1$* and *Coxsackie B$_4$*. Perhaps it is the toxins of the *Ascaris* larvae or *Bacteroides* or *Coxsackies* that induces the seizures. Maybe it is something else about the infestation that induces them. But by killing *Ascaris*, *Bacteroides* and *Coxsackies* (zapper or frequency generator at 408, 325, 364, 362.5 KHz) you have eliminated the first essential link in the chain of developments that causes seizures.

The brain does not quietly tolerate these invaders. It fights back with its immune system. But the wormlets are already too big to be eaten by white blood cells. The brain fights back by producing **inflammation**.

Inflammations are intended to attract calcium so a wall can be built around the intruders. Inflammations are negatively charged regions so the positively charged calcium can find its way to the inflamed site. But lead and mercury are also positively charged! Perhaps this is how these **toxic metals** are attracted to the brain. All metals are positively charged. Perhaps this is their fateful poisonous attraction to living things. Perhaps they do not poison when no inflammations are present! In seizure cases we see many tooth metals in the brain. These must be removed so the inflamed site can heal.

Other toxic substances have also found their way to the inflammation at the seizure center: **vanadium** from leaking household gas; **PVC** from new carpets; **titanium** from face powder; **zirconium** from deodorant; **asbestos** from the clothes dryer belt or hair blower; **lead** from tainted drinking water. Do a good clean up of your environment.

Solvents accumulate here, too. Especially **toluene** and **xylene**. These are found in paint (persons with seizures should never be around fresh paint) but are also found in trace amounts in carbonated beverages. A person with seizures should drink no commercial beverages: see the Recipe section for homemade carbonated and other beverages. There are several other specific brain irritants that accumulate at the seizure center.

The food fungus, **ergot**, is always seen in seizure cases. Perhaps it can act alone to produce seizures. After all, seizures are an ancient malady, existing long before chemicals and solvents were manufactured.

MSG, which is *monosodium glutamate* should never be used in food. It was already banned in infant food in Europe a decade ago. Why are we still allowing it? Are our children not as precious? Healthy adults may tolerate it better than young children. But what about sick adults? Specifically, adults with a brain illness? Glutamic acid is a natural constituent of protein in our foods. And the sodium glutamate it must form in the body does no harm. But MSG is not biologically produced. It is lab-made. Lab-made amino acids are not the same as biologically made. Perhaps it is these "isomers", perhaps it is the simple overdose of a natural thing that is brain-toxic. Whatever the mechanism, MSG should not be consumed by anyone, let alone a seizure sufferer. Fortunately, you can ask at restaurants, where (not whether) MSG is used so you can avoid these foods.

BHT and **BHA**, standing for *bishydroxytoluene* and *bishydroxyanisole* are food preservatives and also seizure triggers. They are often put on the boxes of cereals, rather than the cereals themselves, so the cereals can be pronounced preservative-free. Imagine how much the box must be drenched with to prevent oxygen leakage into the interior?

A more insidious seizure trigger is a perfectly natural substance, **malvin**. Malvin is the natural dye found in grapes, strawberries, plums and blueberries. Stop eating strawberry and grape jam or juice. Chickens and the eggs they lay, have <u>lots</u> of malvin too, stop eating chicken and eggs.

Here are foods relatively free of malvin: artichokes, asparagus, almonds, barley, beans of all kinds, green beans, broccoli, Brussels sprouts, cantaloupe, celery, nectarines, citrus, dates, mango, pears, kiwi, pineapple, Granny Smith apples.[14]

To Summarize

To stop your seizures on a dime, and not have another one:
1. Avoid malvin in food. Eat nothing colored red or blue, chicken, eggs, MSG, BHA & BHT. Boil all dairy products or don't eat them.
2. Avoid ergot in food. Eat no whole grain products; take niacinamide 500 mg three times a day to help the liver detoxify tiny bits in other foods.
3. Kill *Ascaris*, *Bacteroides* and *Coxsackie* virus and stay on a maintenance program of killing them. Avoid reinfection. It would be wise to have only outdoor pets.
4. Replace dental metal with metal-free plastic (See Dental Clean-up).
5. Clean up the home environment and body products of toxic substances.
6. Keep your fingers sanitary: spray them with 10% grain alcohol or vodka after bathroom use.

You can often tell by how you feel whether you are near to having a seizure. But some people get no warning. Don't take

---

[14]Taken from *A Guide to the Identification and Treatment of Biocatalyst and Biochemical Intolerances*, 1988 by J. A. Krohn, Los Alamos Medical Center, 3917 West Road Suite 136, Los Alamos, NM 87544.

chances. Keep your drugs <u>with</u> you, even though you no longer need to take them. Drugs like Tegretol™ and Phenobarbital™ are not harmless. Once you can tell that you're better, try reducing your drug dosage slightly. See how you manage. If you have a breakthrough seizure you could fall and break a bone. Don't take chances. Even a year after your last seizure you should carry your medicine with you and have some in your house. This is because it is <u>so easy</u> to pick up *Ascaris* again. The highway to the brain–its seizure center–is still open. They will travel it again. It might only take two days from the time of accidental swallowing of animal filth, to having little larvae in the brain. Use a frequency generator every day at first, or zap daily to guard against this. Notice that killing parasites the first time may actually start a seizure coming. Simply stop zapping if you feel one coming. Do shortened zapping until you can tolerate a regular treatment. Have someone with you while zapping.

Say good-bye to seizures forever. But don't forget your susceptibility. I believe you should be extra careful for two years. If you have a recurrence, repeat the whole procedure. This time it should be curable in a single day.

Doug's mother was distraught when she brought him, age 8 months. Her doctor only <u>seemed</u> sympathetic with her purpose to keep the baby's temperature down the next time he catches a cold. But her doctor had referred her to the county social worker. She had been completely honest with her doctor, because she was that kind of trusting person. Since her baby had only experienced one seizure (which was during a fever), she didn't see why her beautiful first born child should be on medicine "the rest of his life". She wanted her baby to be perfect. But the social worker had called her, talked about "the law" and being an unfit mother. She was all apart. The baby was supposed to be on Phenobarbital™ twice a day. Our tests showed Doug had *Ascaris* plus lead toxicity. He was also getting home made strawberry and grape juice. She promised to put the three cats outdoors, keep the baby off the floor, keep Doug's fingernails short and <u>always</u> wash his hands before eating. The parasites were easily killed. The lead was sporadically present in the water. She planned to move, and until then would filter all the drinking water so her breast milk would be free of it too. His diet was changed to eliminate eggs, chicken and the red and blue fruits. We recommended leaving the state in order to be able to peacefully raise her child. We promised to treat her child free of charge if another seizure should occur. Two years passed and we heard she was doing fine with her child.

Clara Scruggs, 50ish, was losing control over her seizures and had to be hospitalized while a new medicine was tried. It changed her personality (again!) which upset her husband, too. She was started on the herbal parasite program but could only increase by one drop of Black Walnut Hull Tincture a week, instead of daily, since each new increase would give her a seizure. In half a year she was fairly free of seizures in spite of being off drugs. After each seizure, a checkup showed she had picked up *Ascaris* again sometimes with additional parasites. She could not bear to put her cat outside; Boots had been a friend in need many times. When she finally got Boots onto a regular parasite program she improved enough to go to church and church events again. When Boots finally "wanted out" she didn't mind. She decided to do a liver cleanse—this, too, gave her two seizures the next day but paid big dividends in other ways. She eventually improved to an incidence of one small seizure ("spacey" time or incoherent speech) in two weeks.

Chun Yee, age 28, has been on Dilantin™ from age 15. Now he was up to five pills a day and it didn't control his seizures. Any activity would trigger it. He was put on a low malvin diet and started on the kidney cleanse. His blood test showed he was anemic with a high MCV (104 cu microns), suggesting the *Ascaris* worms were using up all his vitamin B_{12}, too. In six weeks he was down to one or two seizures per week, although he had not yet started the parasite program. He had beryllium built up in him, probably from a kerosene heater. When the pets and family were all treated for parasites he had no more breakthrough seizures and could cut his medicine in half which gave him much more energy. He was no longer in danger of losing his job.

Shiresse Nobel, age 7, was having minimal seizures but the mother did not want to start her on medicine. Shiresse had high levels of mercury in her body, although she had no tooth fillings. The whole family cleared their Ascaris infestation and in three weeks the seizures were gone but aggressive behavior remained. There was mercury in the air of some rooms but it was not in the paint. The bathroom was the worst. When everything in the bathroom was removed, the air cleared and so did Shiresse's behavior problem.

Drew Seaton, age 8, had his first seizure lasting nearly a minute. The parents were very fastidious and extremely conscientious about diet and habits. They were distraught. They all had *Ascaris*. A baby was still being diapered. Drew had arsenic (pesticide under kitchen sink), formaldehyde (some remodeling) and PVC (a new carpet) accumulated in his body. The carpets had to be steam cleaned to get rid of the arsenic. He was started on parasite herbs at once, since he was on medication that would shield him from having another seizure while killing *Ascaris*. Two weeks later everybody, except the mother, was free of *Ascaris*. In another two weeks they were all free and had cleaned up house toxins. They dared to stop his medicine. This let Drew's former happy personality come back to everyone's delight. Two years later there was still no recurrence.

Cosmo Maser, 30ish, was in a hospital across the country. He was having continuous seizures, although he had been there a week. It seemed impossible to transport him but, against doctor's orders, they got him into a station wagon. He had nothing to eat or drink that had any malvin in it (he ate four very well done hamburgers, plain, with lettuce on his trip) and his seizures stopped immediately. They felt a bit sheepish upon arrival 20 hours later since he could sit up, could tell his own story and no longer looked ill. He was without medication, too. They had left in a hurry. They immediately removed all the metal from his mouth; this cleared his mercury problem. He was started on parasite medicine and weathered the small seizures each increase gave him. He could return home in five days with his new diet and thioctic acid daily as a supplement. He occasionally had a seizure (2 a month) until they moved away from the busy street below their apartment. About a year later he could hold a job and go off Social Security support.

Weight Problems

Overweight is not the same problem as *obesity*. In fact, I do not have the answer to either problem, only a part of the answer.

In **obese** women, the ovaries, pancreas and thyroid are all involved. Perhaps the adrenals, the brain satiety center, and the liver are also involved. Maybe it's as simple as gold accumulation in all these places. Perhaps it is bacteria in all these places. When you weigh close to 300 pounds obviously some organ isn't working right. Try several things, but not a starvation diet.

The cause is not eating too much. Try removing all gold: gold teeth, gold jewelry and gold rings. Replace them with non metal varieties. After removing the gold, pull the remaining gold out of your tissues with thioctic acid (2 or 3 a day for several months). Make sure kidneys are able to excrete the gold instead of making crystals by doing a kidney cleanse. Gold accumulates in the pancreas, the brain (possibly in a control center here) and the ovaries (causes some infertility here). Also try clearing the body of all bacteria and parasites by regularly using a zapper. Use the Bowel Program (page 546) to evict the last of the *Shigellas*. Be very careful to avoid nonsterile dairy products. Try cleansing your liver by doing liver cleanses. Get 3,000 stones out.

Make sure you are getting enough nutritious food; make carrot and vegetable juice; use no commercial beverages. Avoid moldy food—don't take risks. If all these measures bring your weight down to the level of mere overweight give yourself good grades.

Overweight is a low energy condition. Your food is being turned into fat instead of energy. The decision not to make energy is being made in the liver mainly, but perhaps other organs as well.

Try cleaning the liver (page 552) until no more stones come out: get at least 2,000 stones. Notice that as the liver gets cleaner you get more and more energy right after each cleanse. Some cleanses have a dramatic effect. Others do not. This suggests that a certain part of the liver is the responsible part. Soon after the cleanse–within a week–the same old lassitude sets in. But during these few days notice how your body feels. It feels light. Your abdomen feels tight, like it's a part of you again. You're mind isn't on food throughout the day. It's very easy to lose weight, in fact you may lose five pounds in these few days without dieting or exercising. Definitely, your long-lost weight regulation is back in force. But then it vanishes. Fortunately, a bit of the weight loss stays with you, and by repeating cleanses (only once in 2 weeks, though) you can shed the pounds you want <u>and</u> gain energy in a permanent way. It is probably the way nature intended.

Try increasing your bowel movements. Notice how cats and dogs seem to derive energy from emptying their bowels. A cat <u>walks</u> to its litter box; after emptying its bowels and carefully covering it up, it <u>jumps</u> from the box and <u>runs</u> away. It now has its playful mood. A body chemical, *acetylcholine*, plays a role in emptying the bowels. Acetylcholine is a necessary operator for many of our muscles. Is there a disturbance in our acetylcholine metabolism in overweight conditions?

Coax your body to release more acetylcholine, at least in the intestines, by using a herbal laxative like Cascara sagrada. Other varieties are useful, too, but don't use a drug laxative: it burdens the liver more. Try to have three bowel movements a day.

Shigella bacteria can cause dreadful constipation. Immediately, the body feels sluggish, abdomen feels disconnected or hanging out. A nameless hunger sets in. Keep a close watch on dairy foods to make sure they are sterile. Zap when in doubt and do the Bowel Program.

Exercise helps as long as you keep at it. Strict dieting works as long as you keep doing it. But there's the problem. When you stop, you lose ground. It doesn't solve the problem of an inefficient body metabolism.

Raising thyroid levels helps but this can be dangerous. Raising thyroid levels naturally, by removing toxins is a very effective method—provided it was low to begin with. Overweight people often have a low body temperature, showing that the thyroid is involved: it is under producing. **But giving the body extra thyroid doesn't solve the thyroid's problem. It only temporarily solves the rest of the body's problem.** The thyroid will have viruses and heavy metals in it. The metal in your mouth drains downward to the stomach passing very close to the thyroid. Perhaps its iodine uptake is inhibited. The chlorine in water and bromine in bread may inhibit iodine uptake by the thyroid, too. After all, they are all halogens. Stop eating bleached bread and filter out the chlorine in your water. If this raises your body temperature you could expect better weight control.

The traditional herb, *Fucus*, was used to treat thyroid problems (and overweight) in days when herbs ruled medicine. Herbalists made a point of discouraging use of plain iodine. Fucus, they said, was much more effective. See *Recipes*.

If all these measures don't work for you, at least you have improved your health trying.

There are some advantages of being overweight. Overweight people seem to weather illness better. They laugh more. But one look in the mirror or at the scales ruins it. Put away the long mirror and scales. Don't ruin your whole life over it. Make a reasonable effort and then let go. Enjoy your stay on this planet.

Underweight can be just as difficult as overweight to correct. Once the stomach has been trained to say "full" or "full enough," even after a few mouthfuls, it is difficult to heal. *Salmonellas* in the stomach wall are often seen. *Giardia* and other common parasites, that don't belong in the stomach, are seen here in cases of underweight.

The stomach is invaded by bacteria and parasites when its immunity is low. The common culprit is tooth metal draining down continuously into the stomach. Remove every bit of mouth metal. Don't cook or eat with metal. Stimulate your appetite with B-vitamins. And, again, the liver plays a role. If it is toxic with mold, it may say "eat no more" and the body obeys.

A stage of cancer illness is weight loss. This is called *cachexia*. The victim believes he or she is eating enough. They may not even have a poor appetite. Yet weight drops steadily. This metabolic problem has been studied scientifically. A chemical, **hydrazine sulfate** (prescription only), can reverse it to some degree. Use 65 mg three times a day for 30 days. Perhaps a lesson taken from cachexia metabolism could be applied to obesity. For the cachexia sufferer, life would end

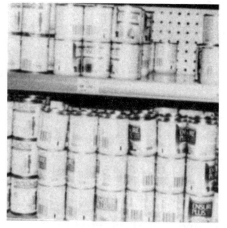

Fig. 33 I found all calorie boosters to be polluted with wood alcohol. Make your own.

sooner if high calorie supplements were not used. But don't use canned "calorie boosters". They are polluted—often with the very solvent that makes the condition worse. Instead, make an eggnog: ½ cup boiled milk, ¼ cup boiled whipping cream, a raw egg (exterior carefully washed), 1 tsp. olive oil, a banana, honey, cinnamon, cloves, nutmeg to taste. Mix all in a blender. Drink 1 cup a day. Vary it daily to keep it interesting.

If all this fails, give yourself credit for achieving health improvement and shift your focus to a different project. Underweight is <u>not all bad</u> either.

Sleep Problems

All big animals sleep, but some sleep by day instead of night. When humans do this, that is, work the night shift, they don't feel as well. Humans need about seven hours of sleep out of the twenty-four. Younger ones sleep more; newborns sleep much more. When we are deprived of sleep we are grouchy, think less clearly next day and have less energy. In spite of lots of research at "sleep labs" sleep problems are not understood, except for sleep *apnea*. Breathing should be even. When breaths are missed it is called apnea. It is especially disturbing when a baby shows apnea.

Sleep Apnea

Since breathing is regulated by acid levels in the blood and this is influenced by air quality, air toxins should be searched for first. **Cigarette smoke** is an air toxin. **Vanadium** from a gas leak is a very serious air toxin and can go unnoticed. Do your own checking since gas companies give wrong answers four out of five times. Ask a home construction company to check for gas leaks or the Health Department. **PVC** from new carpeting may be polluting the air. **Arsenic** from "treated" carpets and drapes and furniture also pollutes. **Asbestos** from clothes and hair dryers may be the toxin responsible. Perhaps even **fiberglass**, **formaldehyde**, or **freon**.

Adults with sleep apnea show swollen throat tissues: not necessarily pain. This makes the air passage smaller; long gasps of air are taken to try to make up for the missed oxygen and the carbon dioxide build up.

Swelling of the throat is a common allergic reaction. The possibility of allergy should get second consideration after air quality. Drug reactions, even in a nursing baby, where only the mother is using a medicine could be the problem. Allergy to food chemicals has been suggested, as well as a simple lack of vitamin C (implicating mold and medicine which consume vitamin C in the detoxification process).

A third possibility is infection. Many bacteria and viruses can cause throat swelling. Redness of the throat is a telltale sign. It doesn't necessarily hurt. Kill all invaders with a zapper and try to understand the basis of low immunity in the throat.

Keeping metal in the mouth constantly, is a cause of low throat immunity since it must drain past the throat.

If you snore, you can deduce that your throat is swollen, even if you don't have sleep apnea. Pursue all three possible causes (air toxin, allergy, infection).

Overweight and obesity have been emphasized as causes. This may apply to some cases but certainly not to babies.

Whatever you do, <u>don't do nothing</u>. Keep removing bad things until you find the cause of irregular breathing.

Chester Fannon, 50ish, was quite overweight and wore a mask at night with an air blower to assist his breathing. He had been referred to a sleep center for sleep apnea. He had extreme dryness of his throat at night and some hearing loss in one ear. He was toxic with arsenic (roach killer), bismuth (cologne), tin (toothpaste), and thallium (polluted dentalware). He was infested with both species of *Ascaris* and had a hacky cough. He had four solvents accumulated in his tissues. He was growing nine pathogens: *Mycoplasma, Haemophilus inf., Streptococcus pneu, A-strep, Nocardia, Staphylococcus aureus, Bacillus cereus* and Flu virus, over half of them in his throat. These were killed with a frequency generator and a general cleanup was done. After two teeth were pulled he no longer needed his mask, he no longer had apnea.

Peter Day, middle age, was set for throat surgery in a few days. He had a couple of scary nights when he thought he was dying and couldn't risk many more nights with his obstructed airways. He was overweight. His throat was red and swollen, although he felt nothing. He never even had colds. His diet was completely changed, to things he rarely ate (bananas, milk, soup, oatmeal) and off things he ate daily (hamburgers, fries, tea, pancakes with genuine maple syrup). In two days, his throat was quite clear, the tissues having become unswollen. Maybe it was the molds in the maple syrup, maybe it was the oxalic acid in the tea, or something else he could not detoxify in these foods. He was certainly happy not to live the rest of his life with an artificial voice box.

Insomnia

Another sleep disturbance is waking in the night and not being able to go back to sleep for hours. Or not being able to get to sleep.

I believe these problems are caused by a high ammonia level in the brain. This belief is based on two observations. **Ornithine**, an ammonia reducer, induces a wonderful sleep in sleep-deprived persons. It is also observed that after killing parasites, which produce ammonia, sleep is much improved. Our metabolism does not produce ammonia. We produce <u>urea</u> which is excreted by the kidneys along with water and then called urine. When we are parasitized, our metabolism is burdened with ammonia, though, made by the parasites. We have to turn it into urea in the liver and kidneys so we can excrete for them. But this can't be done in the brain! The brain lacks an essential enzyme, *ornithine carbamyl-transferase*, for this bit of biochemistry. The brain was never meant to be parasitized or infected and has no defense. Most of our parasites come from animals we associate with. We weren't meant to live with horses, cows, sheep, pigs, monkeys, guinea pigs, cats, dogs and chickens nor to come in contact with dozens more at a zoo. We do so at our own peril.

It is known that ammonia is a strong brain irritant. In fact, a person can be awakened from a coma by being made to smell ammonia "smelling salts." Ornithine reacts with ammonia, mopping it up like a sponge. **Arginine**, another amino acid, also reacts with ammonia, but does not put you to sleep. So there is more to insomnia than mere inability to reduce ammonia levels. Arginine results in alertness and therefore should be used in the morning, when needed. Ornithine, given at bedtime, may take ½ hour to do its magic. Both are perfectly safe, since they are natural to your body, and a food constituent.

Start by taking two ornithine capsules (each 500 mg.) on the first night. Take four the next night. Take six the night after and choose the dose you like best. Sometimes it takes five days to "catch up" on everything that needs to be done for the brain and get you sleeping. Meanwhile, of course, you are planning to kill your parasites and be done with insomnia in the most effective way of all.

Another sleep aid is herbal. A couple of herbs, **valerian** and **skullcap**, are known for such action. The mechanisms are not understood and this makes for nonuniform action. Some persons sleep well with them, others do not. Simply try them to find out. We are all so different in our metabolism details, we respond differently to herbs. But it is a blessing that the mechanism is <u>not</u> understood. Herbs, a tradition that precedes civilization, need to be forever off limits for intervention by government agencies.

Tryptophane, another amino acid, is about twice as powerful as ornithine, but was taken off the market a few years ago. Some persons taking it daily were seen to become quite ill and some deaths ensued. Since tryptophane had been used in prior years without noticing toxicity, something unusual should have been suspected. My tests showed extreme pollution of tryptophane capsules. They contained PCBs, mercury, ruthenium, strontium, praseodymium, aluminum, and benzalkonium. I can only speculate that a mixing vat broke, dumping its precious load onto the floor—but it was salvaged. Or that the mixing vat wasn't cleaned thoroughly from it's last use.

Persons with illness due to taking tryptophane developed an extremely high eosinophil count in their blood test—an index of parasitism, too. Parasitism, that would have led to insomnia in the first place! Were these unfortunate victims seeing the cause or the result of their tryptophane use? This tragic event should have led to a discovery of the heavy pollution, a revelation of the industrial manufacturing process, and a safeguarding against any repetition. It has not been done (certainly not publicly).

Foreign countries' manufacturing processes do not come under U.S. scrutiny or jurisdiction, although some imported products must pass tests. There are no safeguards against repetition of the tryptophane experience. It behooves us to demand safe supplements and medicines. It is not the list of ingredients that informs. Lot analysis, after bottling, would give us the necessary safeguard. The presence of filth contamination and toxins cannot be completely avoided but the consumer can make informed choices if he or she knows it is there. Disclosure, of course, is the bane of the manufacturing business. Interest rate disclosure was the bane of the money lending business. Such important matters can't be left to "self-regulation" policies. The consumers must simply demand to know what they are consuming.

Ruby Adair, 14, ached all over, had ringing in her ears, sinus problems and chronic fatigue. She couldn't get to sleep, ever; and had been half a year out of school already. She had intestinal flukes in her stomach. In three weeks she had eliminated them with parasite herbs and she could go to sleep naturally.

Yeast Infections

The most common yeast in humans is *Candida albicans*. *Candida* has always been around. It flies in the air, searching for a place to land and reproduce. It can invade a variety of human tissues like the mouth (called thrush), skin (including some kinds of diaper rash), vagina, and the digestive tract. We all have some yeast in our digestive tract, but when it gets out of hand, it's called *candidiasis*.

Yeast is a **fungus**. It needs dampness to survive and sugar to grow.

Our immune system, white blood cells, are capable of eradicating yeast provided it isn't growing too fast. And provided the white blood cells aren't immobilized or preoccupied with something else.

Diaper Rash

A baby's rash is an example of the white blood cells being preoccupied. When chemicals are used in the diaper, the white blood cells go after the chemicals and let the yeast grow. Drying the baby's skin helps since the yeast must have dampness. This should be done with air, sunlight and a heat lamp, not with more chemicals! Certainly not with cortisone containing salves that further reduce the immune competence of white blood cells.

Use a heat lamp for five minutes at a time, several times a day. Switch to cloth diapers; do not bleach them with chlorine bleach, the residual chlorine trapped in the cloth is a chronic irritant, setting the stage for another rash and future chlorine-allergy. Cloth diapers should be sterilized, not bleached. Use the hottest water your laundry system is capable of producing. Add ½ cup borax for the washing process. If you have homemade Lugol's iodine (made by your pharmacist or by yourself, see *Recipes*), add a tsp. to the wash or rinse. Vinegar is a yeast in-

246

hibitor, add it to the rinse. Dry diapers at the hottest setting. Dry to kill. Kill all the yeast spores in the diapers.

To strengthen the baby's skin against future infection, do not put chemicals on the skin. Do not use any soap, fragrance, bath oil, ointment or lotion. Do not use cotton balls or baby wipes. Do not give a daily bath. Wash bottoms gently, with borax followed by a vitamin C rinse. Vitamin C is acid and is our natural healing agent but it will sting on a broken skin surface. Use it as dilute as necessary to be tolerated. Zinc oxide is another natural healer because it competes away the iron that fungus and bacteria need for their reproduction. Never use commercially available zinc compounds though, simply purchase your own zinc oxide powder, mix it with cornstarch and keep in a large old salt shaker, dust it wherever there is moisture or fungus growth.

Treat Yeast or Fungus the Same

Other fungus growths, like *Tinea* (crotch itch), ringworm (not a worm at all), athlete's foot, along with *Candida*, can be similarly eradicated:
1. Deprive the fungus of moisture.
2. Deprive the invaders of iron.
3. Deprive the fungus of sugar.
4. Strengthen the skin's immune power.
5. Strengthen the skin's healing ability.

It may be impossible to deprive the fungus of moisture, for example if your feet sweat and you must wear socks. Take your socks off as soon as you are at home, treat your feet with a heat lamp. Use zinc oxide or cornstarch to powder and dry the skin. Boil your socks when laundering. Dry them to tinder-heat (too hot to touch). Launder with borax only (soaps and detergents contain aluminum which pollutes the skin). Rinse skin with vitamin C water. It takes <u>all</u> these measures used simultaneously to clear up athlete's foot fungus. And great persistence. They may have developed a foothold underneath the toe nail where a steady supply of moisture, iron and sugar is available to them. Nevertheless, your white blood cells will eventually gobble them up if you let them.

In thrush (yeast infection of the mouth) you must again outwit its growth by doing everything possible <u>at one time</u>. Eat no sugar, drink no fruit juice, stay off antibiotic. Avoid trauma like eating abrasive foods (crusts, popcorn, nuts, lozenges) or sucking on things. Floss teeth only once a day (using monofilament fish line), followed immediately by brushing with white iodine (or Lugol's, but this may temporarily stain). Hydrogen peroxide is not strong enough. Remember to sterilize your toothbrush with grain alcohol or iodine. You may also rinse your mouth with Lugol's (6 drops to ¼ cup of water). Or apply 6 drops directly to the tongue and rub it in lightly with your lips.

Do not use Lugol's iodine if you have been told you are allergic to iodine.

Kill *Candida* daily with a frequency generator or zapper. Since reinfection is constant, you must continue to do all the treatments given to permanently cure yourself of fungus disease.

Since *Candida* grows right into your living cells (which you are not attacking!) you cannot kill it all at once. Only surface fungus can be accessed by either Lugol's or electrical "zapping". But as the top layer is killed, exposing the next layer, you will make progress. It will take a month of daily treatment to clear it.

Clearing up fungus at one location but not another will not bring you a permanent cure, either. Damp locations like under the breasts, under the belly fold, groin and crotch need to be kept dry with cornstarch daily. Keep it up long after it seems to be cured.

Fluke Disease

Flukes, or flatworms, have a complex life cycle with many stages. Although sheep, cattle, pigs and humans can be "natural" hosts to the **adult** stage, the other stages are meant to develop outdoors and in secondary hosts. When fluke stages other than the adult are able to develop in <u>us</u>, I call it *fluke disease*

Or, when an adult that "normally belongs" to another species is able to develop in us, I also call that fluke disease Or even with adult flukes in their "normal" host, when they move from the organ that they "normally" colonize to other organs in the body I call this fluke disease, too.

Four fluke varieties engaged in this extra territorial pursuit are the **intestinal fluke, sheep liver fluke, pancreatic fluke,** and **human liver fluke**.

As you can see from their names, scientists have studied them well, and know exactly which animals are the "normal" hosts, and which organ in that animal is the adult fluke's "normal" home. Fluke disease is when any of these is "wrong."

Flukes don't have eyes to see with or legs to walk with, so how can they find and travel to the organ they want in the middle of your body? Scientists do not know for sure. However it's concluded from many scientific studies that the liver fluke, *Fasciola,* for example, has no trouble seeking out and colonizing the liver.

Here are some examples of what can happen when flukes go "wrong:"

- Adult flukes (any of the four mentioned) in the uterine wall causes cramping and bleeding when it is not menstrual period time. If an adult crosses the wall to the inside and then manages to get out through the fallopian tubes to the abdominal cavity it takes some endometrium with it—causing **endometriosis**.

- If adults develop in the kidneys, it can cause **lupus** or **Hodgkin's disease**.
- If adults complete their cycle in the brain, **Alzheimer's** disease and **multiple sclerosis** result.
- If the <u>intestinal fluke</u> (*Fasciolopsis buskii*) becomes adult in the liver it causes **cancers** of many (hundreds) kinds.
- If the pancreatic fluke <u>completes its cycle</u> in the pancreas it leads to **diabetes**. This is not an example of flukes straying into the wrong organs, but of having its stages reproducing where they never could before.
- If flukes develop in the thymus, immunity is lowered. If it happens to be the <u>intestinal fluke</u>, **HIV** (Human Immunodeficiency Virus) is released there. In turn, HIV invades other tissues, like penis and vagina.
- These four flukes can also invade the muscles, causing **dystrophies**.

As dissimilar as we always thought these diseases to be, it's obvious to me that they are but one disease—fluke disease

---

Considering the size of these flukes (adults are easily visible), it is not surprising that they can quickly lay waste a human's organs. Yet a human is big and makes a valiant effort to kill the stages, block access to tissues and otherwise battle them.

But only the human's intelligence can be counted on to defeat them. The intelligent approach is to discover what enables these mighty monsters to do their reproducing in our bodies instead of the pond with its snail/minnow secondary hosts.

Flukes and Solvents

The explanation I have found for two of these flukes is the presence of solvents in our bodies. The presence of *isopropyl alcohol* is associated in 100% of cancer cases (over 500 cases) with reproduction of the intestinal fluke stages in a variety of organs causing cancers in these organs.

The presence of *benzene* is associated in 100% of HIV cases (over 100 cases) with reproduction of intestinal fluke stages in the thymus.

The presence of *wood alcohol* is associated in 100% of diabetes cases (over 50 cases) with reproduction of pancreatic fluke stages in the pancreas.

The presence of *xylene* and *toluene* is associated in 100% of Alzheimer cases (over 10 cases) with the reproduction of intestinal fluke stages in the brain.

Much more work needs to be done to examine the relationship between fluke reproduction, the solvent and the chosen organ. But it seems probable that the solvent allows it all to happen. And our intelligence, to save us, must find a solution.

Stopping use of these solvents seems to me to be the most urgent advice. Finding which foods and products are polluted with them is the first step. It is imperative that you test everything you use or eat for solvent pollution. The Syncrometer makes that an easy task. Ideally, we should all pool our results, adding to the body of knowledge I have begun.

In my observations, when the big sources of solvents are stopped, the body's levels go back to zero. In other words, the minute amounts that we inhale here and there do not accumulate to the point of serious damage. We have to eat, drink or absorb them on a daily basis to injure us! So where can they come from?

The sources of benzene and propyl alcohol that I found are given in special lists (page 354 and 335). The sources of wood alcohol are not as well known, but include commercial beverages, cold cereals, artificial sweetener, vitamins, and drugs. Other solvents are even less studied. But a pattern is emerging: foods and products that require sterilization of bottles and machinery to fill these bottles are polluted with propyl alcohol or wood alcohol. Foods and products containing flavorings or oils are polluted with benzene. Let the buyer (you) be wary! Test your own products if possible. If not, do not purchase them.

There are many other flukes and many other diseases. Are there other fluke/solvent/disease trios? Has fluke disease been going on for a long time or is it a recent phenomenon? Certainly cancer is 100 years old, so is the use of propyl alcohol. Diabetes is quite old as an illness, too, and so is its associated solvent, wood alcohol. But HIV, AIDS and Alzheimer's are recent diseases. Should we conclude that benzene, xylene and toluene were used much less in the past?

Fluke diseases could be eradicated with some simple actions: monitoring of solvents in foods, feeds and products. Hopefully, this will begin. It is in the interest of the consumer to have her or his own independent way of monitoring too. Chemical ways can be devised, besides the electronic way presented in this book. Imagine a small test strip like a flat toothpick which turns color when in contact with propyl alcohol. Keep a pack in your pocket and never be unknowingly dosed again...all in tomorrow's world.

Flukes Not Alone

There are other families of parasites. The roundworms and tapeworms are gaining ground too. Are they associated with solvents? Or with yet undiscovered factors? Are they changing their life cycles to take advantage of our lowered immunity? These are important questions. But you are armed with excellent technology. The answers will be found.

And along with answers there will surely develop a new industry. An industry that not only proclaims purity for its products but provides the proof to your satisfaction.

Burning And Numbness

Burning sensations in the skin let you know that nerves are involved. Mercury is the most common offender. Mercury may have started the trek of a host of other toxins as well into your nervous system: pesticide, automotive chemicals, household chemicals, fragrance and even food chemicals. Some people can get a burning sensation after a car trip, some when exposed to perfume, some when walking down the soap aisle in a grocery store. When the affected nerves don't go to skin but instead go to an organ like toes, you might feel a toe cramp or finger cramp instead. Remove your mercury sources.

Burning skin is an ancient malady—maybe even the basis of concepts like "hell." St. Anthony's fire was caused by *ergot* (food fungus) ingestion. Molds don't necessarily come singly. Maybe other mold toxins can go to your nerves, too (see Moldy Food, page 381). Maybe the mold toxins interfere with **pantothenic acid** used by your body, because giving pantothenate (500 mg three times a day) can sometimes relieve the condition and, of course, this is good for your body.

Monosodium glutamate (MSG) can cause burning, especially of the face and lips. Sometimes swelling occurs too. MSG is used as a flavor enhancer. It was found decades ago to be a brain toxin and was taken out of baby food. But what about adults? Especially those who already have a brain problem. Throw it all out of your kitchen. Ask at restaurants which foods have it.

Numbness has a similar cause. Numbness of fingers or feet has become quite common since thallium and mercury toxicity has spread so widely.

If you have burning and numbness, can multiple sclerosis (MS) be far away? Remove all the metal in your dentalware immediately, replacing with composite (see Dental Cleanup, page 409). Hopefully, your immune system is still strong enough to clear the bacteria growing around the metal and in pockets in the jaw. Check and clean cavitations. Start your jaw healing with the milk, magnesium, vitamin D diet. Use thioctic acid to help clear your tissues of remaining metal (3 to 6 a day).

The most common nervous system bacterium is *Shigella*. Its beginning can already be seen in cases of burning and numbness. It is deeply entrenched in cases of MS. Three kinds of *Shigella* are readily obtainable on slides: *Shigella dysenteriae, Shigella flexneri, Shigella sonnei. Shigella flex* causes depression and irritability. All can cause gas and bloating. Zapping doesn't kill all of them because they inhabit the bowel. You must empty your bowels frequently, two or three times a day. And do the Bowel Program until all symptoms are gone. Be very careful not to put contaminated dairy food in your mouth again. Boil all milk products. They must be at boiling point for 10 seconds. This includes cheese, cottage cheese, buttermilk and regular milk. Eat only home made yogurt or home made buttermilk. Butter and whipping cream need this treatment, too. Never use raw dairy products.

Nana Hughes, 48, had numbness of the whole right arm, hand and right side of her head; it was particularly bad in the last four months. She was toxic with PCBs, titanium and dysprosium (paint). She was on thyroid, Xantac™ (for stomach) and chlorazipate medicines. We also found dog heartworm (she had chest pain over the heart). She started on the parasite program, stopped using nail polish, and stopped all detergents for dishes or laundry. In three weeks her numbness was greatly reduced. She still had titanium buildup from dental metal (a partial bridge). Seeing she was on the right track, she stopped use of MSG in her food, switched from concocted beverages to milk and cut down on her smoking. She brought her arm pretty near to normal.

Marla Santana, 45, had numbness in both arms; they would tingle and "go to sleep" a lot. It was spreading to one leg. Her muscles were toxic with thallium. It was in some very old pesticide, still effective and still in use in the house. It was also in the well water, probably, from pesticide seepage. She went off all commercial body products, did a kidney cleanse and killed parasites. She had difficulty getting rid of *Prosthogonimus* but in two months she had everything cleaned up. Her legs, arms, sleep problem, urinary tract problems were all gone and she could focus on her last problem, digestion.

Candy Donaldson, 44, had numbness from her shoulder to the wrist of one arm, it started a year ago. She was toxic with iridium, lithium and vanadium from a gas leak. She was advised to stop caffeine use and switch to milk (her calcium level was low: 9.0 mg/DL) and a magnesium tablet (300 mg daily). Her triglycerides were high, implying a kidney problem. She had urate and phosphate crystals in her kidney. She decreased the phosphate in her diet (meat, nuts, grains, soda pop) and started the kidney cleanse. When the gas leak was fixed, both her lithium and vanadium toxicity disappeared. In six weeks she had also killed parasites and her periods became regular for the first time. An ovarian cyst had disappeared, too, as checked by ultrasound. Soon her PMS was gone, including hot flushes. After four months she had done three liver cleanses and suddenly her numbness improved. After a few more there was no numbness at all.

If cleaning cavitations brings you immediate improvement you <u>know</u> that these bacteria were part of the problem. Have them checked again if problems return; dental bacteria are notorious for returning. If kidney cleansing makes it worse for a day and then better, you <u>know</u> kidney bacteria are partly responsible. If liver cleanses (page 549) make matters worse for a day and then better, you know bacteria are entrenched in the liver. Continue cleansing until none of these sources exist any longer. Kill all bacteria at least once a week electronically. Burning and numbness can be cured, not just arrested. In other words, your nerves can be cleaned up and healed.

Depression

All persons I have seen with clinical depression had small roundworms in the brain. Is it any wonder the brain can't make enough neurotransmitters or gets them out of balance? The usual worms are hookworms (*Ancylostoma*), *Ascaris* of cats and dogs, *Trichinellas* and *Strongyloides*.

Although it is commonly believed that hookworms penetrate the skin when walking barefoot on earth, this appears to be a negligible route. The important routes are eating animal filth and inhaling filthy dust. Our pets pick these worms up daily. We get them and give them in constant exchange with our pets and family members. Diapering babies is an especially hazardous, though necessary, business. Letting little children clean up after their own bowel movements is even more hazardous. Hands should be sanitized with grain alcohol after dealing with bowel contents, whether your own, your child's, or an animal's. If you clean up a messy diaper and then your hands well with soap, then go to make the chopped salad for dinner, you're sure to give each family member a dose of whatever the baby has. It was hiding under the fingernails. Animals clean up the easy way: they simply lick the youngster's bottom. But, we humans are not strong enough to take on a dose of bottom with each meal. **We must sanitize our hands.**

Cleaning bathrooms is also dangerous. Wear gloves. If nobody suffers from depression, you can use bleach (stored in the garage) to disinfect the stool, otherwise use alcohol (50% grain alcohol). Keep doorknobs and faucet handles wiped with alcohol, too.

If you suffer from depression use your zapper to immediately kill these four roundworm species: *Ancylostoma*, *Ascaris*, *Trichinella* and *Strongyloides*.

Other family members should be cleared of these four worms on the same day or as close to it as possible. Reinfection always occurs. In the depressed person, the microscopic parasites travel immediately to the brain. In others, they may simply reside in the intestine or lungs or liver, or other organs. Pathways (routes) to the brain have become established for the depressed person. These must heal before there is any tolerance to reinfection.

Solvents and other toxins, also in the brain, slow down or prevent healing. For this reason the depressed person should do the *Four Clean-ups*.

The bacteria of the *Shigella* family are always seen in depression cases. Kill all *Shigellas* and avoid reinfection by boiling dairy products and not eating those that can't be boiled. Go on the Bowel Program (page 546). Do not eat deli food or hand prepared salads at salad bars. Finally, do the Liver Cleanse, repeating every two weeks. Depression, even of long standing, can lift within days after the brain finally has its territory to itself. Look in the mirror and smile at yourself for your success in vanquishing your invaders. Never again, let these creepy crawlers into the happiness-center of your brain.

Manic Depression

This variety of depression is associated with *Strongyloides*, as the main parasite in the brain. Plus **chlorine** as an allergen! *Strongyloides* is the same worm that causes migraines and other severe types of recurrent headache. It probably depends on where these tiny worms have set up their "housekeeping" which symptoms you get: manic depression or migraines. Maybe chlorine is the deciding factor.

These tiny wormlets can pass the placenta into the unborn fetus. Is it any wonder that these brain disturbances seem to be inherited? Of course, there is ample opportunity to simply eat them off hands, other people's hands, and off floors during childhood. The amazing truth is that some family members do not get infected with it or at least do not get brain symptoms! It is very difficult to eradicate *Strongyloides* in a whole family and thereby let the depressed person get well. It is, in fact, impossible if there is a pet or other animal connection. Getting rid of the chlorine allergy is also very challenging. Step one is to zap all parasites.

I usually see an accumulation of **bromine** as well. Since bromine, fluorine and chlorine are all *halogens*, maybe getting too much of any one could saturate the liver's ability to detoxify chlorine. Stop eating brominated (bleached) bread. Stop taking drugs containing bromides. That is the easy part. You must also stop even washing your face in chlorinated water (use a pure carbon filter system). You inhale it as you wash. Never drink it or use it for any purpose. Of course, there should be no bleach container in the house, even when tightly closed; nor should bleached clothing be worn.

Do the *Four Clean-ups*. Sometimes the cloud lifts and the mind clears on the way home from the dentist. Recovery can be very rapid—less than a week. And recurrence just as rapid when a tiny bit of chlorine is inhaled or drunk. But your careful vigilance pays off. In half a year you can expect no recurrence.

Humans, it seems, must lick fingers with the same compulsion that cows lick their noses and cats lick their rears. The single, most significant advance in human hygiene would most assuredly be stopping the hand to mouth habit. We must always eat with utensils. And never leave a bathroom without washing. These are difficult changes but the new age of parasitism makes it necessary. Together with the new pollutants, solvents, and heavy metals, parasites will overtake us unless we change.

Don't go off lithium and other medicines until your doctor agrees you are ready, about a half year. After this, make sure you still keep it handy. Although you may be free of manic depression in a day, reinfecting yourself weeks later will attack your brain like a hurricane; it has not yet healed, the routes are open. Be patient; healing will happen as it did for these happy persons.

Lena Constantine, age 39, had a history of migraine, TMJ, heavy clotting with periods and numerous pains but it shouldn't have made her try suicide 1½ years ago. She was put on Prozac™ afterward. She was parasitized by intestinal flukes (in the intestine), dog whipworm, *Strongyloides* and human liver flukes. She was started on a parasite program and kidney cleanse. This made her feel so good she took herself off Prozac™ and landed in the hospital for reasons she couldn't remember. After 42 days spent there she got out, wiser than before. She set to work again, leaving no detail undone, because she could remember how good it felt to be free of depression (not drugged out of it). Three months later she still had *Strongyloides* (she had a cat) but she did her first liver cleanse anyway. She got over 500 stones out. Her depression was gone. She substituted 4 ornithine and 2 ginseng capsules daily (more if tension was not relieved) for Prozac and cured her problem.

Mona Zabala, 33, was extremely depressed over her job. She was full of mercury, arsenic, PCBs, chromate from eye liner, wood alcohol from drinking colas and she had *Ascaris*, pancreatic flukes, *Trichinellas* and *Strongyloides*. She thought she was a hopeless case. But in less than three months, when only half her clean-up chores were done, she was already saying positive things about her job.

Acey O'Hara, a young graduate student, was very careful to avoid junk food, caffeine, fragrance, and body products because he had learned the hard way that he didn't tolerate them. When "crying" depression hit him he was not only surprised but angry that his good health habits "hadn't paid off." He was buying his drinking water; it came in clear plastic containers. He had cesium in his tissues and brain. When he switched back to plain tap water (filtered in small quantities) the depression lifted in a week and he was no longer crying over anything.

Leisa Underwood, 46, was clinically depressed and in therapy. She believed it was due to going through menopause. She had a heavy burden of *Strongyloides* but no other worms. Only one of her two dogs had *Strongyloides* (saliva test) and the cat was free of them also. She was full of cesium (from drinking refrigerator water) and vanadium (from a gas leak). In two months she had accomplished the impossible: all pets and herself were free of *Strongyloides*, they had repaired three gas leaks and her depression was just a memory.

Roland Greeley was diagnosed as manic depressive a few years ago and was put on Ativan™ and Prozac.™ This controlled him but did not relieve depression. He had a prominent tremor. He had *Ascaris* and sheep liver fluke stages in the brain. Also *Trichinella*, *Strongyloides* and human liver fluke stages. Styrene (from styrofoam cups), methyl ethyl ketone (beverage) and carbon tetrachloride were in his brain also, probably setting the stage for parasite reproduction. He had high levels of mercury and silver but highest of all–throughout his body–was chlorine (from bleach and tap water). In four weeks he had all the metal removed from his mouth. He stated that this "unchained" him. He could already tell on his way home from the dentist that something special had happened. His depression was simply gone "the way you lift a blanket off a bed". He resolved to clean up his whole body and recover from his illness using logical methods, like ours. Staying away from regular chlorinated water was a fine challenge to his resolve but with whole house filtering now available he may have done it.

Darren Knox, age 48, had been on Thorazine™ for 36 years but was recently changed to Desyral™ and Valium™ and lithium. He had *Ascaris* and hookworm and two dozen more assorted parasites including fluke stages. His brain was also hosting *Bacteroides* and *Nocardia*. All parasites were killed in half an hour by frequency generator at his first visit whereupon he immediately announced himself free of depression; better than the last eight years. He had many metals in his brain, also chlorine. In four weeks his tremor was way down, after dechlorinating his tap water. His depression never came back after dental work was done.

Schizophrenia

Much more mold toxin was seen in schizophrenic families than in other kinds of illness. They usually had four or more kinds of mold toxins at the same time, meaning that one toxin was not detoxified before the next was already eaten. It may reflect on the liver as much as the food selected. The initial injury, though, to the liver may have occurred in early childhood.

Schizophrenia does not require mercury or other dental metal pollution for its expression. This pattern is logical when it is seen that young children can have schizophrenia. Schizophrenia is an ancient illness, being described in some very old literature, before dentistry existed. But parasites existed. And moldy food existed. And copper existed!

Ergot is always seen in sick persons. Other mycotoxins are also present, including *sterigmatocystin, cytochalasin B,* and *aflatoxin.* As the mycotoxin panorama changes, brain symptoms can change from compulsive hand washing to paranoia or from hearing voices to meanness in disposition.

It is my belief that the current increase in violent crime in U.S. society can be attributed to the especially high levels of mold consumption in foods and beverages, with the resultant effect that behavior erupts into violence with almost no provocation, merely some frustration. It would not be difficult or expensive to experiment with a mold-free diet in our prisons.

A bacterium, *Mycobacterium phlei*, may also be a cause because I have seen a high correlation between it and schizophrenia cases. What its specific effects are, I don't yet know. This bacterium may be hiding under teeth. It is also seen in dogs.

Shigella bacteria from nonsterile dairy foods are part of the problem, too. They produce brain and nerve toxins resulting in irritability, depression, anger. In fact, anger can be so intense, it erupts in violence.

Lead and copper are commonly seen in schizophrenia sufferers. The usual source for these is the household water (household plumbing may have lead solder joints). Change plumbing to PVC, then take thioctic acid (100 mg, twice a day).

Parasites always found in schizophrenia are hookworms (4 *Ancylostoma* varieties) in the brain.

Instructions:

1. Stop eating all grain products, nut products and syrups immediately.
2. Sterilize all dairy products.
3. Search for lead and copper in the water.
4. Stop drinking commercial beverages, including bottled water.
5. Zap the parasites in the whole family for three days, followed by repetitions twice a week.
6. Eliminate *Shigellas* with the Bowel Program (page 546).
7. Give away pets. Schizophrenia is too serious to risk reinfection.
8. Do the dental cleanup (page 409).

The need to zap repeatedly arises from reinfection. Nothing needs to be killed twice. But reinfection from self, family members, pets and food happens every hour. One cannot rely on zapping to stay well. Do a thorough diagnostic search of all foods eaten at the last meal, the water drunk, the air breathed. Only when all these are clean, will the brain heal.

When can you eat grains again? When you are well. Find a cereal or pasta that has no mold. Test it for the mold frequencies (77, 88, 100, 126, 131, 177, 188, 232, 242, 277, 281, 288, 295

KHz). Search especially for ergot (295). Remember, ergot makes *lysergic acid diethylamide* (LSD), not a good thing for a schizophrenic brain. Honeys, too, have ergot. Ergot takes longer (up to 20 minutes) to detoxify with added vitamin C. (Read the section on Moldy Food, page 381). If you become ill again after starting grains, go off again. Take 500 mg. niacinamide 3 times a day to speed up ergot detoxification by the liver. Avoidance is much easier.

Healing of the brain is very rapid; in less than one week feelings and behavior are more normal. Perhaps there are herbs that hasten healing; considering how old the illness is, there must surely be several useful herbs. But considering that herbs, too, can be moldy, be very careful to search for molds electronically before using any herbs. Blue vervain, sage, and ginseng are herbs worth trying.

A question may have popped into your mind as well as mine. If the whole family is eating moldy food, why aren't they all schizophrenic? In fact, family members usually do suffer from some symptoms that are similar to the victim. But every person's collection of parasites and pollutants is unique. Certainly, the whole family should obey the moldy food rules, in order to function better.

Autism

Childhood brain disorders suggest an inherited genetic defect. Yet numerous parasites and pollutants are able to pass into the unborn child through the placenta. Even some bacteria and viruses can.

Lead accumulation is always seen in children with autism. Was it acquired before birth?

Mercury can be transmitted from mother to child, too. If mercury fillings were not removed before pregnancy, have them replaced as soon after delivery as possible (never during pregnancy since the removal itself causes a surge of heavy metal to enter the body).

The common tiny worms such as *Ascaris*, hookworm, *Strongyloides* and *Trichinellas* easily enter the brain. They are present in dirt. Dirt enters buildings via shoes. Shoes carry animal filth. Don't let children put their own shoes on until they have learned to avoid touching the soles. Don't let your child crawl on the floor of a public building, even though it looks glossy. Don't set shoes on furniture or table! A preferred habit is to leave shoes at the door.

Once wormlets have found a pathway to the child's brain it is difficult to reroute them. They must all be killed repeatedly since there is daily reinfection from putting hands in mouths. All family members should kill these parasites weekly to protect the child with autism. When lead and parasites are gone consistently for several weeks the pathway to the brain heals and reinfection no longer sends them to the brain and your child can resume a normal life.

I have not treated enough cases to point to a particular parasite or pollutant. For this reason you must do a total cleanup: body, environment, dental, diet (especially solvents and molds).

Leon Dickson, age 10, appeared normal at birth but he crawled and walked late. At age 3½ he began having seizures and was also diagnosed with autism. (Seizures are caused by *Ascaris* larvae, they probably began the routing to the brain). He was started on Phenobarbital™ by his clinical doctor; switched to Dilantin™; then two other drugs were tried. Now he was on Tegretol™ plus Depacote.™ The mother used no anti nausea medicine during pregnancy, no caffeine, no alcohol or nicotine, not even a single aspirin. In spite of his medicines he seemed to have headaches, continued to have seizures which disturbed his sleep and he wasn't trying to talk. He vomited a lot. He would take no pills or drops (no herbs even mixed with honey) and our frequency generator method was not discovered at that time. He couldn't kill his parasites and *Shigellas*. His brain was full of thallium (not mercury!)

besides the roundworm larvae. He must have gotten this from Q-tips™ or cotton balls or some other mercury-sterilized product. Leon's favorite food was grilled chicken which he ate nearly every day, as well as two eggs a day.

His diet was changed to exclude chicken, eggs, bacon, chips, preservatives and colors in foods, grape jelly and strawberry jam. One month later he had not improved, nor had they been able to kill his parasites with the herbal recipe. The diet change was extremely difficult; he was screaming for his favorite junk food and the whole family was upset over his restrictions. But we encouraged the mother to stick to her purpose, get a different baby-sitter who would obey her, and to try to get some parasite herbs and thioctic acid (100 mg. daily, stirred into honey, to take out lead) down him. The first week the new baby-sitter succeeded in getting him to take thioctic acid. He had only one seizure that week. This encouraged the mother to enforce the parasite program and the diet rules. He became attentive in one month and tried to voice sounds.

The problem with eggs is that they are contaminated with *Salmonellas*. I find, however that it is the <u>outside</u> of the eggshell and the carton that is contaminated. The safe way to handle eggs is to remove them and return the carton to the refrigerator, then wash the eggs and your hands before cracking them. Eggs also contain malvin, a known seizure trigger.

Kirk Peeples, age 5, did not have any words yet but he would point to something and voice M-M-M to mean he wanted it (usually food). He was in a special school and "doing well." He had the brain toxin MSG, and antioxidants BHT and BHA accumulated in him. In other words, his liver was not able to detoxify these common food chemicals. At that time, I had not found the mold toxins yet; I would now surmise that they were responsible for the liver's disability. Besides going off these food additives he was "desensitized" to them with homeopathic drops by an alternative allergist. The result was immediate. In one week he tried several new sounds and managed his first word: "box." After killing parasites with the herbal program over a four week time period he could speak 19 words. The parents were bewildered with joy. They cleaned the toxins out of their home so thoroughly, there was no place to sit and nothing familiar to eat. But their son could say things and the parents loved each new sound as if it came from a newborn baby. In two months he was saying two-syllable words and putting phrases together. He needed us no more (he was on homeopathic thyroid drops, too).

Geoff Berkely was diagnosed autistic. He went about his business of examining everything in the office without a word. He was infested with both species of *Ascaris* (there was a pet dog) and was started on the herbal parasite program: just a little less than the adult doses. (Children's' syrups are not as effective.) He was toxic with mercury, too. He had 2 or 3 "baby" root canals. These were to be pulled out. He was also taken off food color, MSG, chicken and eggs. The parents accomplished all this very quickly and called to say their child had become normal but they didn't want us to spread the good news to the "autism" club they attended for fear of criticism for doing unorthodox things. Only in the USA could such thinking occur!

Digestion Problems

Burping, bloating, and being gassy are signs that your digestion isn't perfect. What has gone wrong? Burps are gases escaping upward. Bloating is due to bubbles of gas causing pressure. Your body does not make gas! Gas can only be made by bacteria. The immediate conclusion is that bacteria are growing in your digestive tract (stomach and intestines) that should not be allowed to do so. They are likely to be the common enteric (digestive tract) bacteria: *Salmonellas*, *Shigellas*, *E. coli*, *Bacteroides fragilis*.

You may wish to identify them before killing them with the zapper. Or you can sweep through the whole bacterial and viral range killing all with a frequency generator. The good effects can be felt in an hour, although the last gases may take days to get rid of. *Salmonella* and *Bacteroides fragilis* are two bacteria that can eat bile, and can do without oxygen, so they are commonly seen in the liver. *Bacteroides* probably escaped from its roundworm host, *Ascaris*. *Salmonella* probably came with non-sterile dairy food.

If you have an intestinal problem involving digestion or pain, start immediately to boil all dairy foods. Stop eating those that can't be boiled: cheese sandwiches, yogurt, ice cream. It must be boiled for 10 seconds. The bacteria are in the liver because your liver attempted to strain them out of your blood and lymph in order to kill them with bile. Instead, they turned around and "ate" the bile, turning it brown as evidence. Now, every time the liver lets down bile into the intestine (and stomach), a population of these bacteria goes with it. The intestine becomes a seething mass of bacteria, bubbling away as they produce CO_2, SO_2, H_2S, CO (carbon dioxide, sulfur dioxide, hydrogen sulfide, carbon monoxide). Some of these gases are quite toxic.

Help your liver expel its bacterial overload with liver cleanses (page 552) until all the bile is a beautiful bright green. This is evident as dark brown bowel movements. Without the green color of bile added to your intestine, the bowel movement remains light colored, such as tan, yellow or orange! By stopping eating polluted food, killing bacteria and cleansing the liver, digestion becomes normal again.

Of course, there must be enough acid in the stomach and digestive enzymes produced to make good digestion possible. Otherwise, leftover food goes to <u>feed</u> the waiting bacteria.

Persons with a chronic digestion problem may also find they harbor lead, cadmium, or mercury in the intestine! This is very good in a sense. Your body has kept these toxins <u>in the intestine,</u> preventing it from getting into your vital organs. The bad news is that their presence in the intestine could start an intestinal disease. Toxins in the intestine would inhibit your immune system (here the white blood cells are in clumps called *Peyer's patches*), from gobbling up the "bad" enteric bacteria. Maybe the "good" bacteria found your intestine too toxic to live there. Clean up your dentalware. Search for lead and cadmium in your drinking water. After improving your lifestyle, continue to do liver cleanses. Keep your goals high: a flat tummy that feels energetic, no burps or gas.

Stomach ache (page 98) and **hiatal hernia** (page 133) are also digestive problems but are dealt with under pain. (See also lower abdominal pains, page 97, and appendicitis, page 100).

Alan Barth had his two young sons with him. One of them had a very sensitive stomach, a poor appetite, wanting nothing but sweets or chips to eat. The 16 year old had aches and pains that were keeping him out of sports. The father had a tonsil problem; they swelled if he drank milk. One problem was obvious. Their milk was tainted with *Salmonellas* and *Shigellas*, setting up throat problems for the father, stomach problems for one child and a pain syndrome for the other child. Boiling all their milk, not bringing raw chicken into the house (*Salmonella* source) and stopping eating yogurt and cheese was the solution. There were traces of lead in their tap water and the house air had vanadium in it, announcing a gas leak. They were all heavily parasitized. When these problems were cleaned up, the whole family's health improved.

Kae Nakajima, middle age, had a history of ulcers and stomach problems. She took a lot of Zantac™ and Tagamet™ over the years. She was drinking coffee, tea and colas. She had *Ascaris* and cadmium in her stomach. Five months later she had cleaned up everything except dentalware and was feeling very good. She didn't need any medicines. She still had arthritis and sinus problems but felt so encouraged she had the dental work scheduled.

Sven Lippencott, age 4, had been tube fed for several years due to weak stomach action. He was quite underweight for his age. He had a population of intestinal fluke in his stomach along with arsenic (pesticide). The rest of the family also had intestinal flukes. After killing parasites and washing the upholstered furniture, Sven's appetite went up so he ate more by mouth and grew immediately. But he soon picked up *Ascaris* and cat liver fluke (there was an indoor cat). Then the whole family got intestinal flukes again. They all, including Sven, drank carbonated beverages *ad libitum* (whenever they wished). With both parents working it would not be possible to discipline the habit. Sven had wood alcohol, methyl butyl ketone, hexanedione, methylene chloride and toluene buildup making his recovery hopeless.

Alzheimer's

What was once a rare disease has become a household word because it now affects so many. Two new pollutants of the brain, inviting an old parasite to a location it would not normally be, is the explanation. The new pollutants are solvents that seek the brain.

Xylene and **toluene** are pollutants of popular beverages, decaffeinated powders and carbonated drinks. At first, the body can detoxify these but with a steady stream of solvent arriving, detoxification slows down and parasites begin to build up in the brain. Common fluke parasites which we eat in undercooked meat and perhaps get from our pets, can now reach the brain and multiply there.

Other toxins are also present, such as aluminum, mercury, freon, thallium, cadmium. Aluminum buildup is seen in all Alzheimer's sufferers (100%). This is undoubtedly part of the true cause. Did it come before or after the parasites?

Whatever the answer, your job is clear. Remove every bit of aluminum from the food and environment. Throw out the pots, the aluminum foil, the cookie sheets, the tea ball. Throw out the kitchen salt, the pickles, the baking powder. Buy things made with baking soda (not baking powder), use a plastic salt shaker, buy salt without added aluminum. Stop using commercial soaps and lotions. Make the soap recipes in this book. Finally, tape over all aluminum handles in the bathroom and elsewhere (e.g. the walker) with masking tape. Then find a chelating doctor to help remove aluminum from the brain. Also use thioctic acid (100 mg; take 2 three times a day).

Kill the four common flukes with the first frequency generator or zapper you can get your hands on. Prevent reinfection from meats and pets. Stop all commercial beverages, including water. The processing has left xylene and toluene in them. They are not put in intentionally. For the same reason, health food beverages are similarly polluted. Only milk is safely bought from the store. You must still sterilize it, however. Make your own fruit juices. Select beverages from the list of recipes given. Drink water from your cold water tap, filtering it with a small pure carbon filter as in a filter pitcher (see *Sources*).

As much as xylene and toluene are brain-seeking solvents, *Shigella* is a brain-seeking bacterium. The symptoms it causes are not always the same since they depend on the location of infection. Sometimes they cause tremor, sometimes loss of balance, sometimes speech problems. But they are very serious problems. Kill *Shigellas* every day at bedtime with your zapper. Start the Bowel Program (page 546). When improvement is lasting you know you have stopped reinfecting from your own bowel or from polluted dairy products.

Remove dental metal and use thioctic acid as a help to clear tissues of metal. Use vitamin C (3 grams) and B_2 (300 mg) to assist the liver with detoxification. Use B complex (2 a day) to assist the liver generally. Avoid food molds; ergot especially has strong mental effects (see Moldy Food, page 381).

Start a kidney cleanse (page 549) as soon as you can. Follow this with a liver cleanse (page 552). Clean up environment and diet. Your beloved family member or friend with Alzheimer's can regain her or his mental function to a considerable degree. **Most important is stopping the mental deterioration** before it is not reversible.

Lisa Anne Reed, 60ish, was tentatively diagnosed with Alzheimer's 10 years ago. She needed complete care at present but was able to walk (could disappear quickly) and eat. She could occasionally say her name. Her brain had intestinal flukes and their eggs and was toxic with aluminum (cooking pots) and aluminum silicate (salt). One week later she still had the parasites because nobody could skillfully give her the parasite program. She was also toxic with benzene so reinfection was occurring. In addition she was toxic with bromine (from brominated bread?), chlorine (chlorinated water?) lithium, bismuth, vanadium, and tungsten, all known to have strong brain effects. She was also toxic with moth balls and iridium. She harbored *Naegleria*, another brain parasite. In another week there still were no changes due to inability to administer the treatment.

Isabelita Ufford, 77, was in a wheelchair, brought by her two daughters who took turns caring for her. She was on Clanopin™ medicine, did not try to speak and needed total care, including feeding. She had been ill about seven years. She had intestinal flukes and their stages in her brain (the cerebrum) as well as intestine. She also had isopropanol solvent, aluminum, chromate and high levels of arsenic in her body. She was given the parasite herbs plus instruction to get rid of solvents and metals but the plans could not be carried out. The parasites could not be killed without considerably more help than was available. She was a dear, sweet person. The daughters were highly motivated but were overwhelmed with the size of the task.

Beth Hamm, 60ish, arrived led by her ever-vigilant, ever-caring husband. She was started by medical doctors on EDTA chelation to remove aluminum from her brain. My tests showed aluminum, toluene, sheep liver flukes, asbestos and *Shigella* bacteria. The parasites and bacteria were zapped immediately and her husband began the difficult task of excluding non-sterile dairy products from the diet provided. In four days she was able to walk by herself, knowing where she was going. She could finish a short sentence and comply with directions to sit down and get up. Then she had a set back—she had acquired *Salmonellas* in the brain from a bit of dairy food that had slipped by his attention. She was given Lugol's and she improved further. In ten days she was a new person; an interview of twenty minutes length did not reveal Alzheimer symptoms. Will she be able to hold on to her gains? Only if the aluminum and asbestos are removed from her home environment, his vigilance with dairy food keeps up, and she stays on a maintenance parasite program. But her husband appeared intent on her recovery. She is a person again. And there seems to be a delightful companionship.

Ruben Camberos was brought by his wife and a friend for Alzheimer's. The first day he arrived, the intestinal flukes in his brain were found and killed. He was started on EDTA chelation. They were warned about non sterile dairy foods. His *Shigella* was zapped. Four days later he spoke his first meaningful sentence: it was three words long. He could pay attention to the appointment proceedings. Two days after that he was reading a newspaper. This was utterly shocking to his wife. In another three days, he could hold a conversation consisting of very short sentences. Larger ones became hopelessly garbled. He was started on ornithine (4) and valerian capsules (6) at bedtime: this produced a beautiful nights sleep (especially for his caretakers!) and his days were less agitated. There were still setbacks later but his wife was determined to get him well.

Dementias, Memory Loss

Memory loss is progressive with age but not <u>due</u> to aging. There are plenty of nonagenarians and centenarians with clear minds and good memories to prove that age is not the deciding factor in the dementias. Why do some people deteriorate much sooner? Could you prevent personal deterioration of mental abilities? You probably can. You will know it by noticing memory <u>improvement</u>. Telephone numbers that left you with no recall, unless you wrote them down, number by number, now form groups as you hear them, and you can jot them down the way you always did! This is a good sign of memory improvement. Your writing can improve. The jagged, crooked, misaligned words can be smoothly written again! You can remember things that happened earlier in the day and talk about it later, at mealtime. You can finish your thoughts in conversation.

Mental deterioration of the elderly is not as complicated as is generally believed. Although circulation and blood pressure play a role, **the effect of toxins is much greater**. The action of toxins is greater in age than in youth. The same polluted water and food causes disorientation in the elderly when it only gives a young person a stomach ache.

The liver's detoxification capability may be the real issue. Indeed, the liver may age, in accordance with the calendar date. Perhaps the liver is the only truly aging organ. It may even determine your life span. The answer, then, is to stop giving it toxic substances and shortening your life span.

As the liver is less able to detoxify them, common toxins are allowed to roam the body with the circulation, doing harm to all the organs. The brain feels disoriented or dizzy; there is memory loss. At first, the liver can "catch up" its work and finally clear the toxin for excretion. But, eventually, it can't catch up or keep up. The body, notably the brain, is bathed in toxic chemicals that interfere with its functioning. Now, the elderly person must use a cane for stability, must walk very carefully not to fall, must write everything down to remember it, calls people by their wrong names, can't "find" the right words to speak with, can't finish sentences, must write on a calendar to keep the days straight, starts talking to themselves to help think of things, develops tremors and unsteady gait, acquires a passive personality, loses weight, gets stooped, stops reading the newspaper.

All these signs of aging (dementias) can be reversed by simply removing the common toxins with which we are already familiar.

273

Of primary significance are <u>food molds</u>. These cause brain hemorrhages. Clean up diet, mouth, body, environment, very meticulously.

Of course, an elderly person cannot bring these changes to herself or himself. If you have a loved one with symptoms of aging, and this person is willing to cooperate with you, you can honestly promise them numerous improvements. Spend a good deal of your effort on persuasion since living longer or being healthier may not seem worth giving up a coffee and doughnut breakfast. On the other hand, they might respond to the goal of needing fewer pills, getting into their own apartment again or becoming freed from a walker.

Walter Heffern, 64, had been to various neurologists but could not find any help. He appeared to have the same kind of mental deterioration as his mother, but at a much earlier age. He couldn't understand an ordinary conversation; he constantly spoke about winning money, walked hesitantly and had to be left undisturbed to accomplish anything—even eating and dressing. He needed a lot of care. We found he had *Ascaris* larvae in the brain—in the cerebrum, where you <u>think</u>. He also had *Acanthocephala*, *Dipetalonema* (a chicken roundworm), amoeba (*Entamoeba histolytica*) and *Fischoedrius* in the thinking part of his brain. He had been in the poultry business all his life: his mother probably shared this exposure, as well as other lifestyle habits that gave them solvents and pollutants besides parasites. He had constant ringing in his ears, this could affect hearing an ordinary conversation. He had a water softener that would have supplied a daily dose of aluminum to the brain, too. There always were dogs in the house. Perhaps the marvel is that he was no worse off, a tribute to human strength in general.

Pushing Back Age

This chapter is a tribute to Jimmy, Nazy, Michele, Suzanne, Marlena and all the others who achieved excellence with daily care-taking of Mary Austin, deceased at 97.

It's true that we have to die sometime. But why die before our life span is up? If many people can live to 100 years, then surely this is the human life span, not three score and ten. Some scientists think the true human life span is closer to 140 years! And that we all lead shortened lives. The shortening is due to failure of some organ in us. Other organs are dependent on the failing organ and begin to fail also. When the brain fails, death occurs, sometimes in five minutes.

If we knew which organ is failing, we could come to its assistance and prevent the collapse of the whole body. Often it is easy to see which organ is failing. But whether this is the true beginning of the body's problems we cannot know. Before death there may have been appetite loss. Before the appetite loss there may have been a broken hip. Before the broken hip, dizziness. Before the dizziness a blood pressure or blood sugar problem. Before these, an episode of "flu" or a dental "repair." Sometimes we know what started it all. But often we don't. Just make a guess and begin somewhere.

Diet

If your aging friend or relative is in a home for the elderly, you may be able to persuade him or her to choose a diet that is wiser than the average diet people eat there. This can help a lot. Just stopping drinking the coffee, decaf, iced tea and carbonated beverages that are served, and switching to the recipes in this book could get them off some of their medicines.

The beverages to encourage are sterilized milk and hot water—delicious with whipping cream, honey and cinnamon. This gets them away from solvents, oxalic acid and caffeine.

Old age is not a time when you "no longer need milk." Calcium losses <u>increase</u> in old age. Milk has the organic form of calcium, chelated with lactic acid, and it has the cream to promote absorption. For this reason, milk should never be reduced in fat content (not less than 2%). The cream is <u>necessary</u> to improve calcium absorption.

In old age it is downright dangerous to be taking many calcium <u>tablets</u>. The stomach does not have the acid necessary to dissolve them. They pass into the intestine, disturbing its function and acid levels. With tablets, too, one must be careful with dosages, while food is self limiting. No elderly person would be able to drink more than one cup of milk at a time. This contains 250 mg. of calcium.

Milk, however, requires stomach acid to curdle it as the first step in digestion. If there is not sufficient acid, it will pass undigested into the intestine, causing new problems. We must <u>listen</u> to the elderly when they say milk gives them gas or other troubles.

Having the milk warm to hot helps in getting digestion started in the stomach. Milk served hot with cinnamon accomplishes two purposes: it will stimulate acid secretion and the cinnamon is an insulin aid. Milk served hot with honey adds the nutritive value of honey, displacing the need for other unnatural sweets. The meal should always include something <u>sour</u> to curdle the milk. It does not have to be added to the milk; it can simply be included with the meal somewhere.

Lemon juice or vinegar can be put in certain foods but the most reliable way to get it into the diet is to put 1 tablespoon into the water glass along with a teaspoon of honey. This gives the water a "sweet and sour" flavor, enough to make it interesting throughout the meal. The fresh lemon juice or white distilled vinegar and a honey dispenser that is easy to use should always be on the table. Bring these two items to your loved one at the "home" if it cannot be provided regularly and reliably. Pop in at mealtime to check up on it. Powdered vitamin C (¼ tsp.) is another useful acid if the first two are not effective enough.

The lemon and honey habit, alone, can add years (healthier years) to an elderly person. The extra acid taken with lunch and supper (the stomach has its own best supply of acid in the morning, for breakfast) improves overall digestion and helps dissolve the calcium, magnesium, iron, zinc, manganese, and other minerals in the food so they can be absorbed.

The habit of using vinegar and honey in water as a beverage was made famous by Dr. Jarvis in his book *Folk Medicine*, circa 1960. He recommended apple cider vinegar for its extra potassium. In those days, vinegar was made of good apples. Now, all the regular vinegars have mold in them. The toxin, *patulin*, in moldy apples has been carefully studied by scientists. It taints the vinegar as well as apple juice and concentrate made from them. I have not tested patulin to see if it can be detoxified by vitamin C. We must use only white distilled vinegar, even though it lacks potassium, aroma and popularity. Using a variety of honeys can make up for the need to vary the flavor. Get orange blossom, linden blossom, buckwheat, wildflower, and sage honey, besides clover blossom.

But honey is not perfect food. It usually has *ergot* mold, a very serious toxin. To detoxify the ergot, you simply add vitamin C to the honey as soon as it arrives from the supermarket. This gives it plenty of time to react with the ergot before you eat it. Bring your "fixed" honeys to the home.

If your elderly loved one has not tolerated milk in years, start with the vinegar and honey beverage, or lemon and honey, and be patient until that is accepted. Then add only ¼ cup milk to the day's diet, (in the morning, on homemade cereal). Go up very gradually and only when digestion allows it. <u>Of course, the milk must be sterile</u>.

If it is not sterile, the final warming will only <u>increase</u> the bacterial count. You must be sure of its sterility. Boil the milk yourself. Near-boiling is not hot enough. It must be heated until it bubbles up and almost goes over the container for ten seconds. Use a non-metal pot that holds one to two quarts. You may throw away the skin. Then cool and refrigerate. Supply it to the home, too.

Milk that is marketed in paper containers that need no refrigeration has been sterilized; it is safe.

Once the body, even an aged body, finds a nutritious food that does not cause troubles of its own, it asks for more. Your loved one will accept it and drink it without forceful coaxing, if there is no problem with it. As long as your loved one tries to avoid drinking it, your challenge is to find the problem and solve it. It is <u>not</u> a matter of taste or habit. It is a matter of digestibility and lack of toxicity. When your loved one is drinking three cups of milk (or buttermilk or whey) a day and three cups of water, there will be no room (nor request) for the usual coffee and tea and other bad beverages.

We all must die of something. But it needn't be a stroke, or heart failure, or cancer. Choose what seems to be the most pressing problem to work on. Common problems that plague the aged are brain problems, incontinence, bad digestion, diabetes, tremor, weakness, feeling cold, sensitivity to noise, losing the sense of taste and smell, hearing loss, insomnia, kidney and heart failure.

Increase Oxygen

Brain problems include memory loss, communication deficit, dementia (calling things by inappropriate names and saying

278

inappropriate things). The brain is simply not getting enough oxygen and food to work right. It is like having a pocket calculator with rundown batteries: it will give you wrong answers (without telling you they are wrong). Not enough oxygen to the brain is the main cause of memory loss, inability to find the right words, getting words mixed up and not being able to speak in sentences. You can prove this by providing oxygen from a tank; modern equipment is very easy to use and inexpensive. If your loved one responds well to a few hours of oxygen, you have proof of the problem.

How can you increase oxygen in the brain?

1. Open the blood vessels wider.
2. Increase pressure of blood running through the blood vessels.
3. Raise the oxygen level in the air that is breathed. Less carbon dioxide, tobacco smoke and auto exhaust. All these, including a gas leak from the pipes in the house, compete with oxygen.
4. Increase the oxygen delivery system to the brain by raising hemoglobin levels. Cure anemia and low iron levels.
5. Raise oxygen saturation of blood by keeping body acidity down.
6. Correct a slow and irregular heart beat.

Niacin

Open blood vessels wider by giving **niacin**. Give it early in the morning, upon rising, as soon as the feet are set on the floor. Keep it at the bedside, use small capsules or tablets and combine this chore with water drinking. The water should not be cold and should have nothing added to make it a beverage. (Drinking water within minutes of sitting upright may also move the bowels soon.) A 250 mg. time-release niacin tablet (see *Sources*) is a good choice. The elderly have little side effects. Even the niacin-flush, which reddens the face and neck is welcomed since it gives a sensation of warmth.

The flush is intensified by giving hot liquids or acids (even vitamin C) to drink. The flush is reduced by giving cold liquids. The opening of blood vessels by niacin only lasts a few hours. If you see it has a good effect on your loved one, give several a day. Do not use a prescription variety, since they are polluted with heavy metals; use only the brand in *Sources*, or a brand that you have tested pure. You can freely experiment with niacin to find the best dosage and variety; it is not toxic in this amount; but the size of the tablet should not turn it into an unpleasant chore. Reduce it if it seems too large to swallow. Don't cut tablets in half, the rough edges can scratch the throat.

Hawthorn berry is an herb that opens blood vessels, particularly to the heart. Carefully watch the effect on blood pressure when using it.

Food mold, particularly ergot, has the <u>opposite</u> effect of niacin. Brain blood vessels are made narrower, cutting down the oxygen supply. Ergot is a common contaminant of grains: don't provide rye or pumpernickel breads or crackers. Don't provide wine or other alcoholic beverages; they are too contaminated with ergot and aflatoxin. Narrowing the blood vessels in the brain can lead to stroke. If you notice an attack of dementia coming, try a niacin tablet (100 mg, not timed release) immediately.

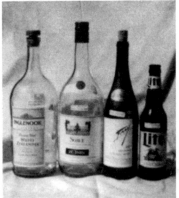

Fig. 34 Alcoholic beverages contain ergot and aflatoxin. Add vitamin C (1/8 tsp.) upon opening and wait 10 minutes for it to act.

TIA's, Strokes and Purpura

Sometimes, the elderly person is aware of the onset of a brain attack; they may see stars or peculiar shapes or lose vision temporarily. These are called *temporary ischemic attacks* (TIA's). Immediately give a 100 mg tablet of niacin, 1 gram vitamin C, and a B-complex in this order of importance.

TIA's are caused by spasming in the brain blood vessels. If this causes them to spring a tiny leak somewhere, a part of the brain will not get its usual oxygen and nourishment. A stroke results.

The spasming was probably caused by sorghum molds. Cooking during the manufacturing of sorghum syrup kills the mold but its toxic byproducts (mycotoxins) are still present. Other syrups may have sorghum added, polluting them. Brown sugar is also polluted with sorghum molds, but fortunately you can detoxify this mold with vitamin C as usual. Mix well ¼ tsp. powdered vitamin C with each new (1 lb.) box of brown sugar.

Purple patches, like bruises, on the hands or arms of an elderly person are called *purpura*, and is also caused by sorghum molds. It weakens blood vessels so they break easily.

When an elderly person has purpura or TIA's and the mold source isn't obvious, you must track it down. Test in a saliva sample for all the sweetenings used recently (at least an hour ago). At the very least, keep notes on all the sweeteners being used. Look for a common one at the next attack. Never let the trigger food be eaten again.

Blood Pressure

Increase blood pressure if it is habitually too low. Blood pressures below 110 may prevent strokes but ruin the quality of life. Low blood pressures are often due to toxins from foods. But severe salt deprivation in the diet can also cause this. If the adrenal glands are not conserving salt properly, too much sodium is allowed to leave the body with the urine, resulting in low sodium levels in the blood and a blood pressure drop. Adrenal performance is improved by taking the kidney herb recipe.

The kidney herbs (page 549), at half dose level (½ cup a day instead of a whole cup) can be given daily for three weeks and then on alternate days indefinitely. Be very careful to keep the herbal tea sterile by reheating. Elderly people seem to sense the improvement given by kidney herbs. Try other kidney herbs from time to time: **shave grass, cedar berries, juniper berries, butcher's broom, cornsilk**. None interfere with drugs. Remember, they also have a diuretic effect. Be prepared to use extra paper padding in underwear to help catch the extra urine output. The first few nights may be disturbed by extra urination. Interpret this positively.

After the blood pressure comes up to 115 (systolic) mental performance will be greatly improved. Don't try to bring it up to 120 since this raises the stroke potential without giving you much improvement in performance. Use an electronic device to measure blood pressure, one with a <u>finger</u> cuff, not an <u>arm</u> cuff which can itself induce broken blood vessels. Purchase a device that needs <u>no</u> adjustments of any kind and has automatic cuff tension control (see mail order catalogs if your pharmacy does not have one).

Air Pollution

Improve the quality of the air by lowering the pollution level. Check into carbon dioxide, carbon monoxide, fumes from a gas stove pilot light, auto exhaust from an attached garage or nearby highway, arsenic from household pesticide, PVC from new plastic curtains or carpeting, formaldehyde from wearing new clothing before washing it, asbestos from hair dryers, freon from a refrigerator, fiberglass, and chlorine from running tap water. Some of these displace oxygen, some are simply toxic to the body and lungs. Clean up the air according to the general principles of environmental cleanup (see Four Clean-ups, page 409).

For the elderly pay special attention to **chlorine** in the air. Shower water puts a lot of chlorine into the bathroom air which then distributes itself through the rest of the house. Notice whether your elderly person goes into the bathroom in fair shape mentally but comes out confused, unreasonable. Not every day's chlorine exposure will have the same effect. Trust your judgment. Attach a carbon filter to the shower head (see *Sources*). Purchase a variety that has very simple-to-replace cartridges. Figure out how long it should last and write the date for replacement on the outside of it for your own convenience.

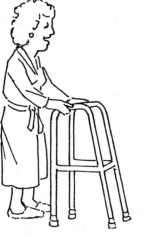 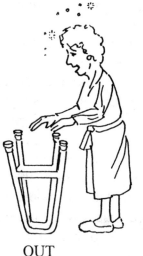

INTO | OUT

When into and out of the bathroom is a different performance suspect chlorine. Put a filter on your faucets.

Fig. 35 Chlorinated water can cause mental symptoms.

Washing hands and face in chlorinated water can give off enough chlorine to trigger a manic episode in a manic-depressive person. Certainly, it is enough to cause mental effects in an elderly person. Of course, the chlorine bleach bottle should not be kept under the sink. It should be kept in a closed plastic bag in the garage. It should not be used while the elderly person is in the house and never for his or her laundry. Use chlorine-free bleach.

Don't pollute the air with fresh flowers, potpourris, or room fresheners. These can induce a dizzy spell.

Room air conditioners may have a <u>fiberglass filter</u>! This fills the house with tiny particles of glass to be breathed by everybody. The body makes tumors out of them in order to stop them from cutting through your tissue. Replace the filter with a foam sheet. This sheet is 1/8 inch thick and washable. I have not found these types of foam filters to emit formaldehyde.

Room air <u>filters</u> are not the answer to polluted air. Removing the pollution <u>source</u> is. Air filters may remove some of the toxic elements but by blowing the air (and dust) around vigorously the remaining toxins are made much more vicious in their effect. The noise of a filter motor and fumes it may put out itself adds misery to the simple job of breathing. Using a <u>non-fiberglass</u> filter at the furnace is a better idea.

Make sure all fragrances are removed from the air, even though family members "like" them. They don't belong in air. The lungs treat them like toxins to be coughed up or removed by the kidneys and immune system. This includes colognes, scented tissues, soap and shampoo and shaving supplies. If you can walk into the bathroom blindfolded and know you're in the bathroom, it's not clean enough. Everything in the bathroom pollutes the air of the whole house. People who must use fragrance should apply it outdoors to keep the indoor air less polluted.

Anemia

Oxygen gets to the brain on a carrier system of tiny rafts called *red blood cells*. They were meant to be an exact shape and size to fit the most oxygen molecules onto them.

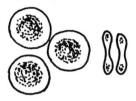

Fig. 36 Red blood cells, top and side view.

Each red blood cell is shaped like a doughnut without the hole. This fits a lot more oxygen, O_2, than round balls would. Yet, if there isn't enough vitamin B_{12}, the dimple isn't put into them to make them doughnut shaped. This reduces the body's oxygen supply and the disorder is called *"pernicious" anemia*. The changed shape of the red blood cells is reflected in a bigger volume called *mean cell volume* (MCV). The correct volume for red blood cells is about 90 cubic microns. Many elderly persons have a MCV over 100!

I have seen pernicious anemia to be associated with *Ascaris* infestation. Kill *Ascaris* on a frequency generator (408 KHz) or zap. The source of *Ascaris* is usually a pet, owned in the past. Once infected, the tiny worms do not leave your body on their own. The infestation may date back to childhood. What a relief for the bone marrow whose job it is to make red blood cells to have enough vitamin B_{12} again! What does *Ascaris* do with your B_{12}? B_{12} is a beautiful rose colored vitamin. Some worms are actually <u>pink</u> from absorbing your B_{12}! Giving B_{12} shots is the current clinical treatment for B_{12} deficiency. Killing *Ascaris* twice a week by zapping and taking B_{12} lozenges (see *Sources*) is a better solution. (If your loved one is getting shots, make sure that no isopropyl alcohol is used on the skin beforehand. Provide vodka yourself in a small pocket flask or 70% grain alcohol for this purpose. Unfortunately, the shot itself may contain traces of this harmful solvent—take a sample home for testing.)

285

Other kinds of "anemia" can deprive your elderly person of oxygen. A low red blood cell count (under 4.4 million/mm^3) is the "garden" variety. Sometimes iron levels are low and can explain the low red blood cell count. Sometimes they are not.

Most regular anemias, including low iron levels, are associated with <u>hookworm</u> infestations.

Kill all *Ancylostomas* along with *Ascaris* twice a week. It is not wise to take iron pills, even if they do raise hemoglobin levels, except in life-threatening situations. Remove the tiny creatures that cause microscopic bleeding instead. Iron in the form of pills is too easily snatched up by bacteria who also need it, making them more virulent to the body. Use grain alcohol rinse in the bathroom to kill *Ascaris* and hookworm eggs under fingernails. Don't have pets in the house or keep them on daily parasite killing herbs.

It takes nutritious food to build the blood back up to its normal hemoglobin level. Eggs and meats (all very well cooked) are the richest sources of iron and other minerals used in blood building. B_6 and other vitamins are also involved and can be given as a B-complex (see *Sources*). Do not use black strap molasses as an iron source, or any molasses, since it contains toxic molds. (The molds could be detoxified with vitamin C the same way as honey. However, I have not tested enough molasses for solvents and you cannot risk these.) In the past, when the nutrient properties of molasses were discovered, the molasses manufacturing was a small, carefully conducted business. Now it has molds which cause platelet destruction, (purpuric spots) internal bleeding, and immune failure.

Acid Levels

Oxygen must first jump onto its raft, the hemoglobin, in the lungs. Later, in the brain, oxygen must jump off again to enter the brain cells. A difference in acid levels makes this possible. Acid levels operate the latching system that decides whether oxygen will be attached to hemoglobin or let go! Acidity un-latches oxygen. There should be no acidity in the lungs so oxygen can attach here. Sometimes, the entire body is too acid! Diabetics, asthmatics, arthritics, especially, suffer from total body acidity.

Acid was meant to be removed from the blood and loaded into the stomach at mealtime for digestion. When this isn't happening, it was meant to be shipped out of the body with the urine. But the kidneys may be doing a poor job because they are clogged with tiny crystals and because not enough water is drunk, so the body's acid levels rise. You can test total body acidity by measuring the pH of the morning urine. It should not be under (more acid than) 5.5. If the body acid level is too high, help the kidneys excrete it by adding more water to the diet and more minerals to neutralize the acid. The main minerals for this purpose are calcium and magnesium.

Increase Minerals

Adding water to the diet could be the most difficult of tasks if your elderly loved one "doesn't like it." Calcium should be in the form of milk, magnesium as a tablet. When tablets cannot be swallowed; use magnesium oxide powder (see *Sources*). Use 1/8 tsp. added to cooked cereal, soup, stew, pudding. Magnesium, being a mineral, does not get destroyed as vitamins may. You can add it anywhere in the diet where it won't be tasted. Notice how calming it is to have extra magnesium in this gradual way. And how much better the sleep is at night.

When water "doesn't taste good," there is probably a valid reason. The body may be trying to reject chlorine or other toxins in it. In this case, filter it with a small <u>all-carbon</u> unit that is changed right on schedule. A plastic pitcher (not clear plastic or flexible plastic) with a carbon pack fitted into the top is best. <u>Sterilize it once a week</u> by putting a cup of water and one tbs. of grain alcohol in it and turning it upside down so the filter can soak for 15 minutes. Flush out the alcohol with two pitchers of water. Make sure the temperature suits the person. Temperature can mean everything to the never-thirsty person. Don't allow ice cubes, however, nor beverage making, with the essential water. Adding lemon or vinegar (white distilled) and 1 tsp. honey is probably the best way to stimulate both thirst and appetite.

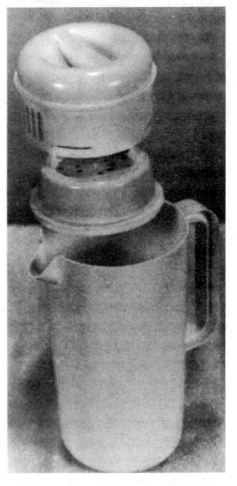

Fig. 37 Water pitcher with filter.

When blood is properly oxygenated it takes on a bright red color, unoxygenated blood is more purple. A chelation doctor can easily see the state of oxygenation.

Chelation

Chelation is a powerful way to quickly improve oxygenation of blood. The most important rule to observe, though, is to take the treatment slowly. Especially if *ethylene diamine tetra acetate* (EDTA) is being used to remove heavy metals, it is important to take the treatment over a two hour time period. Mini doses may be given in a shorter time. Generally, you are in charge of the flow rate. Discuss it with the nurse. Weekly chelations can correct many problems of the elderly that no other treatment could.

Because of hostility from insurance companies who do not wish to add another cost to their ledger and doctors indoctrinated with misinformation, bad publicity is given to this wonderful, life-prolonging mode of treatment. Clinical doctors who have no time to really investigate the statistics of chelation treatments and for whom this is purely competition may feel antagonistic to these treatments. Your loved one should not be the one who must suffer from medical politics. Go to see for yourself what chelation is all about. The receptionist should be glad to show you around. The secret is to talk to the patients themselves. They are usually sitting around a room, eating their lunch and reading as their IV's drip. The pulse, blood pressure and blood chemistry is also carefully monitored. Sit down with them to find out their stories. Get a realistic picture of benefits and costs.

Pulse

The pulse reflects the heartbeat. A **slow pulse** can give weird brain symptoms besides great fatigue. The cause is usually a drug that is being taken to correct a **fast pulse!** Check with the nurse. Read the insert included with packaging for all drugs used. The drugs responsible are usually "beta blockers", used for the purpose of smoothing out the heart beat, that is, making it regular. Often the drug can be changed.

Less than 60 beats per minute will lead to trouble. For a young person it is a good sign to be as low as 60, provided no drug is involved. But for the elderly it does not reflect a strong athletic heart beat.

The heart is made of four separate "chambers" or compartments each pulsing in turn. They are like four horses pulling a wagon. Unless they pull evenly, the wagon feels jerky, and irregular. The wagon will wear out sooner with jerky pulling. To smooth them out you simply slow them down. Apparently they sense each other better and can pull evenly now.

A heart that is beating 100 times per minute, not unusual for a weak old heart, can be so irregular that it misses every fourth beat. That creates a terrible deficiency of oxygen. Imagine your four cylinder car or lawnmower missing one out of four engine strokes! Beta-blockers have some quite undesirable side effects but heart regularity has a higher priority. So drugs are the immediate choice. Later, when heart health is improved, the heart will beat regularly without drug use. In the meantime, watch over the pulse. When the pulse drops below 60 the new danger is slowness. Take the pulse daily when a new drug has been added, or when you are working on heart health, without getting your loved one anxious about it.

Heart Health

To improve heart health, the first steps of course would be to go off caffeine and to kill parasites and bacteria. This alone could drop the pulse from 120 to 80 in a few days. Obviously, the need for a drug is gone. Cut the drug dosage in half immediately. Don't wait for a doctor's appointment to O.K. it. If you waited another day the pulse could be below 60.

Many common bacteria, especially *Staphylococcus aureus*, choose the heart as their favorite location. Their nesting place, though, will be under a missing tooth in the jaw (cavitation). Heartworm and *Loa loa* are two very common heart parasites. You can have all these killed in a day, without side effects and your heart is once more free to beat regularly. Don't take a chance on over-medicating. As soon as the beat is regular and under 100 per minute, reduce your heart drugs. Stop them when you are regular and under 80. Fatigue will leave and the brain will work better.

Raising potassium levels slows the pulse. Try to do this with diet by eating more potassium rich food and by conserving on potassium losses. The adrenals are in control of losses. Give them a thorough cleaning. The adrenals are situated right on top of the kidneys where all toxic things are being excreted. Being this near to the urinary tract will result in shared toxins. Urinary tract bacteria, small kidney stones, moldy foods and metal from dentalware are the chief offenders. Switch to composite tooth fillings. Use non-metal jewelry. Cook and eat with non-metal ware. Don't handle metal unconsciously throughout the day. Aluminum objects that must be touched should be wrapped in masking tape: this includes walker, shower door, bathroom supports.

Door knobs, taped walker handles, and cane handles should be wiped daily with a grain alcohol solution.

Treat the adrenal glands to 5 supplements

1. **Vitamin C:** shake some into all foods that can absorb a bit of the sour taste, even cooked cereal and vinegar water.
2. **Pantothenic acid:** 500 mg., one daily.
3. **B$_6$:** 250-500 mg. daily.

4. **Folic acid:** 800 mcg. daily.

5. **B$_2$:** 150 mg. daily. These are minimum dosages.

If no capsules or tablets can be swallowed put a three day supply in a heavy plastic bag. Pound with a hammer; then roll finer with a big glass jar. Use about 1/3 of the mix each day. If you are trying to do all this in a nursing home, feed it to your loved one while visiting. Put the powder mix in a plastic (not styrofoam) cup, add honey and stir until you get a paste. Feed the paste directly by spoon. Often the elderly prefer it this way in order not to bother with pill taking at meal time. Remind them it will turn the urine yellow.

When the brain problems are corrected for an elderly person, be sure to relate the improvement to him or her. Improvements should not be dismissed lightly. Keep notes. This encourages the elderly, letting them know their existence and quality of life is important to you. Improvements are not merely steps to yet further improvements. Enjoy each bit of progress; it is often too subtle for your loved one to notice even when it is glaringly obvious to you. Before and after a chelation treatment can show a dramatic change in mood, energy, appetite and communication ability, yet get no comment from your loved one. Point it out explicitly so your loved one can look forward to it, too.

Aging is no fun. The elderly long for a brisk gait, laughter, and a picnic at a park again. They dwell on dying, though, because they know it isn't far away and wonder what to do about it. They dare not talk about it because it is too painful a subject for the loved ones. And the immediate problems are too pressing to allow much contemplation of future problems. Talk about aging in its positive aspects. Let your loved one express feelings about it.

Incontinence

plagues most elderly persons. It begins to plague women much earlier—after childbirth, for instance. Surgically shortening the bands that hold the bladder in position (called bladder "lifting") can give temporary relief, but the surgeon may be the first to tell you that it is a temporary fix. Still, it is so shocking not to be able to run a few steps or sneeze or cough without wetting the underwear, that anything seems better than doing nothing. Surgeons will tell you that the bands have been "overstretched."

The real reason why nothing, not even surgery, is permanent is that the support bands are <u>weak</u>. Bacterial invasion causes most of this weakness. Low potassium levels (due to excess potassium losses by the adrenals) causes more weakness. When you kill bacteria (and *Schistosomes* and *Ascaris* and other parasites that bring in bacteria) and blood potassium levels go up, the problem is solved. Overnight you may throw those pads away. Even though you needed three pads to be "safe" you will not need <u>any</u>. Whether you have killed bacteria permanently determines whether you have permanently cured the condition. Make sure all dairy foods are absolutely sterile. Ask that the milk be boiled for ten seconds and other foods that can't be sterilized are not on the menu, like sour cream. Sour cream has too much *tyramine* to be safe. Tyramine is a bacterial by product that is quite toxic; it is rather high in aged cheese, also. With the food bacteria, *Salmonellas* and *Shigella*, out of the way and parasites being killed regularly, you can focus attention on the adrenals which control potassium levels.

Be careful not to rave about the foods that your loved one cannot eat.

Eating more potassium in food is a good nutrition project. Bananas are the top choice. Fresh fruit salad and baked potatoes and soup also provides a lot. Mixing potassium salt with regular salt, half and half, for the shaker is another easy trick, even if you only use it in cooking where the taste cannot be detected. Potassium by prescription is often used by clinicians to conserve body potassium during diuretic use. This need not be stopped (if the pills are not polluted) although taking potassium pills is less useful than salting it in because the adrenals will let any big dose escape anyway. A sign of <u>too much</u> potassium is a slow pulse.

It may be necessary to wear some kind of incontinence underwear. Try to avoid them at night, though, so the skin can breathe freely. Bring a commode near the bed for the night, rather than diapering your loved one (but don't call them diapers; say "underwear"). Absorbent pants of all kinds are heavily chemicalized. This is absorbed by the skin and adds to the toxin level. Less will be absorbed if you powder the skin with cornstarch first. Use them minimally and line them with tissue or paper towel. Chair and bed pads, too, are chemicalized. Don't sit on them with bare skin. To facilitate getting to the commode quickly in the night, dress the elderly in a short night shirt, no pajamas or long gown. Bed socks on the feet help with warmth.

Wash the body parts daily, around the urinary and rectal outlet, using borax water. Follow with 5% grain alcohol. Put washcloth in laundry after a single use. Nothing, not even brain improvement, impresses and encourages an elderly person as much as seeing the incontinence lessen. This bit of progress will put him or her solidly on your side. When they believe in you, it makes your task more rewarding. Remember to enjoy and celebrate your achievements together; don't make a grim business out of it.

Bad Digestion

with its excessive gas and burping is another plague of the elderly. They would rather not go to church nor visit a friend than embarrass themselves in that way.

Chewing

It all begins with the stomach although chewing food well is essential for really good digestion. Dentures should fit perfectly so the mouth does not develop sores. Using denture cream is not a good substitute for correct fit and is toxic. Denture plastic is often toxic, even containing mercury in its composition! Toxins in plastic can seep! Such toxins lower the immunity of the mouth and throat and stomach since it all flows down into the stomach. Low immunity in the mouth permits throat infections to be chronic. If your elderly loved one has a red-looking mouth or throat, instead of pink, an infection is going on in spite of no coughs and no complaints.

It will do no good to keep zapping bacteria when reinfection is so easy. First kill the bacteria in the dentures by soaking in 70% grain alcohol. Then test the dentures for <u>toxins</u>. Soak the dentures in water for several hours. Rinse and soak again in fresh water. Repeat a third time to insure that any toxin found came from the dentures, not the saliva. Save this water for testing. Search for heavy metals in the denture water. If you find any, you know the dentures are toxic! <u>Get new ones</u>, made of uncolored methacrylate (see Dental Cleanup, page 409).

The denture-soak should kill bacteria each night. Plastic has tiny pores where bacteria can hide. Use 70% grain alcohol which you make yourself or plain vodka which is about 50% alcohol. Since alcohol evaporates and is expensive, use a wide mouth jar with close fitting non-metal lid for all this. Fish them out with your toothbrush so it gets sterilized too. It only takes minutes to kill everything. Commercial denture cleaners are much more toxic than grain alcohol; don't use them.

Use food grade hydrogen peroxide or salt water to brush teeth in your mouth, **never toothpaste**. Toothpaste has toxic metals (tin, fluoride, strontium) besides benzene pollution. See the section on brushing teeth (page 532) for details and sources. If you are responsible for this daily chore, use homemade floss (2 pound to 4 pound nylon fish line) first; then brush. If your loved one is seated they may be able to handle the brush by themselves, giving them pride in the achievement.

If an elderly person refuses or can't wear dentures, provide food that is soft and without chunks since this decides whether the stomach can digest it. The stomach is the weak point of the digestive process for the elderly because nearly all don't produce enough acid to get the job done.

Stomach Acid

The body produces hydrochloric acid (HCL)which gets pushed into the stomach from the blood! The enzyme, *carbonic anhydrase*, a zinc enzyme, is involved. Not many ways are known to stimulate this whole process. Drinking water before meals stimulates it in unknown ways but is hard to do for the elderly. Next best is to provide acid.

Because strong HCL would dissolve teeth it is not available as a solution to aid digestion. Ask a pharmacist to make a 1% HCL solution and use 10 drops of it in a beverage at mealtime once a day. HCL as a tablet ("Betaine HCL") is available but doesn't have enough HCL in it.

Using a lemon or vinegar and honey beverage helps with digestion although this provides <u>citric or acetic acid</u>, not hydrochloric. These acids are completely metabolized so they don't add to the body acid level. But the fact that it is not hydrochloric means that it can't kill bacteria and parasites in the stomach like regular hydrochloric acid could. The stomach becomes a haven for *Salmonellas* and other bacteria and this is **the biggest digestive plague of the elderly.** *Salmonellas* dig deep into the stomach wall, safe from antibiotics and stomach acid and aren't washed away with the food. When they take over the region near the top of the stomach, it weakens the esophageal sphincter and food keeps coming back up a bit—a most uncomfortable development, especially after supper or when lying down.

When the Salmonellas spread out further to invade the diaphragm around the sphincter, the diaphragm weakens, and lets a bit of the stomach up through the hole.

This causes *hiatal hernia* distress. Don't settle your loved one in an easy chair after supper. This presses the stomach upward and the food up, too. Leave them sitting at the table a while, then walk a bit, to get the food down lower. The food will sink lower if some of it can leave the stomach at the lower pyloric end. But if *Salmonellas* are entrenched here, too, the lower end does not have enough action to push the food through the valve. Drugs like Reglan™ are given to speed this up.

What helps most is getting digestion completed. This sets up the natural cues for emptying. Digestive enzyme tablets have been in popular use to help digestion. But they may not be safe since they have not been sterilized. Always try the vinegar and honey method first. Coughing during eating is a sign that the diaphragm is irritated (by a hiatal hernia). If drinking water starts the coughing, omit it at the beginning of meals. Work in sips during the meal.

Salmonella and Shigella

Some *Salmonella* infections can bring dizziness to your elderly person. Dizziness is another plague of the elderly, keeping them from going shopping, getting to church and even from getting around their own homes. Drugs such as Antivert™ are given but only take the edge off the problem. Feeling dizzy can make your loved one home bound and stuck to a walker for every move.

Salmonellas, along with *Shigellas,* produce very toxic substances that cause dizziness. There are three common *Salmonella* varieties: *Salmonella enteriditis, Salmonella paratyphi,* and *Salmonella typhimurium* (386, 380, 354 KHz). Kill *Salmonellas* daily for a month by taking Lugol's iodine (6 drops in a half cup water, after meals and bedtime, see *Recipes*). Unfortunately, this will not kill *Shigellas*; follow the Bowel Program (page 546) to get them.

During this time set up a system of sterilizing all dairy products (see Milk, page 425) since this is the source of reinfection. Set up a system of rinsing fingers (and fingernails) in 10% grain alcohol in the bathroom. Deli food and restaurant salads carry *Salmonellas* and *Shigellas,* too. Kill them, routinely, after eating such food due to necessity. A warm stomach full of food at a neutral pH is just the right culture condition for these bacteria. It's like putting yeast into a bowl of warm water, flour and sugar. In half an hour it is overflowing with growth.

Once *Salmonella* is entrenched in an organ it is difficult to eliminate. Only an electric zapper can kill them all (in an organ, not the bowel). If your body has the right conditions (like a low acid stomach) to let them grow you dare not swallow another one! *Shigellas* arrive with dairy foods, too, but prefer the lower intestine as their headquarters. Indigestion that starts right after eating is probably due to *Salmonellas.* If your indigestion comes in the night, this suggests *Shigellas,* since they've had time to reach their favorite place further down.

Campylobacter and *E. coli,* other digestive bacteria, are sometimes the culprits. The Bowel Program is effective against these also. Besides getting digestive improvement you get mental improvement, less depression, less dizziness, less irritability after clearing these up. Remember that eating bacteria and killing them later will not solve the problem. Stopping eating them will.

Other Clues

Digestion problems that remain after eliminating bacteria can be diagnosed in a rational way. Ask these questions:

- Is the stool orangish-yellow, or very pale, instead of greenish brown? If so, bile isn't getting delivered to the small intestine from the liver.
- Is there abdominal pain? (More about this on page 97). It may be due to *Ascaris,* flukes, or other parasites.
- Is there constipation? This will let wastes accumulate, all the longer for bacteria to thrive on them.
- Is there bloating? This is due to gas made by bacteria.
- Does the stool float? If so, it must be lighter than water and contain fat or a great deal of undigested material.

Liver Bile

Bile is necessary for digestion. Absorption of fat and calcium depends on bile mixing with the food. When fat isn't absorbed, it stays in the intestine. Fat is lighter than water; it makes the stool float. Feces should not float. When the stool floats you can assume that calcium isn't being absorbed either, leaving the blood in a deficit which will be taken from the bones.

If the stool floats or is orangish in color prepare your elderly person for a liver cleanse (page 552) to clear a bile duct of obstruction. They get quite fond of these cleanses and will ask to have one. Liver cleanses are completely safe, even for persons in their 80's. One of the stones pictured on page 554 came from a woman age 97. The general rules apply to the extremely elderly: kill all parasites first by zapper if possible, otherwise by herbal parasite killing. Do a kidney cleanse (page 549) first, using half a dose instead of the regular dose, for three to six weeks. Attend your loved one in person for the liver cleanse, have a commode at bedside, protect bedding from accident: use paper underwear if necessary. Share the joy of getting gallstones out painlessly with your loved one; let them see and count them if they wish before you flush them (use a flashlight).

Be extra careful with the skin cleansing. Hot water soothes and heals. Use starch skin soother to dispense onto the wet paper towel, besides borax solution and alcohol. Don't use ordinary soap. The starch skin softener gives the smoothness of soap, and prevents the pain of friction. An elderly person may have no diarrhea at all with the Epsom salts! Evidently the body absorbs all the magnesium so eagerly, none is left in the intestine to absorb water and create diarrhea. It is especially important though to rehydrate your elderly person after a diarrhea. This time they do not balk at water consumption. The liver cleanse, it seems, gives them new thirst as well as new appetite. But it doesn't last long. As the stones from the far corners of the liver move forward, they compact into larger stones and plug the ducts again. Their previous symptoms return. Try to give a cleanse once a month until the dark color of the stool returns and it no longer floats.

The benefits of a liver cleanse will last longer if **valerian herb** is taken the day after the cleanse and from then forward. It may be preventing spasm of the bile ducts. Use 2 oz. of the herb (cut) in 3 cups water. Simmer for 5-10 minutes, let settle or strain. Add honey to sweeten. Give a few tbs. every 4 hours (or 6 capsules) for several days followed by a daily dose at bedtime.

Constipation

If constipation is a problem, use an herbal product rather than a drug until you have removed the cause. **Cascara sagrada** (half dosage) or **prunes** work for many people. Adding **roughage** to the diet is a good solution but often doesn't work. If you try bran, you should add vitamin C and boil it, first, because it is very moldy. But even eating tree branches for supper won't move a bowel that has the wrong bacteria in it.

Bacteria are part of the cause; and part of the result! Constipation increases the bacteria level which causes further constipation! You may solve the constipation problem immediately by zapping. Even though this kills some "good" with some "bad" bacteria, no harm is done. The stool is recolonized in one to two days.

Poop Your Troubles Away

Two bowel movements a day are the minimum necessary for good health. The first one should be in the morning. The morning cup of water, drunk at the bedside has the magical ability to move the bowels. Cold water may fail. But the water effect only works in the early morning. Waiting until after breakfast may not work. Notice the energy lift your loved one gets from this most primitive body cleanse. Take advantage of this to exercise them. Go immediately for the morning walk. This might be the only time of day they can <u>enjoy</u> their walk.

Walking and **liver cleansing** are <u>the most</u> health-promoting activities you can do for your loved one.

Make walking as essential as eating. Walking is not merely walking about the house or shopping. Walking should be done outdoors. Walking is a brisk exercise, done as speedily as possi-

301

ble and lasting at least ½ hour. Only if the weather doesn't allow outdoor walking can an indoor walk be substituted. Don't let your elderly person choose whether they will walk that day. To overcome resistance, find a cheerful neighborhood person willing to do this task for pay. The need to respond to a new stranger energizes the elderly more than your persuasion can.

Sugar Regulation

Diabetes is a common development in the elderly. If your loved one is already on a pill for beginning diabetes, take this as your challenge never to let it get worse. It is not a chronic metabolic deterioration. It is a destruction of the pancreas (specifically the islets) by the pancreatic fluke which is attracted to the pancreas by wood alcohol. Zap flukes and eliminate wood alcohol as described in the section on diabetes (page 173).

Use no artificial sweetener and no beverages besides milk, water and the recipes given in this book. This is one regimen your loved one will not resent. They are well motivated to prevent the need for giving themselves daily shots of insulin. Use this motivation to acquire the taste for new foods and beverages.

Elderly Person's 7 Day Diabetic Diet

Daily supplements: 4 chromium (200 mcg. each), 1 or 2 B-50 complex, vitamin C (1,000 mg. or ¼ tsp.). Take with food.

Breakfast

Choose any one; they need not be in order.
1. Two eggs, (replace carton and wash hands and eggs before cracking), wheat-free, corn-free bread, not toasted (special breads can be found in the freezer section of natural food

302

stores), with butter and 1 tbs. orange blossom honey. 1 peeled pear, raw, with whipping cream. One cup hot milk with cinnamon.

2. Old fashioned oats, with 1/4 tsp. cinnamon and 1/8 tsp. vitamin C, stirred in just before serving. Mix whipping cream with sterilized milk to make a "half n half" for the cereal. 1 tbs. honey. 1 banana. One half cup milk, one half glass water with honey and vinegar.

3. Fried potatoes with 2 eggs (use only butter, olive oil or lard), 1 cup hot or cold milk. A quartered orange (wash the orange before quartering).

4. Cream of rice, with homemade "half n half" or whipping cream, cinnamon and vitamin C stirred in. 1 cup milk, 1 banana.

5. Cottage cheese, cooked in covered skillet to sterilize. Add chives or peeled fruit (not canned). Wheat-free, corn-free bread, or rice bread with 1 tbs. honey. 1 nectarine or piece of melon. 1 cup hot milk. Water with vinegar and honey.

6. Pancakes or waffles with butter and eggs (no sweetening). Fruit (peeled), hot milk, water.

7. Fruit cup, large bowl of peeled, chopped mixed fruit with whipping cream and 1 tbs. honey and rice bread or other wheat-free, corn-free bread with unsalted butter. 1 cup hot milk with cinnamon.

Remember, all honey must be pretreated with vitamin C. All fruit is peeled and free of blemishes and soft spots. All milk, cream, butter must be sterilized for 10 seconds at full boiling point. Butter must not be "raw". Get wheat-free, corn-free bread at a natural foods store.

Lunch

It is better to have most of the day's calories in the middle of the day than at the end. Arrange for <u>dinner</u> at noon if possible.

Dinner

Choose any one.

1. Green beans with potatoes, meat dish, cabbage apple salad, water with lemon juice and honey, 1 cup hot milk. Water.

Fresh green beans, especially fava beans contain a substance that is described in old herbal literature to be especially beneficial to diabetics. Don't overcook them—it might harm this substance.

For the same reason, don't use canned green beans. If "fresh" isn't possible, choose "frozen" but rinse the chemicals off before cooking. Potatoes (not overcooked), peeled to make sure there are no blemishes (contain mold and pesticide) can be cooked with the beans. Cook with onions and oregano for flavoring. Add fresh chopped parsley to the sauce or butter for both green beans and potatoes. Fresh parsley has special herbal goodness (high magnesium, high potassium, diuretic.)

The meat dish should be overdone. "Fast food" is plopped from the freezer into the boiling grease which browns the outside nicely but can easily leave the inside undercooked. Meat must never be "rare." There should be no redness near bones! Canned meat is safe from parasites but may have smoke flavoring added (contains benzopyrene) or nitrates. Avoid these chemicals. Avoid MSG too. Whenever a meat dish is not accepted, substitute sardines. Let them choose from a display of six kinds. Purchase the flip-top cans to avoid eating metal grindings from the can opening process.

Cabbage for salad should be chopped fine enough to be digestible. Add finely chopped apples (peeled) and a few apple seeds and whipping cream for the dressing.

Sweet things are reserved for dessert. Since a diabetic's tissues are not absorbing sugar, they crave it more and more. As the diabetes improves they crave it less. For dessert, serve 1 tbs. of honey to satisfy this craving without endangering their blood sugar regulation. It can be used in the hot milk or in other ways. Undercooking the vegetables also helps slow down the sugar release. Never serve mashed potatoes for this reason.

The drinking water should always have a little vitamin C, lemon juice or vinegar added, and 1 tsp. honey if desired.

2. Asparagus, potato, raw salad, fowl dish, fruit, water with vinegar and honey, 1 cup hot milk.

The asparagus can be fresh or canned. Bake the potato: not in aluminum foil, not baked until fluffy. Don't let the skin be eaten. Use genuine butter, only, or a homemade sour cream dressing (see *Recipes*). Fresh chopped chives may be added but no regular sour cream since this is very high in *tyramine*, a brain toxin.

The raw salad should be chopped small enough to be edible by dentures. Use homemade salad dressing with a preference for oil and vinegar styles.

The fowl dish should be very well done, never "fast food".

For dessert, fresh fruit chunks dipped in a homemade honey sauce (honey, water and cinnamon). Less sweets are consumed if you dip the fruit rather than pour the sauce over. Limit the total to 1 tbs. honey. Don't serve grapes or strawberries due to the intense mold problem.

3. Soup, sandwich, fruit, hot milk, water.

Soup should be homemade from scratch. Add bones and 1 tbs. vinegar (white distilled) or a tomato to the kettle to ensure some calcium leaches out of the bones. A fish chowder serves this purpose very well, too.

The sandwich has lettuce, real butter, and whatever else tastes good (no cheese, bacon bits or condiments). The bread is wheat-free, corn-free, stored in freezer. Homemade salad dressing can be added.

The fruit may be chopped with whipping cream, cinnamon and honey sauce (not more than 1 tbs. honey).

The water may be plain if there was vinegar in the soup.

4. Fish, green beans, potatoes, other greens, fruit, hot milk, water.

Fried or baked fish is served with lemon or lime. Green beans are served with a cheese sauce so a lot will be eaten. (Cheese sauce: add milk, olive oil to a block of cheese. Melt and cook at least 10 seconds.) Serve au gratin potatoes or scalloped potatoes or any kind of potatoes that will be enjoyed. The extra greens can be beet greens, collards, mustard greens or spinach served with a favorite dressing to make sure it's eaten. (No croutons or bacon bits, though.)

Never serve dessert if the plate has not been cleared. Your loved one isn't hungry enough. If appetite is very poor, sweets will only worsen the problem. Try to change the menu to stimulate the appetite. Acid foods stimulate; spices and B-vitamins (especially B_1) stimulate; hot foods stimulate. Much appetite is controlled by the liver and brain. Toxins at either location (especially food-derived toxins) tell the body to <u>stop eating</u>. Suspect food molds first, bacteria and chemical additives next.

5. Asparagus, meat dish, white rice (brown rice contains mold), coleslaw, milk, water, ice cream.

A hot meat dish (no pasta, no wheat flour, no regular gravy) can be fried, cooked or baked, but not grilled. Asparagus is fresh, frozen or canned. Rinse if frozen. Fix it differently than last time. Season rice with parsley and minimal salt and pure herbs like thyme; no MSG or mixed seasoning, make butter sauce. Dessert is homemade ice cream (see *Recipes*).

6. Fish or seafood hot dish. Green peas or peas and onions. Peeled sweet potato with butter (not canned). May switch sweet potato with rice on asparagus day. Sliced tomatoes or cucumber or other raw vegetables with or without dressing. Milk, 1 tbs. honey (can be used on sweet potato).
7. Chili or stew with unlimited rice-bread and butter. If chili produces gas, stay away from it. Serve no canned varieties. Grated carrot salad with stewed raisins added and heavy cream. Milk, water as usual. Blueberry pie, sweet potato pie, custard pie.

If more bread is requested, provide a wheat-free, corn-free variety; but limit bread eating to "after main dish" eating. If not enough milk is drunk: make custard pudding or rice pudding so the daily amount (3 cups) is consumed.

Supper

1. Tuna with salad dressing or tuna salad (no pasta). Non-wheat raisin bread (from natural foods store) and butter. Milk, water.
2. Custard, cooked greens, baked potato. Rice-bread and butter. Herb tea with milk added (single herb only, not mixed herbs).
3. Vegetable soup, homemade, from scratch. Leftover meat sandwich with rice-bread (no deli or cold cuts or luncheon meat). Milk, water.
4. Baked squash with butter, rice pudding with cinnamon, raisins, and honey. Canned salmon or sardines with wheat free, corn free bread. Milk, water.
5. Chili or stew leftovers with wheat free, corn free bread. Custard pudding sweetened with honey, and nutmeg/cinnamon mix. Milk, water.

6. Sardines and rice bread or other wheat free, corn free bread. Homemade tomato juice with celery, strained. Milk, plain water. Pie a la mode (homemade pumpkin or squash pie and homemade ice cream).

7. Potato salad. Leftover meat dish and beans, stewed tomatoes, squash. Baked apple with cinnamon, cream and honey. Milk, water.

Many diabetics lose 50 points (mg/DL) of blood sugar in a few days on this diet. This is why: there is less bread than a diabetic would prefer. There is very little cheese (it must always be boiled in a sauce to sterilize). There is no fruit or vegetable juice except homemade, and not much of that because it crowds out milk and water. If your elderly loved one can't eat all this, make sure there are no snacks consumed between meals that are forbidden.

There is no pasta anywhere. Pasta is mold-ridden. Even after cooking, it may be toxic. There is no wheat or corn bread. The menu is heavy on green beans and asparagus and cinnamon. If by chance, your elderly person hates these and starves themselves to get your sympathy, add a lot more potatoes and rice (never brown) to raise calories.

There is no sweetening other than honey (5 kinds). There are no syrups or sugars. Honey is self limiting—the taste for it is all gone after 1 tbs. Not so for other sugars. The heavy use of cream and butter is offset by no deep fat fried food and little cheese.

Keep in mind that this diet may reduce the need for insulin almost immediately. You may have to cut it in half! But how would you know this? The morning blood sugar test is essential to keep track of changing circumstances. Don't neglect it. Be careful <u>not to use rubbing alcohol</u> when making the finger stick (use vodka or grain alcohol). Your elderly person will feel it is all worthwhile (doing without coffee or pie) if one less insulin shot is needed or if they can go back on tablets instead of insulin. Or even just the knowledge they are staying well controlled and will never have to take insulin shots. Remember to give yourself the credit for a fine accomplishment when your loved one's diabetes improves.

Diabetic Supplements

Several supplements are especially good for diabetics:
- Fenugreek seeds, 3 capsules with each meal.
- Fresh vegetable juice made of raw green beans and carrots (½ cup total).
- Bilberry leaves. Maybe they have something in them that helps detoxify wood alcohol, since bilberry leaves are good for eyes, too. Get in capsules or make a tea.

Diabetic Eating Out

Since the rules are always somewhat relaxed when "eating out" a diabetic loved one will badger you to go out with them. If rules are sure to be broken, calculate it into the rest of the day so you can compensate for it.

Extra Diet Tips For The Elderly

Food should taste good.

Eating is a fundamental pleasure of living. In old age there is no other pleasure that can equal enjoyment of food. It is a time when we long for the foods of our own childhood, too. Ethnic foods often had to be given up when children were raised (switched to hot dogs and pizza) but with this diversion gone, a return to family food would be most welcome and most healthful. Ethnic foods were made from scratch. And they certainly were made at home where cleanliness and "persnickitiness" are at their finest! A speck in the batter gets noticed. Not so in a commercial mixing vat. Pots and pans are sanitized with hot water, not chemicals.

Good advice is to return to old fashioned home cooking: with its flour and butter, lard and cream, homemade pasta, olive oil and soup, coarse cereal grains and plain fruit. Gone are the fruit juices, flour mixes, crackers and sweets that fill grocery shelves. What about convenience? Old fashioned cooking took most of the day. It does take 3 or 4 hours to make a soup from scratch. But you then get 3 days off! Each day you reboil it, it is sterile again. Or freeze half of it (take the potatoes out first). It does take a whole morning to make pasta or some ethnic dish. Freeze it in plastic sealed containers so the delicate flavor isn't spoiled. Baking homemade bread is automated now. Do at least this much to get away from the mold-ridden grocery store loaves. Make your own ice cream and nut butters. They last many days and free your schedule.

Time is the great inhibitor but if you have the means or the help, the best advice, nutritionally, is a return to old-fashioned cooking and recipes. Use your new insights to improve them where you can. Don't use your mother's aluminum ware; use her enamel ware or the new glass and ceramic ware. Don't use her copper-bottomed tea kettle or gold-rimmed cups or "silver". Use her wooden spoons, glass glasses, and plain dishes, her wooden and straw bowls and enamel pots and pans.

Salt

Should you avoid salt? No. But a good salt rule is to either cook with it or have it on the table, but not both. Use aluminum-free sea salt, and make sure the salt is sterilized by heating five minutes at 400°F in a glass pie plate to kill mold. (Sea gulls fly over the salt flats where sea salt is gathered. Their droppings provide a medium for mold.)

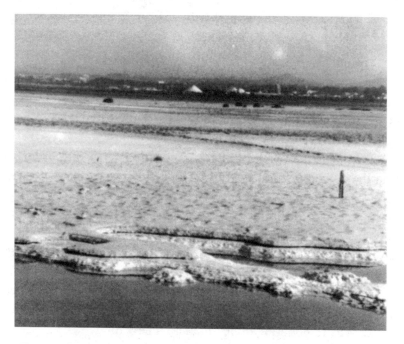

Fig. 38 Sea salt flats are often roosting places for sea gulls.

The <u>best</u> salt is a mixture of 1 part of your aluminum-free, sterilized sea salt and 1 part potassium chloride (another kind of salt, see *Sources*). Potassium ousts sodium (salt) from your body, so you can use twice as much of this kind of salt! Also, the extra potassium helps lift fatigue and has other benefits.

Always use a non-metal salt shaker with a closable lid to keep out moisture. Don't put rice in your salt because it invites mold.

Since you, the cook, know where the salt is, (mostly in soups and stews), don't serve as much of these when there is heart and kidney illness or high blood pressure. Don't put salt in cereal, cooking vegetables, or other dishes. Just leave it out! Use herbs instead. **Tip:** encapsulated herbs stay fresher and are more potent. Fenugreek and thyme are the most beneficial of the common cooking herbs. Just open a capsule and season.

Tremor

Tremor is a symptom, not a natural part of aging. The nerves controlling the hands and arms are poisoned. The nerves originate in the brain where the poison has accumulated. What is the poison? Did it happen long ago? No! It could have happened as long as two weeks ago <u>but not longer</u>!

Tremor is the result of <u>ongoing</u> poisoning! It is important to find the poison as soon as you can since the rest of the body will soon be affected, too. Search your memory for the new things that happened in the last two weeks. It is a herculean task but only gets harder each day, so keep notes as you ask: Is there new carpeting? Is there a new furnace? Is there a different water supply? Is there a new hair dresser? Did somebody bring a vase of fresh flowers? Is there a new laundry person? Was the place sprayed for insects? Is there a new medicine (drug) or supplement? Was remodeling done? Is there a new food?

The list is endless and the situation looks hopeless because so many new things can happen in two weeks.

Rather than asking individual questions like these, let's ask only **five general questions** and have the assurance that one of them will catch the culprit.

1. Is it in the **air**? This will catch insecticide, flowers, carpets all together.
2. Is it in the **water**?
3. Is it in the **medicines** or **supplements**?
4. Is it in the **clothing**?
5. Is it in the **food** or on the dishes?

To answer each question, test the item using your Syncrometer searching technique. Make a test substance. Then search a saliva sample for it.

To test the air, take a dust sample off the kitchen counter or table (this gives you fresh dust). Pick up the dust with a few wipes by a small, two inch square of damp paper towel. Place in a resealable baggy.

To test the water, make samples by putting about a tsp. of hot, cold, or filtered water into a resealable baggy with a bit of paper towel in it. Try to get the first morning water before it has run.

To test the medicines and supplements put one of each in resealable baggies.

To test clothing (laundry) use a bit of it, (such as a sock) rolled up tightly.

Testing food is the biggest job. If there are leftovers in the refrigerator or freezer, this helps. You can combine all the leftovers in a single baggy. Frozen things don't need to be thawed for testing. Still, the chance of missing a food culprit is quite high. Be sure to test everything eaten in a two week time period: unusual things like popcorn, candy, crackers, cookies, health foods and special powders. A consolation is that you will find a number of <u>bad</u> foods that are <u>not</u> necessarily the tremor causes but which cause other health problems.

Tremor Remedies

1. Let us imagine that the air (dust) sample proves toxic (resonates with the saliva sample). What is it in the air that is toxic? These are the biggest suspects:

- CFCs (from leaking refrigerant, check refrigerator and air conditioner by removing them from the house and retesting the dust after three days, or simply buy a non-CFC variety)
- vanadium (from leaking house gas from a fuel line—repair)
- arsenic from pesticide (switch to boric acid)
- solvent from a lamp or can of lighter fuel (take them out of the house)

- chlorine from water (use carbon filters; remove bleach bottles)
- asbestos (clothes dryer belt)
- paint thinner, carpet cleaner (remove from house)
- fiberglass from bare insulation somewhere (fix holes in ceiling or wall)
- formaldehyde (new foam bedding, new fabric or clothing)

2. Suppose the water proves toxic (appears in your white blood cells); search for lead, copper, and cadmium. Although municipal water tests occasionally detect small amounts of propyl alcohol, benzene, or wood alcohol, I have never detected them—you need not search for them.

3. If the medicines are toxic just change brands. Your pharmacist can help you find a replacement brand. Find which ones are toxic and stop using them. (Don't use up any of the polluted pills or supplements.) They do more harm than good.

4. If the clothing or dishes are toxic (appear in the saliva), suspect

- cobalt   • PCB   • aluminum

Stop all detergent use. Use borax, or washing soda, or use paper plates and plastic cups (not styrofoam).

5. If the food is toxic, suspect

- food molds   • aluminum   • bacteria

Don't eat that food any more.

6. Any bacterium or toxin that invades certain brain centers can cause tremor. The most common culprits are *Shigella*, mercury, thallium and arsenic. Try to identify these for your sake as well as your loved one.

The *Salmonellas* and *Shigellas* will have come from some food. Be sure all dairy foods, including butter and whipping cream, are sterilized. Parasites come from meats. Be sure no undercooked or fast food meats are eaten. Kill all bacteria, viruses and parasites with a zapper. Sterilize fingernails with grain alcohol to prevent reinfection. Use Lugol's (see *Recipes*) and the Bowel Program (page 546) to clear them up.

Bacteria, coming from teeth and jaw (bone infections, called *cavitations*) may not seem as recent as two weeks. Indeed, they may have been there for ten years. But something recent may have aggravated them, so they now can enter more easily into the blood and brain. You may never find out what caused this. It is wisest to check this possibility with a dentist before doing weeks of other testing. See a dentist who can find and clean cavitations. Do dental repair according to the principles described in the dental section.

Going after a tremor problem in this logical way <u>always</u> finds the cause of tremor

whether its a simple short attack or a situation of long standing tremor with head shaking and drooling. If your situation is extra difficult, <u>you will at least improve it</u> and stop its progression. **This includes Parkinson's cases.**

In cases of Parkinson's disease I often find the bacterium *Clostridium tetani*, well known for causing stiffness. It hides under tooth fillings, too.

Remember, there is a consolation for doing all this work. When you find the culprit, you not only will be stopping the tremor, you will be improving a lot of other conditions along the way. Conditions like hesitant speech, shuffling walk, getting up stiffly and slowly from a chair. These are <u>extra dividends</u> for your loved one. And you have learned which things to avoid for <u>yourself</u> too.

One more thing, <u>don't take no</u> for an answer.

If the problem is a drug, don't accept "No, it can't be changed." Everything can be changed. Go to higher levels of authority. Doctors are very understanding and sympathetic with your intent. If the problem is leaking house gas, don't accept "We can't find a leak," implying there is none. Go to a building contractor or the Health Department. Their equipment is better. If you get nowhere, change to electric utilities. If the problem is auto exhaust, don't accept "But we have to use the kitchen door to the garage, because it's cold outside." Conveniences vs. tremor is no contest. Everyone benefits by excluding auto fumes from the house. <u>Lock</u> the door and cover it with plastic. By the time you have identified the culprits (probably 20 hours of work) surely you have won the right to make changes.

Often others are not impressed. Even when the tremor lessens and the elderly person plainly states they feel better, family members may disregard your recommendations. **Get tough!** It's your loved one. You have something at stake too. Be sympathetic with negative responses. But very firm. Make their choices clear:

- Either the inside door to the garage gets sealed off or the cars and lawn mower get parked outside and anything containing gasoline or solvents gets put in a detached shed.
- Either the girls use their hair dryers in their bedrooms with the door closed or you'll get them all new ones that don't contain asbestos.
- Either the clothes dryer gets a new belt or it is taped securely shut and the laundry is dried on the line or taken to a Laundromat.
- Either the plumbing gets changed (to plastic) or each faucet in the house gets a filter. (If your plumbing is corrod-

ing, not even filters are a good idea—you would have to change them every week!)

Weakness

should not be taken for granted in the elderly. Especially if they themselves complain about it. It isn't normal for them. Sometimes they will describe "spells" of weakness. This is an important clue. Check the pulse immediately. Count for 30 beats at least. Are there missing beats? There should not be! Missing two beats in a row certainly can produce a weak or "sinking" spell. The brain and body need every pulse of blood sent out right on time.

Check into caffeine use first. Take it all away. Caffeine speeds up the heart; then the overworked heart has to "take time out" for itself by missing a beat. Don't switch to decafs because this introduces solvents and new problems. If no other natural beverages appeal, serve hot water with cream and cinnamon. After stopping caffeine use ask: Is the pulse too slow or too fast? The pulse should be between 60 and 80 beats per minute.

If it is lower than 60, a medicine may be at fault. Ask the clinical doctor about it immediately. A slow pulse could certainly bring about weakness. A young athlete may have a slow pulse legitimately, due to having a very strong efficient heart, but your elderly person does not fit this category. The cause must be found.

If the pulse is quite high, over 100 perhaps, this will wear the heart out much sooner than necessary. Ask why it is beating so fast? A probable answer is that it is so weak that it has to beat faster to keep up with its job of circulating the blood. What is making the heart so weak?

Heart Disease

When the heart is enlarged, the valves don't quite close where they should, making the work harder for it and weakening it. It may be called "congestive heart failure." Why is it enlarged? Possibly because it is so weak! Yes, it becomes a vicious cycle, getting worse and worse. But you can break into this cycle and get it all reversed again. The real culprit is parasite invaders and toxic pollutants.

The most common parasite heart invaders are *Dirofilaria*, heartworm "of dogs" and *Loa loa*, another small filaria worm. At one stage these worms are so tiny that they can slide through the smallest blood vessels. They are very contagious. Even persons who don't live with a house dog can pick up heartworm. *Loa loa* is thought to be a tropical parasite but it is alive and thriving in the USA! The source of *Loa loa* <u>seems</u> to be tapeworm stages; this is not a certainty.

Both heartworm and *Loa loa* are very easy to kill with a zapper and both are very easy to pick up again. Treat your elderly person twice a week if there is <u>any</u> heart problem. It makes no difference that the house dog is getting monthly preventive treatments for heartworm. They pick it up daily and have thirty days to develop it and give it to others between treatments. Killing the dog's parasites twice a week with a zapper would be very helpful to you. These heart parasites may not cause any pains, yet disturb the rhythm or the pulse of the heart and cause it to enlarge.

Staphylococcus aureus is a bacterium hiding out in far away places like pockets left under teeth when they were extracted or along root canals. Make sure extractions heal and don't leave permanent cavitations where bacteria can live. Ask a dentist familiar with cavitations to do a mouth search. Once the mouth source is cleaned up, the bacteria do not come back to the heart (after one last zapping). If they do, go back to the dentist!

Killing these three invaders (heartworm, *Loa loa*, *Staphylococcus aureus*) should cure an irregular heart beat immediately (within a day).

If the elderly person is on a heart-slowing drug, check the pulse twice a day after zapping to make sure it doesn't drop too low. They may need to be <u>off</u> their heart medicine. Nobody will notice the relief of going off this medicine as much as you. The sunshine breaks out! Your loved one can smile again at little things! Even interest in sex returns so watch out! Life is normalized when drugs, especially beta blockers are gone. (Other heart medicines, such as Digitoxin,™ don't have this depressive effect. They are used to make the heart beat stronger, not to affect the <u>rate</u> of beating.)

The pulse should be around 70 beats per minute and <u>perfectly</u> regular.

If it isn't, there is still something wrong. Get rid of toxic body products and house pollutants. Test your air for gas leaks frequently. Gas heat, gas stoves and gas water heaters are notoriously leaky. Weather changes, namely temperature changes make pipes expand or shrink—leaving cracks! The gas is toxic and a small amount can't be smelled. What a predicament! Delivering poisonous house gas to our homes in pipes that are not fail-safe is an archaic practice. Especially when the blood test shows a high "total CO_2" level, near the upper limit, search for an air pollutant like house gas or auto fumes. And read the sections in this book on pulse (page 289) and brain problems (page 278) very closely for more things to check.

With the heart regular again, it will be much stronger, too, since it doesn't have to work against itself. This strength is necessary to push the blood into the farthest "corners" of the body, especially the hands and feet, and warm them up! If your loved one constantly has cold hands or feet, try to improve circulation. Dissolve phosphate crystals with the kidney herb recipe. Give niacin (page 279). Give cayenne capsules (one with each meal). Blood thinning drugs to improve circulation are dangerous—use only if the doctor insists. Monitor blood clotting time if your loved one is on a thinner.

Heart/Kidney Relationship

A strong heart is necessary, too, to push the blood through the kidneys. Often a kidney problem is linked to the heart disorder. Kidneys are made of tubes that get finer and finer. It takes pressure, namely strength, to push the blood through them so wastes and extra water can be let down the kidney tube. Think of the kidneys as a colander full of tiny holes of various sizes that let certain things through them but not bigger things. These holes are constantly being adjusted by the adrenals which sit right on top of the kidneys and "supervise".

If the elderly person is not producing four cups of urine in a day (24 hours), it is not enough. The body cannot get enough cleansing action from less than four cups. More liquid must be consumed. If most of the urine is passed in the night this reflects on unhealthy kidneys. Use the kidney herb recipe—but only half a dose (so it will take six weeks instead of three to see good effects). As the tiny "colander" holes open up there is freer flow and many more trips to the bathroom result. The urine loses its awful odor (no ammonia, acetone and bacteria!) and gets a clear look that shows no sediment. Now that water and wastes (urea and uric acid and other acids) can leave the body quickly through more holes, it takes less pressure from the heart to get blood pushed through the kidneys. This brings relief to the heart because its work is easier. The heart and kidneys work together. Like horse and wagon the heart provides the power and the kidneys follow.

This is why heart medicine and diuretics are commonly given together. *Diuresis* (urine flow) helps the heart and a stronger heart helps the kidneys. Similarly, they fail together. In the old days this was called *dropsy*. Urine that should have left the body is backed up in the tissues. Sometimes it shows up in pockets that hang like giant oranges from the skin.

Even (especially) when the strongest diuretics (Maxzide™, Lasix™) fail to work, even when coupled with strong heart medicine (Digitoxin™), the kidney herb recipe can bail you out of the emergency.

The secret is in the varied actions of different herbs. This makes them work together. Be very careful to keep the herb tea sterile by reheating every fourth day. Freeze unused larger amounts. If too much is drunk at once, especially on the first day, a stomach ache can develop and a pressure felt in the bladder that is most uncomfortable. Go extra slow on the first few days, even though you find it quite tasty, so there is no discomfort (only lots of bathroom visits).

Diuretics

As soon as urine is flowing better, blood pressure may drop. Keep track of this twice a day with a modern electronic finger device (not an arm cuff that itself can break blood vessels). Cut down on drug diuretics gradually, using only ¾ dose the first day, then ½ dose, then ¼ dose. The amount of urine produced or the weight of the person can be used to assess how effective your method is. **Your goal is to not need any drug diuretics.** Again, mood will improve dramatically when diuretic drugs are removed for your loved one. The sense of humor comes back:

be prepared for some new jokes and new laughter. Give yourself good grades for this accomplishment.

Don't throw out the drug diuretics. After being off them for a while, they become more potent again. So if an emergency (sudden edema) should arise they could again be useful.

With a parasite and pollution-free heart and a low-resistance, freely flowing kidney, some reserve strength will soon be built up. Weak spells are gone and forgotten. Your loved one is walking better, needing less sleep, and a "golden age" finally arrives. It is free of pain, free of medicine, free of shots and doctor visits, free of dementia, free of the dreadful weakness that demands so much help. They are free to enjoy family and friends again. Seeing themselves gain strength and be able to do more for themselves gives the elderly a sense of pride.

Give them the credit for improving their health. When they balk at having to take herbs or vegetable juice, remind them of the days they were on a handful of pills and still had heart failure, pain and kidney disease.

Feeling Comfortable

If all this improvement doesn't warm up their feet or hands (feel them yourself) put extra socks on. Warming up their feet might have the effect of warming up hands, too. But if it doesn't, raise the room temperature.

Being forced to feel cold is an undeserved misery of the aged.

Others must accommodate to the elderly's need for body warmth. The thermometer does not tell all. Comfort is paramount for each of us. Younger persons can undress for comfort. The elderly can't make changes for themselves. Usually, by the time they are complaining of cold, they have suffered a long time, feeling too guilty to request a temperature hike. <u>Ask</u> your loved one. They will appreciate it. A shawl, a lap-blanket, woolen sweater, long underwear and fleecy thermal outerwear help a lot. But if your hand still senses cold feet, the thermostat must still go higher. Cold body temperature is an invitation for fungus and viruses to multiply. Viruses escape into the body daily. Don't give them the advantage.

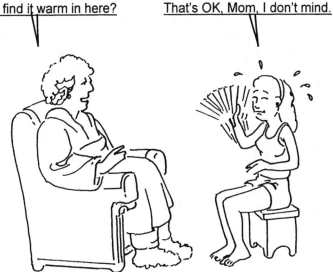

Fig. 39 Too hot and too cold.

But unless all these things are tried, <u>don't</u> raise the temperature. It is much healthier to be warmly dressed and breathe cool air than to be lightly dressed in an 80°F room. The heart, especially, benefits by the cooler air temperature.

For this reason, it is important to have air conditioning during the hot season. Keep your elderly person warmly dressed, away from air conditioner or fan drafts, but keep it cool. As cool as their body temperature and comfort will allow. Don't seat an elderly person under a fan in restaurants. The blowing air not only chills them, but brings filth in dust that blows in the air currents. Bacteria and viruses are soon to follow.

Being comfortable, knowing you are there to care for them, brings out the best in your elderly person. They might get well enough to long for a genuine relationship again. And put you to the test. The test of listening. This can be very rewarding if they are still able to communicate and distill their life experience into wisdom for you. If you can listen and be interested in their distillations or their ramblings their longing for relationship will be fulfilled. There's just one catch, if the new found interest in communication can't be expressed. If they haven't communicated much for a long time, it would be easy for you to miss a simple fact. <u>They can't hear!</u>

Hearing Loss

The hearing deficit in an elderly person is always much greater than they or you realize. Try to understand these communications:

What you (caregiver) say	What the elderly person hears	What they think	What they respond
"Look at the sunshine, isn't it a nice day?"	"Look at something, isn't it a nice bay?"	What a stupid sentence. But she wants an answer. So here goes,	"MmmHmmm" (Meaning, "yes.")
"We'll have such a nice walk."	"Have a...rock."	Rock what? I'm not in a rocking chair. I better not say anything.	
"What kind of soup should I make?"	"What kind of hoop should I make?"	I haven't used a hoop for embroidery for a long time. Why is she digging that up. I better say I don't know.	"I don't know."

Don't let this ruin your relationship. It takes the fun out of their life as much as yours. **Get hearing aids.**

324

Don't ask your loved one if they need a hearing aid. The answer may be "I'm not deaf." You can go about it more persuasively. Every time you talk, come quite near to the person's ear and speak loudly. They can <u>see</u> that you must come near. If they are fighting against the whole business, they will say things like, "You don't have to shout. I can hear you." (It's what you're saying that's wrong!)

Arrange for a hearing test. It is free. That will appeal. The results of a hearing test, as it is told by a salesperson, is much more persuasive than you can be. Let the salesperson use his or her special talents to sell your loved one on hearing aids. But you make the choice on quality. Both you and your elderly person deserve the best tone quality that is made. Plus a regular <u>cleaning</u> service. Most companies do offer this but don't tell the customer because of the dreadful amount of time it would take if everybody took advantage of it. <u>You</u> take advantage of it. Clogged hearing aids are the most troublesome feature of any of them—and never mentioned! Make it a rule to buy your batteries at the same hearing aid office where they are cleaned free of charge. This repays them and serves the elderly best. Hearing loss is too subtle to leave to chance; have the hearing aids cleaned each time you buy fresh batteries (about three months). Take your loved one to a nurse for ear cleaning every six months after hearing aids are begun. Wax and debris accumulate behind the aid because the channel is stopped up.

With hearing aids that hear, and kidneys that flush and a heart that beats strongly, your elderly person may choose to attend concerts again, go to church or gatherings—and leave you out of the picture. Give yourself good grades for this achievement. Get them incontinence pants, get regular taxi service. **Do whatever it takes to get your loved one out into the world again!**

If the excitement of a night out keeps him or her from sleeping use **ornithine** and **valerian** capsules. They are good for the health anyway. Hot milk and a piece of cake (homemade, never chocolate) may do as much.

But if insomnia is the rule, not the exception, you need to go after it as a special problem.

Insomnia

is <u>always</u> associated with high levels of parasites and bacteria. This leads me to believe it is their waste products, namely ammonia, that really causes insomnia. Read the section on Insomnia under Sleep Problems for more on this (page 243).

A sound sleep refreshes as nothing else can. Your elderly person will have more energy throughout the day and a better mood if sleep was good.

Of course you must guard against daytime napping if nights are sleepless. Sleep at night is more important than sleep by day. They are not equal. Try to turn your loved one's cycle back to night-time sleeping if it has become turned around by bad kidney function (frequent urination at night) or too much daytime napping. Sleep can be disturbed by taking vitamins at bedtime too. Sleep is enhanced by taking magnesium. Limit bedtime supplements to magnesium, ornithine, valerian (6 capsules) taken with hot milk.

Healthful Habits

If your loved one had his or her way, they would drive the car forever, wear the same cosmetics forever, smoke or chew tobacco forever and eat their favorite dessert forever.

But if you are the caretaker, you know that some things must stop. You also know that gentle persuasion is useless; it merely erodes your relationship. Here are a few tips.

1. Ask your loved one to <u>ask</u> their doctor (clinical doctor or trusted medical advisor) the following question: "Would it be better for my lungs to stop smoking?" Be present so the question does not turn into "Will smoking a few cigarettes once in a while kill me?" Hearing it from the doctor is what's needed.

2. <u>Don't ever</u> purchase something you believe is detrimental to your elderly person. Whether it's coffee, cigarettes, beer or lipstick, say "That is something I can't buy for you; it's against my principles." Don't be surprised if you cave in a few times to some super ruse they use on you. But the next time, have your answer ready.

3. Let your family and other caretakers know you are no longer supplying these items (the car keys, the wine bottle, the codeine-containing pain pills). Try to get cooperation. Discussing it with your loved one may do more harm than good. If they start the discussion, you end it. This is not a task for the timid! After it's done, you'll wonder what was so difficult.

4. Don't buy a wheelchair if your loved one can still walk with your help. Stay with a cane as long as possible. Then the walker. Stay with a walker as long as possible. Then your personal help. Once a wheelchair has been accepted, the last bit of exercise, walking, is lost. Fight against it. Hide it in a far away closet.

Aging is necessary but chronic illness and pain are not.

If you have managed to free your loved one from having to take pills or from certain disabilities that would soon require pills, you can give yourself great credit. Perhaps you, too, will find the needed natural help when you are aged and have lost your authority and your way mentally. Our lives are all foreshortened, much like the life of a domestic steer's. Does a captive animal learn from seeing its companion disappear? It does nothing to escape its fate. Should we accept our fate with the same docility? None of us can remember how things were in precivilized times. We are eager to believe the <u>present</u> is the best time that has ever been. The steer, too, has its feed provided, its water provided, its shelter for the night provided, seemingly the best time it ever had. Perhaps the price we pay for civilization, like the steer's price, is simply too high. There must be other ways. As a society, we should search for our lost longevity.

Not Old Yet

For persons merely over 40 and not ill a most important rule is: **don't overdo**.

It's easy to injure tendons and muscles by pulling or stretching them too far. Don't try, with almighty determination to open a jar. Leave it for <u>stronger</u> hands. Don't try to stretch a <u>gigantic</u> stretch to reach something on a high shelf. Wait for someone taller to come along and reach it down for you. Don't do exercises, that have left you with strains in the past. Do different exercises. Don't do new exercises, with a determined approach; start moderately; stay moderate. If you start a new job that uses a foot, leg, hand or wrist a lot, more than it was used before, even though it's in ordinary use, it can feel injured. These stresses and strains invite bacteria toward themselves. Bacteria from the liver or your own intestines find these strained tissues immediately and intensify the pain. Kill the bacteria with a zapper, cleanse the liver, and start the Bowel Program if this has already happened to you.

Don't kneel on the floor to do some cleaning job. Don't sit on the floor at a gathering. Don't let your grandchildren take "rides" on you. Don't bend over as far as you can to pick something up. Let your family know you are aiming to reach 100 years in healthy condition.

Super Longevity

We should be able to live to 140 years of age. Middle age might begin at 65, old age at 90. What is the clue to long life? Surely it is keeping all your cells healthy so they can coordinate the constant tasks of nourishing themselves, removing their wastes, plus whatever job that cell was meant to do.

Since your cells divide and therefore start again at age zero, even though you are 90, why do you age at all? Only the <u>nervous system</u> does not divide. Is it the nerve that ages then, and decides death for each of us?

It would never do to live forever. It would clutter the planet. Are evolutionary forces at work preventing this? But we have never cluttered the planet yet. So how could evolutionary forces have "learned" to establish death to prevent overpopulation? Living to age 140 is not living forever. Wisdom comes with age. Wisdom would serve our society well. Perhaps wisdom is needed more than ever for humans to survive. Part of the human tragedy is war. Wisdom gathered from a knowledge of history, might help end wars! But history can't be gathered and understood in less than 100 years. If centenarians can't think well or express themselves, their perspectives are lost. Longevity seems a very useful trait if only it were accompanied by health!

Dying

Although it can't be avoided it can be helped. Dying <u>alone</u> is the most barbaric of all society's practices.

It is still like death in the forest amongst chimpanzees. Unable to feed, to run, to call for help brings pain, fear, loneliness and finally, death. When your loved one is in the mood to talk about dying, <u>listen</u>. Especially if it is about their own imminent death. This doesn't obligate you to carry out any of their wishes. When death approaches the important thing is simply to <u>be there</u>. They may not have requested this, out of a sense of guilt or masochism, or plain dementia. But it is the most primitive of needs, the same as having a loved one nearby during childbirth. It is just a <u>presence</u> that counts. How can you be there if you have a job or are attending a family's needs? It is a time of great frustration for you. All your hard work and successes are culminating in one grand failure!

The good news is that it need not be you who attends your loved one every minute of the last week. Pay for someone to sit—someone who is recognized. But arrange for immediate privacy when you return. No matter how much your loved one admonishes you to go about your business, you will know when you share the final minute that your presence <u>helped</u>. The loneliness of the last coma, the last silence is unspeakable. Give yourself the reward of knowing you shared the pain, fear and silent cry for help.

Curing Cancer

Cancer is no longer the deadly disease it once was. In fact, you can clear it up in less time than it takes to get a doctor's appointment for a check up. If you notice a lump or think you might have cancer, don't rush to see a doctor <u>first</u>. Rush to clear it up, yourself, <u>first</u>. By the time your doctor's appointment arrives, you can be sure of a negative test.

Another Fluke Disease

Cancer is so easily cured because it is a parasite-caused disease. Kill the parasite and you have stopped the cancer. This does not mean you have also stopped being ill. If the cancer damaged your ovaries or prostate, you still must heal these organs. The Ca-125 or PSA test will <u>not</u> drop to normal unless you begin to heal them. These markers reflect the <u>condition</u> of the organ, not its malignant nature. Remember that killing a mosquito does not remove the lump it caused. That will take its course. It will heal beautifully if you let it. But if you scratch it mercilessly, it will take longer. Removing toxins from the affected organs lets them heal.

Fortunately for us, **cancer is not like a fire, unstoppable once it has started.** It takes only 7 minutes to zap all the parasite adults and their stages which cause your cells to multiply.

The responsible parasite is *Fasciolopsis buskii*, the **human intestinal fluke**, a flatworm. It is a human parasite although it can also parasitize other species. It normally lives quietly in the intestine. (The goal for all larger parasites is to live quietly. After all, your demise is their demise.) They were meant to pass their thousands of eggs with your bowel movement, outside, to some pond where snails live. But when the eggs hatch before they leave your body and are allowed to continue their development inside you, the setting is right for cancer to develop.

If the fluke eggs and other stages go through their development in your breast it can become breast cancer. If it is in the prostate it can become prostate cancer. And so on. Each different kind of cancer means the developmental stages of the intestinal fluke are present there. Only one more thing is needed to bring about an avalanche of reproduction, so that hundreds of little larvae turn into hundreds more in a short time: a growth factor. It makes them multiply and your cells are similarly affected. This growth factor, *ortho-phospho-tyrosine* (and possibly, also, *epidermal growth factor* and *insulin-dependent growth factor*) really begins your cancer.

Teamed With A Solvent

The good news is that this growth factor, which is essential for cancer to develop, cannot be made, without the presence of an abnormal solvent, **propyl alcohol** (or more exactly, isopropyl alcohol).

Without taking in propyl alcohol you could never get cancer. It takes two things, together, to give you cancer: propyl alcohol and the human intestinal fluke parasite.

Since it takes a frequency generator (3 minutes at each of 434, 432, 427, 425, 423, 421 KHz) or zapper mere minutes to kill the fluke and its stages you will be stopping the production of growth factors immediately.

Zap yourself every day for three seven minute periods, until after you are completely well.

After killing the flukes, those growth factors already formed will disappear in one hour. Your malignancy is stopped. It cannot return <u>unless</u> you infect yourself with the parasite again!

Getting rid of propyl alcohol is also a simple task. Once you have stopped using it, the last remnants leave your body within three days.

We must marvel at the body's wisdom and capabilities for restoring health. You are not permanently damaged by this large and hungry parasite. Given half a chance your body will throw the rascals out and restore order in you tissues.

Read the list of foods and products that are polluted with propyl alcohol. It is not, of course, usually on the label. If it is used as an ingredient, it is on the label, easy for you to avoid. It is the pollutants not appearing on the label that pose sinister hazards.

All the store bought shampoo I tested had propyl alcohol. Health brands were no exception

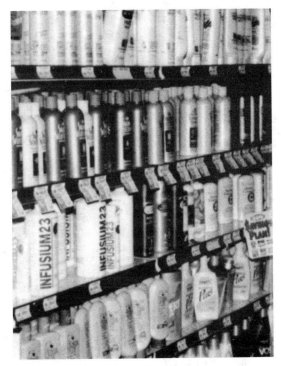

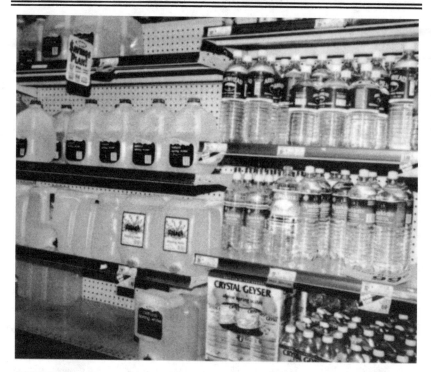

All bottled water is polluted with antiseptics from the bottling procedure. This is a main source of propyl alcohol.

Cosmetics are laced with propyl alcohol. Use the recipes in this book to make your own.

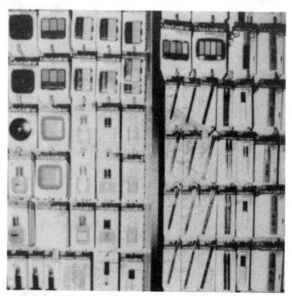

Fig. 40 Products with propyl alcohol.

Propyl Alcohol Polluted Products

THROW THESE OUT

even if propyl alcohol is not listed on the label!

- **shampoo**, even health brands
- **hair spray** and **mousse**
- **cold cereals**, even "natural" granolas
- **cosmetics** (make your own)
- **mouthwash**
- **decaffeinated coffee**, Postum™, herb tea blends (single herb teas are OK)
- **vitamins, minerals and supplements** (unless you test them)
- **bottled water,** distilled water, or spring water
- **rubbing alcohol**
- **white sugar** (brown is OK if detoxified)
- all **shaving supplies** including aftershave
- **carbonated beverages**
- store-bought **fruit juice**, including health food brands

Tear out this page, put it on your refrigerator, and make a copy to stick on your medicine cabinet. Remember propyl alcohol is also called <u>propanol</u>, <u>isopropanol</u>, <u>isopropyl alcohol</u> and <u>rubbing alcohol</u>. You won't drop dead from getting propyl alcohol, but your cancer will flare up with each small addition.

Avoid the entire list, meticulously. Even using one of these, **like your favorite shampoo or bottled water**, will result in failure. Your body will continue to make *human chorionic gonadotropin* (hCG) and the pathology will remain "indeterminate"—not cancerous but not well, either. If you have learned the new bioelectronic technology described in this book, you can <u>test</u> all your foods and products for isopropyl alcohol.

When you find a beverage that is free of propyl alcohol, it may have other pollutants. Xylene and toluene invite parasites to the brain. Wood alcohol invites them to eyes and pancreas. The diseases caused by these are not as frightening, perhaps, as cancer, but entirely avoidable. For this reason, I suggest in this book that you go back (actually "forward") to self made products, unprocessed food and a limited number of tested supplements.

Getting Well After Cancer

The ravages of cancer must be healed once the malignancy has been stopped. This is where *carcinogens* play a role. The lung lesions will not heal unless cigarette smoking, freon, asbestos, and fiberglass exposure is stopped. Carcinogens were thought to be the <u>cause</u> of cancer. Actually, they <u>drew</u> the cancer to the organ. Nickel <u>draws</u> cancer to the prostate. Barium found in lipstick <u>draws</u> cancer to the breast. And so on.

The following toxins can be present in <u>any</u> organ! I consider these to be our most serious threat. Starting with the worst, they are:

1. **Freon** (same as **CFCs** or refrigerant). I have not found a single person to be entirely free of it, including persons without cancer or disease. But in cancer sufferers it is always concentrated in the cancerous organ, and facilitates the accumulation of other toxins. This makes your <u>refrig-</u>

erator, if it leaks even microscopically, the top cancer hazard in the country!

2. **Copper** from water pipes. All cancer sufferers have an accumulation in the cancerous tissue. This makes plumbing the second greatest hazard.
3. **Fiberglass** or **asbestos** is present in about 25% of the cancer victims I see.
4. **Mercury** as in tooth fillings.
5. **Lead** from solder joints in copper plumbing. All colon cancer sufferers test positive.
6. **Formaldehyde** as in foam bedding and new clothing.
7. **Nickel** usually from dental metal. Most prostate cancer sufferers test positive.

At first, tumors are benign—what a relief to find your tumor was benign. Its true nature is still unknown, but it contains freon, other toxins, and later propyl alcohol! Since tumors are often large, many centimeters in diameter, and toxins do not occupy much space, there is much unidentified substance. These tumors can multiply and enlarge, as in fibrocystic breast disease, all without being malignant. But what a convenient place for baby stages of the fluke to hide out and multiply, safe from your immune system. After being colonized by fluke stages, the tumors become malignant. Eventually they also become infected when metastasis sets in.

All malignancies have the same two fundamental causes: intestinal flukes and propyl alcohol. Whether you have a rhabdomyosarcoma or a mesothelioma or melanoma, you can cure it quickly, never to return.

Herbal Parasite Killing Program

Flatworms, roundworms, protozoa, even bacteria and viruses are remarkably easy to kill using a combination of zapping and this herbal program. Thus it is not just for cancer, but a general treatment that can benefit almost every illness

1. **Black Walnut Hull Tincture Extra Strength** (see *Recipes*, page 543):
   Day 1: (this is the day you begin; start the same day you receive it)
   Take one drop. Put it in ½ cup of water. Sip it on an empty stomach such as before a meal.

   Day 2: Take 2 drops in ½ cup water same as above.
   Day 3: Take 3 drops in ½ cup water same as above.
   Day 4: Take 4 drops in ½ cup water same as above.
   Day 5: Take 5 drops in ½ cup water same as above.
   Day 6: Take 2 tsp., all together in ¼ cup water. Sip it, don't gulp it. Get it down within 15 minutes. (If you are over 150 pounds, take 2½ tsp. Do not take more than 3 tsp. because no additional value has been observed.)

   This dose kills any remaining stages throughout the body, including the bowel contents, a location unreachable by electric current. The alcohol in the tincture can make you slightly woozy for several minutes. Simply stay seated until you are comfortable again. You may put the tincture in <u>lukewarm</u> *water to help evaporate some of the alcohol, but do not use* <u>hot</u> *water because that may damage its parasiticide power. Then take niacinamide 500 mg to counteract the toxicity of the alcohol. You could also feel a slight nausea for a few minutes. Walk in the fresh air or simply rest until it passes. You may add more water or honey or a spice to make it more palatable.*

For a year: take 2 tsp. Black Walnut Hull Tincture Extra Strength every week or until your illness is but a hazy memory. This is to kill any parasite stages you pick up from your family, friends, or pets.

Family members and friends should take 2 tsp. every other week to avoid reinfecting you. They may be harboring a few parasite stages in their intestinal tract without having symptoms. But when these stages are transmitted to a cancer patient, they immediately seek out the cancerous organ again.

You may be wondering why you should wait for five days before taking the 2 tsp. dose. It is for your convenience only. You may have a sensitive stomach or be worried about toxicity or side effects. By the sixth day you will have convinced yourself there is no toxicity or side effects.
Going faster. *In fact, if you are convinced after the first drop of the restorative powers of Black Walnut Hull Tincture Extra Strength, take the 2 tsp. dose on the very first day.*
Going slower. *On the other hand, if you cringe at the thought of taking an herb or you are anxious about it's safety, continue the drops, increasing at your own pace, until you are ready to brave the decisive 2 tsp. dose.*

2. **Wormwood** capsules (should contain 200-300 mg of wormwood, see *Sources*):

Day 1: Take 1 capsule before supper (with water).
Day 2: Take 1 capsule before supper.

Day 3: Take 2 capsules before supper.
Day 4: Take 2 capsules before supper.

Continue increasing in this way to day 14, whereupon you are up to seven capsules. You take the capsules all in a single dose (you may take a few at a time until they are all gone). Then you do 2 more days of 7 capsules each. After this, you take 7 capsules once a week forever, as it states in the Maintenance Parasite Program. Try not to get interrupted before the 6th day, so you know the adult intestinal flukes are dead. After this, you may proceed more slowly if you wish. Many persons with sensitive stomachs prefer to stay longer on each dose instead of increasing according to this schedule. You may choose the pace after the sixth day.

3. **Cloves**:
   Fill size 00 capsules with fresh ground cloves; if this size is not available, use size 0 or 000. In a pinch, buy gelatin capsules and empty them or empty other vitamin capsules. You may be able to purchase fresh ground cloves that are already encapsulated; they should be about 500 mg. Grocery store ground cloves do not work! Either grind them yourself or see Sources.

Day 1: Take one capsule 3 times a day before meals.
Day 2: Take two capsules 3 times a day.
Days 3, 4, 5, 6, 7, 8, 9, 10: Take three capsules 3 times a day.
After day 10: Take 3 capsules all together once a week forever, as in the Maintenance Parasite Program.

Take **ornithine** at bedtime for insomnia. Even if you do not suffer from insomnia now, you may when you kill parasites.

Parasite Program Handy Chart

Strike out the doses as you take them.

Day	Black Walnut Hull Tincture Extra Strength Dose	Wormwood Capsule Dose (200-300 mg)	Clove Capsule Dose (Size 0 or 00)
	drops 1 time per day, like before a meal	capsules 1 time per day, on empty stomach (before meal)	capsules 3 times per day, like at mealtime
1	1	1	1, 1, 1
2	2	1	2, 2, 2
3	3	2	3, 3, 3
4	4	2	3, 3, 3
5	5	3	3, 3, 3
6	2 tsp.	3	3, 3, 3
7	Now once a week	4	3, 3, 3
8		4	3, 3, 3
9		5	3, 3, 3
10		5	3, 3, 3.
11		6	3
12		6	Now once a week
13	2 tsp.	7	
14		7	
15		7	
16		7	
17		Now once a week	
18			3

At this point you do not need to keep a strict schedule, but instead may choose any day of the week to take all the parasite program ingredients.

Continue on the Maintenance Parasite Program, indefinitely, to prevent future reinfection.

Maintenance Parasite Program

YOU ARE ALWAYS PICKING UP PARASITES! PARASITES ARE EVERYWHERE AROUND YOU! YOU GET THEM FROM OTHER PEOPLE, YOUR FAMILY,

YOURSELF, YOUR HOME, YOUR PETS, UNDERCOOKED MEAT, AND UNDERCOOKED DAIRY PRODUCTS.

I believe the <u>main</u> source of the intestinal fluke is <u>undercooked meat</u>. After we are infected with it this way, we can give it to each other through blood, saliva, semen, and breast milk, which means kissing on the mouth, sex, nursing, and child-bearing.

Family members nearly always have the same parasites. If one person develops cancer or HIV, the others probably have the intestinal fluke also. These diseases are caused by the same parasite. They should give themselves the same de-parasitizing program.

Do this once a week. You may take these at different times in the day or together:

1. **Black Walnut Hull Tincture Extra Strength**: 2 tsp. on an empty stomach, like before a meal.
2. **Wormwood capsules**: 7 capsules (with 200-300 mg wormwood each) at once on an empty stomach.
3. **Cloves**: 3 capsules (about 500 mg. each, or fill size 00 capsules yourself) at once on an empty stomach.
4. Take **ornithine** as needed.

Day	Black Walnut Hull Tincture Extra Strength Dose	Wormwood Capsule Dose (200-300 mg)	Clove Capsule Dose (Size 0 or 00)
	1 time per day, on empty stomach	capsules 1 time per day, on empty stomach	capsules 1 time per day, on empty stomach
1	2 tsp.	7	3
2			
3			
4			
5			
6			
7			
8	2 tsp.	7	3
9			
10			

11			
12			
13			
14			
15	2 tsp.	7	3
and so	on...		

The only after-effects you may feel are due to bacteria and viruses escaping from dead parasites! Be sure to zap after taking your maintenance parasite treatment. After-effects also let you know that you did indeed kill something. Try to discover how you might have picked up parasites and avoid them next time.

Pet Parasite Program

Pets have many of the same parasites that we get, including *Ascaris* (common roundworm), hookworm, *Trichinella, Strongyloides,* heartworm and a variety of tapeworms. Every pet living in your home should be deparasitized (cleared of parasites) and maintained on a parasite program. Monthly trips to your vet are not sufficient.

You may not need to get rid of your pet to keep yourself free of parasites. But if you are quite ill it is best to board it with a friend until you are better.

Your pet is part of your family and should be kept as sweet and clean and healthy as yourself. This is not difficult to achieve. Here is the recipe:

1. **Parsley water**: cook a big bunch of fresh parsley in a quart of water for 3 minutes. Throw away the parsley. After cooling, you may freeze most of it in several 1 cup containers. This is a month's supply. Put 1 tsp. parsley

water on the pet's food. You don't have to watch it go down. Whatever amount is eaten is satisfactory.

All dosages are based on a 10 pound (5 kilo) cat or dog. Double them for a 20 pound pet, and so forth.

Pets are so full of parasites, you must be quite careful not to deparasitize too quickly. The purpose of the parsley water is to keep the kidneys flowing well so dead parasite refuse is eliminated promptly. They get quite fond of their parsley water. Perhaps they can sense the benefit it brings them. Do this for a week before starting the Black Walnut Hull Tincture.

2. **Black Walnut Hull Tincture (regular strength):** 1 drop on the food. Don't force them to eat it. Count carefully. Treat cats only twice a week. Treat dogs daily, for instance a 30 pound dog would get 3 drops per day (but work up to it, increasing one drop per day). Do not use Extra Strength.

If your pet vomits or has diarrhea, you may expect to see worms. This is extremely infectious and hazardous. Never let a child clean up a pet mess. Begin by pouring salt and iodine[15] on the mess and letting it stand for 5 minutes before cleaning it up. Clean up outdoor messes the same way. Finally, clean your hands with diluted grain alcohol (dilute 1 part alcohol with 4 parts water) or vodka. Be careful to keep all alcohol out of sight of children; don't rely on discipline for this. Be careful not to buy isopropyl rubbing alcohol for this purpose.

Start the wormwood a week later.

---

[15] "Povidone" iodine. topical antiseptic, is available in most drug stores.

3. **Wormwood capsules:** (200-300 mg wormwood per capsule) open a capsule and put the smallest pinch possible on their dry food. Do this for a week before starting the cloves.

4. **Cloves:** put the smallest pinch possible on their dry food.
Keep all of this up as a routine so that you need not fear your pets. Also, notice how peppy and happy they become.
Go slowly so the pet can learn to eat all of it. To repeat:

- Week 1: parsley water.
- Week 2: parsley water and black walnut.
- Week 3: parsley water, black walnut, and wormwood.
- Week 4: parsley water, black walnut, wormwood, and cloves.

	Parsley Water	Black Walnut Hull Tincture Dose	Wormwood Capsule Dose	Clove Capsule Dose (Size 0 or 00)
Week	teaspoons on food	drops on food, cats twice per week, dogs daily	open capsule, put smallest pinch on food	open capsule, put smallest pinch on food
1	1 or more, based on size			
2	1 or more	1		
3	1 or more	1 or more, based on size	1	
4	1 or more	1 or more	1	1
5 and onward	1 or more	1 or more	1	1

Parasites Gone, Toxins Next

Healing is automatic when you <u>clean up</u> your body tissues. Killing parasites and bacterial and viral invaders is fundamental. Removing toxins which invite them into your organs is even more fundamental.

How do you know which toxins are responsible for <u>your</u> cancer? Unless you use a Syncrometer to test, you can not know. So learn to use a Syncrometer, it will save your life.

The only other alternative is to move to a safer environment. Go on vacation. Stay in hotels less than ten years old (so the plumbing hasn't started to corrode) but not in new construction (give the carpets time to outgas). Do not have a freon containing refrigerator in your room. Do not use the hair drier they supply. Do not let them spray your room with <u>anything</u>. Launder the sheets and towels yourself at a Laundromat with borax and/or washing soda. Don't hesitate to drink the municipal water. Get busy with your dental cleanup.

When you get better on vacation, let that be your inspiration to <u>move</u> from your home. All of the toxins come from a civilized lifestyle. Resolve to leave it behind. Select a warm climate where you can spend your time outdoors in the shade most of the day. Have no refrigerator, air conditioner, clothes dryer, hair dryer, new clothing, detergent. Check that the plumbing is relatively new and that no pesticide is being used. Make the Easy Lifestyle Improvements (page 397). Throw away non-essential health supplements (unless tested) and drugs. The risk is greater than the benefit.

Watch For Bacteria

In the later stages of cancer the tumors are more and more infected with the common bacteria *Salmonella, Shigella,* and *Staphylococcus aureus.* Killing parasites prepares a feast for these ubiquitous bacteria. Now, more than ever, must you stay off dairy products (except for boiled milk), do the Bowel Program, take Lugol's. Remove *Staphs* by doing the dental cleanup (page 409). Don't delay.

346

Help Your Family, Too

If you had cancer, your whole family should be freed of intestinal fluke parasites <u>to protect you</u>! They may not be getting cancer (yet!) but your closeness puts you at risk. Kissing on the mouth could reinfect you. Request that family members zap themselves and take at least one 2 tsp. dose of Black Walnut Hull Tincture Extra Strength while living with you.

Pets, too, can be a source of cancer fluke stages (in their drool). They get propyl alcohol from their feed. Use unflavored, uncolored feed for them to minimize pollution from processing. Add 1 tbs. vitamin C powder to the top of a 5 lb. bag; it will stick to the pellets as they pour out. Zap your pet along with yourself by holding them and touching a bare spot such as nose or paw.

Never eat rare meats or fast food chicken. Parasite stages survive heat up to the boiling point. If you have taken a risk, zap yourself as soon as you get home to minimize the damage.

Cancer could be completely eliminated in the entire country if laws required testing for solvents in animal feeds and human food and products. Presently it is allowed in the United States Code of Federal Regulations (CFR) (see page 428)!

Another reason for propyl alcohol pollution (and other pollutants) in our food are the chemicals used by manufacturers to sterilize their food handling equipment.

21 CFR 178.1010 (4-1-94 Edition) Sanitizing solutions.
Sanitizing solutions may be safely used on food-processing equipment and utensils, and on other food-contact articles as specified in this section, within the following prescribed conditions:

(a) Such sanitizing solutions are used, followed by adequate draining, before contact with food. **[Note rinsing or drying is not required!]**

(b) The solutions consist of one of the following, to which may be added components general recognized as safe and components which are permitted by prior sanction or approval.

[Now comes (1) through (43) permissible sterilizing solutions, including several with isopropyl alcohol, like:]

(25) An aqueous solution containing elemental iodine (CAS Reg. No. 7553-56-2), potassium iodide (CAS Reg. No. 7681-11-0), and isopropanol (CAS Reg. No. 67-63-0). In addition to use on food processing equipment and utensils, this solution may be used on beverage containers, including milk containers and equipment and on food-contact surfaces in public eating places.

[Then in paragraph (c)(19) the exact concentration of the iodine is specified. Nowhere is the concentration of the isopropanol specified. It can be as strong as desired.]

Fig. 41 U.S. regulations on sterilizing solutions.

Even if there were regulations governing removal of sanitizing solutions, the overwhelming truth is missed: that **nothing can ever be completely removed after it has been added.** Or perhaps the lawmakers didn't miss this fact. Perhaps they believed that small amounts–too small to measure with an ultraviolet spectrophotometer–could surely do no harm.

Meanwhile, protect yourself by avoiding propyl alcohol. And by observing 2 extra rules:

1. Never eat moldy foods.   2. Always take vitamin C.

Aflatoxin

A common mold found on bread, nuts and fruit and in beer, apple cider vinegar and syrups, produces *aflatoxin*. This is what prevents you from detoxifying tiny bits of propyl alcohol that get into your body!

Buy bakery bread or bake your own. Roast nuts after washing in vitamin C water to destroy aflatoxin and then store in refrigerator. Keep moldy fruit out of the refrigerator where the spores can spread. Use only white distilled vinegar. Use honeys instead of syrups and even add vitamin C to them.

> ## Vitamin C helps your body detoxify all the mold toxins I have tested, including aflatoxin.

Keep powdered vitamin C in a salt shaker. It belongs on the table with salt and pepper, and at the stove. <u>Put it in everything possible,</u> from cereal to soup to rice (1/8 tsp. is enough). Besides this take 1/8 tsp. powdered vitamin C with each meal (500 mg).

Developing cancer is a chain of events. This explains why it is a disease of aging. For ten years or more you poisoned your body with freon, fiberglass, asbestos, mercury, lead, copper, etc. You continually ate moldy food (chips, nuts, etc.) which was toxic to the liver. But the liver regenerated the pieces that died. Eventually a mold toxin prevents the liver from regenerating. Your aflatoxin-ed liver then lets propyl alcohol build up after using it. You use more and more propyl alcohol.

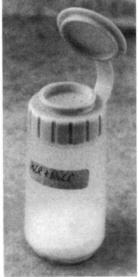

Fig. 42 Keep both salt and vitamin C powders in closable plastic shakers.

Somewhere, over the years, you pick up the intestinal fluke in a hamburger or from a pet or person. The stage is set and cancer is inevitable.

349

But pull out any <u>one</u> of the links in this chain and cancer is <u>impossible</u>. **Pull them all out for a return to good health.**

So cure yourself, prevent reinfection, heal the damage and go through life without this sword hanging over you.

Over 100 consecutive case histories of cured cancer victims are the subject of another book[16] along with more detailed instructions and suggestions.

---

[16] *The Cure For All Cancers*, by the same author, New Century Press 1993.

Curing HIV/AIDS

HIV and AIDS disease are very similar to cancer. That is why cancer is so often seen with HIV/AIDS. It is caused by the same parasite but the solvent is **benzene** instead of propyl alcohol.

**HIV stands for
Human Immunodeficiency Virus**

**AIDS stands for
Acquired Immune Deficiency Syndrome**

Many researchers believe HIV causes AIDS. I observe them both caused by parasites and solvents!

When the body can no longer detoxify benzene it soon may not be able to detoxify propyl alcohol. Food mold, at the base of the propyl alcohol problem, is also at the base of the benzene problem. Zearalenone, a mycotoxin I find in popcorn, corn chips, and brown rice specifically inhibits detoxification of benzene. None of us should be eating these foods untested.

Several common mold toxins inhibit the immune system, too, specifically those white blood cells that are supposed to eat and destroy viruses. Consequently, the HIV virus cannot be checked once it is introduced in the body.

Benzene goes to the bone marrow where T-cells are made, and to the thymus where T-cells are programmed, two big blows to the immune system.

Benzene, a most unthinkable pollutant, is widespread in extremely small amounts. But when **benzopyrenes** are added, the total is entirely too much for the liver and it begins to accumulate <u>in your thymus</u>.

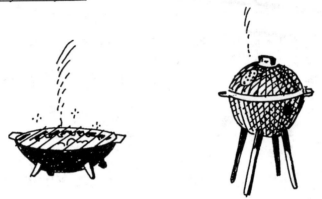

Fig. 43 Grilled food has benzopyrenes as do hot dogs and "smoke flavored" foods.

Benzopyrenes are <u>made</u> right in your food by direct flame-heat. Grilled food, smoked food, hot dogs and lunch meats with "smoke flavor" all have benzopyrenes—even toast has it. Food fried in a skillet does not (even if you burn it black!). As the thymus deteriorates from its benzene burden so does your immunity.

Without benzene in your body
you can't get AIDS.
Without the intestinal fluke in your body
you can't get HIV.

After killing the parasite and its stages the HIV virus will be gone in 2 hours, almost as quickly as the cancer marker, ortho-phospho-tyrosine. It is not necessary to zap the virus itself at 365 KHz.

But the AIDS is not gone. This depends on removing benzene from your body and keeping it <u>out</u> of your body. Keeping it out on alternate days or 5 days of the week will not suffice. It must be out consistently. Only then can your thymus and bone marrow recover.

As your thymus recovers your immunity returns. Immunity to all the diseases that lurk at very low level in our bodies. They are already in us. We have accumulated them in a lifetime. Mumps, measles, chicken pox, CMV, *Staphylococcus aureus*, *E. coli*, are all there. Until now they have been controlled–kept down–by an ever vigilant immune system. If this system fails you are an easy target for any and all of these invaders.

Method Of Treatment

As soon as you find you are HIV positive, don't panic. It was inevitable. It is also inevitable for many others with unexplainable risk factors. If you have a source of infection with the intestinal fluke and at the same time a source of benzene, HIV and AIDS are a logical result. You must stop the source of both.

Purchase or make a zapper or use somebody's frequency generator (434 KHz to 421 KHz giving 3 minutes to each KHz). Kill your flukes immediately. Take vitamin B_2 immediately to help detoxify benzene (three 100 mg. tablets 3 times a day, 9 altogether). Zap daily until you feel completely well: no night sweats, no coughing, no symptoms of any kind.

Remember parasites are all around us. We pick them up daily. And your weakened immune system lets everything gain a foothold in your body. Avoiding benzene will restore your immunity. Use the benzene pollution list to guide you.

Benzene Polluted Products

THROW THESE OUT

Your health is worth more than the fortune you spent on them!

- **Flavored food,** yogurt, jello, candies, throat lozenges, store-bought cookies, cakes
- **Cooking oil** and shortening (use <u>only</u> olive oil, butter and lard)
- **Bottled water,** <u>whether distilled, spring, mineral, or name brand.</u> Bottled fruit juice.
- **Cold cereal,** including granola and health brands
- **Toothpaste,** including health brands
- **Chewing gum**
- **Ice cream** and frozen yogurt
- **Pills and capsules.** At least a third of all I test are polluted. This includes herbal extracts and prescription drugs. Test yours and switch brands until you find a safe one.

- **Vaseline products** (Noxzema™, Vick's™, Lip Therapy™), chap stick, hand cleaners
- **Vitamins** and other **health supplements,** unless tested.

- **Rice cakes,** even the plain ones
- **Personal lubricant,** including lubricated condoms
- **Baking soda and cornstarch** (see *Sources*)
- **Soaps, hand creams,** skin creams, moisturizers
- Flavored pet food, both for cats and dogs
- Bird food made into cakes

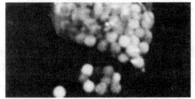

Fig. 44 Mexican made candy with no benzene.

It is impossible for me to have tested every batch of every food and product, but so many test positive you simply can not risk <u>any</u> of the foods and products on the list.

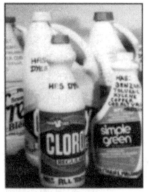

Learn to use the Syncrometer to do your own testing. While you are learning, observe the rules perfectly. There is no half way measure with benzene. Take an attitude of over-compliance, not "getting away" with as much as possible. Over-compliance can bring back

Fig. 45 Pollutants are in unlikely places

<u>radiant</u> health, strength you never knew you had, a beautiful normal body again! You will be able to resume your plans for education, professional life, personal relationships, free of the sword hanging over you. You will not be infectious to anybody. Let over-compliance enthuse you.

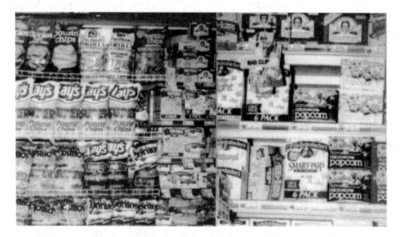

Fig. 46 Every brand of popcorn and corn chips I tested had zearalenone contamination.

There are 2 extra rules that help eliminate benzene buildup:

1. Never eat moldy or grilled foods including popcorn, corn chips, grocery store breads, pasta, nuts, alcoholic beverages, toast, brown rice (white is OK).
2. Always take Vitamin B$_2$ (three 100 mg tablets three times a day) and vitamin C (1/8 tsp. with each meal).

Plan For The Future

After you are well again, you may wish to indulge in some philosophy. How did an obscure virus–a snail virus!–become a human virus? This is not so bizarre. After all, rabies virus comes to us from animals, and many encephalitis viruses come from mosquitoes. How did HIV spread so rapidly? How did a pollutant as dangerous as benzene get to be in our very food? Are other parasites getting set to spring on us? What must be done to protect ourselves and loved ones from future disasters? Would getting away from fossil fuel be a big answer? Would getting away from preoccupation with chemistry be a big answer? Would more disclosure of industrial practices be an answer? Should the government agencies responsible for food and product safety be depoliticized? Should public inspection of food manufacturing be a right? Should disclosure of foreign origins of food ingredients be mandatory? Would communicating with other cancer and AIDS survivors be useful? The computer age would make communication possible. Communication leads to answers. Answers might lead to new policies. Policies supported at the grass roots level can bring about change.

Over 50 case histories of cured HIV victims are the subject of another book[17] along with more detailed instructions and suggestions.

---

[17]*The Cure for HIV and AIDS*, by the same author, New Century Press, 1993.

Curing The Common Cold

Sometimes you can zap *Adenovirus*, the common cold virus, at 393 KHz for three minutes with a frequency generator and be rid of your cold, magically, in five minutes. But magic and luck are not really responsible for this. And most of the time the cold will reappear a few hours later.

Homeopathy, too, can immediately banish your cold symptoms. The reason is not mysterious either. But, this time, the cold reappears later in a different location. Choose the right homeopathic remedy for that, and you can chase it away again.

Tapeworm Stage or Mites

The fascinating story of how we really "catch" a cold kept me spellbound for a year. I was hot on the heels of *Adenovirus* wherever it might be in my body. Sometimes I saw it; sometimes I didn't. Sometimes I had cold symptoms; sometimes I didn't. Sometimes I could zap it; sometimes it did no good.

It is now apparent to me that *Adenovirus* isn't our (a human) virus at all! It belongs to other parasites. Parasites as varied as tapeworm stages and mites. Perhaps it belongs to many other parasites, as well. My evidence comes from a tapeworm stage, cysticercus of *Diphyllobothrium erinacea*, the mites *Sarcoptes* and *Dermatophagoides*, and our own colon bacteria, *E. coli*.

The tapeworm stage flies in the dust as eggs, you can trap these by setting out a pint jar with a little water in it. In three days' time you are likely to find its frequency near 487 KHz in your jar. You are also likely to find it on your kitchen sponge, since you wipe up dust each day. To test it, place it in a plastic bag, wet it thoroughly and search from 510 KHz downward, one KHz at a time. The various tapeworm stages emit between 510 and 440 KHz.

If you have a household pet, you will <u>always</u> be able to find a tapeworm stage in your sponge or in a dust sample you collect from the table or kitchen counter in the morning. Gather dust with a damp bit of paper towel, put it in a plastic bag. Then wash your hands or you may accidentally eat some.

This, of course, happens to every household member. Eating the dust off the tables, inhaling the dust, and eating off surfaces wiped by the kitchen sponge happens to everyone. And everyone "catches" colds. If you search for *Adenovirus*, though, in your dust sample, it isn't there!

Similarly, you can search for the mites in your house dust. Search near the frequencies given for them. There is a good chance you will have one that is not given, because the list is so incomplete. Name it after yourself. Compare notes with others; maybe it is common, maybe it's a rare one. Again, you will not find *Adenovirus* beeping its characteristic frequency out of your mite specimen. Why not? Possibly, it is too faint; it must multiply and create a loud chorus before you can hear it. But multiply it will, if given a chance, in <u>you</u>. You must, of course, first eat or inhale the dust.

Then the tape eggs hatch into the *cysticercus* stage, which promptly gets to the liver. Sometimes it gets to other organs, like the muscles, the spleen, the pancreas. Presumably the liver screened it out of the blood originally.

Soon you will zap them, wherever they are. If you are using a slide specimen of *cysticercus* you can locate it in your body. If you are only listening to its beeps, you can't. If you can do both, you may be able to see which organ allows the virus to replicate after it emerges. Maybe only the respiratory organs do; maybe they start to replicate in the organ where they emerge, such as the liver and <u>then</u> get to the respiratory tract. This is a fascinating avenue I have not yet explored.

Mites are inhaled or swallowed or both, just as tapeworm eggs are. They are on your kitchen sponge, and in any food or dishes that stand uncovered anywhere in the home. Never drink water from a glass that has "stood out" all day. After finding one, you will notice it beeping in you for several days. Then the beep disappears; presumably the mite is dead.

The tapeworm stage beeps may disappear in a few days, too, presumably dead. Except in cases of disease. Muscles that are diseased will take in the newcomer and allow it to survive adding to the parasites and pollutants already there! Evidently the immune power of such diseased locations is way down.

On the day that the mite stops beeping, the day it dies, *Adenovirus* appears!

Not many *Adenovirus* at first. You will need to search several times during the day to find it in your white blood cells. (And you have no symptoms, yet, either!) Is it a coincidence that *Adenovirus* appeared directly after a tapeworm stage or mite died?

You can find out by waiting until a time when you have a tapeworm stage or mite and no *Adenovirus*. Then kill your tapeworm stage or mite by zapping for seven minutes. Within minutes after that, the beeping of the tapeworm stage or mite is gone and *Adenovirus* can be heard, loud and clear at 393 KHz! And minutes later you may feel a stuffy nose, a slight congestion developing, a certain head feeling that is different. You are "catching" a cold!

Will you really get this cold? Will it become a full blown cold of the usual kind? After seeing this happen dozens of times after killing a mite or tapeworm stage I concluded that *Adenovirus* really belongs to them; the virus is scuttling its dying host like people jumping off a sinking ship into the ocean. Our bodies are the ocean for them. They too, immediately swim and search for a hospitable island. Our respiratory tract is such an island; perhaps other organs, too.

Yes, this "baby cold" will develop into a full blown cold if, but only if, you have a mold in you!

Molds and Colds

This is part two of the cold story. You may have *Adenoviruses* quietly slipping into your blood stream and tissues from a tapeworm stage or mite you inhaled, or *E. coli* bacteria that strayed into your tissues, and which is being slowly killed by your immune system. Your immune system can keep up with them quite easily <u>provided</u> you don't have a mold in you at the same time. The significance of the mold is that it lowers your immunity, specifically and generally.

Mold eluded, is health improv-ed.

This has already been studied extensively for a number of food molds. There are a variety of ways that mold toxins lower immunity. Some simply kill white blood cells. Others seem to "bind and gag" them so they just can't go about eating viruses.

So with mold toxins present, *Adenovirus*, fleeing the dead tapeworm stage, mite, or *E. coli* is not gobbled up. It has time to get to its favorite organ and enter the cells there. It may get in your lungs if they're full of arsenic or formaldehyde, in your throat if it's full of mercury from your fillings, in your spinal cord if it's full of thallium. Sometimes you feel the viral attack, sometimes you don't.

When *E. coli* is the source of your *Adenovirus*, a question pops up. Why don't you have a perpetual cold, since these bacteria are always in your colon...and should be! As long as *E. coli* stays dutifully in your colon, no *Adenovirus* is seen. But as soon as any cross the colon wall to invade your body, your white blood cells pounce on them. After this, *Adenovirus* appears and again you are catching a cold. They may go to your internal organs where you don't feel them.

One place you do feel an attack is in your respiratory tract: lungs, bronchi, sinuses, nose, Eustachian tubes, inner ear, eyes or head. And the size of the attack depends on whether you recently ate moldy food.

Human food (in general, in the U.S.) is very, very moldy. We do not taste it because manufacturers have been using more and more flavorings in food. This covers up small amounts of mold or "off" flavor. Measures to reduce mold are not effective enough.

Bread is a good example. Calcium propionate is added to bread-stuff to inhibit molding. That's fine. But then the bread is encased in plastic to hold in moisture and keep it "fresh". The moisture acts to incubate mold spores and overwhelms the inhibitor. Vinegar is used instead of calcium propionate in some breads but, again, the plastic ruins its effectiveness.

Another good mold inhibitor is lime water. This is used in making tortillas. None of the old fashioned tortillas (made with just corn, water, lime) that I tested had any mold, even without propionate added! Other tortillas made of flour and calcium propionate frequently had molds.

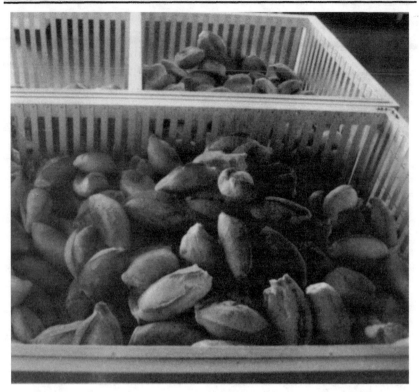

Fig. 47 This Mexican bread had no molds. It is made from white, unbleached flour and is not wrapped in plastic.

Bread is such a staple we must correct its mold problem immediately. The two likely sources for the mold spores are: in the flour to begin with, or just flying about the bakery and landing on the newly baked loaves. Bread flour in the grocery store is quite free of mold spores, so maybe it is the bakery that needs to change. Perhaps it is not possible to bake 24 hours a day in the same building, year after year, without bits of flour and moisture accumulating in the millions of tiny cracks and crevices that all buildings have and germinating mold. Yet bread from small neighborhood bakeries does not have mold!

> **Only buy fresh bread not wrapped in plastic.**

As soon as you feel a cold coming, ask yourself: what did you eat recently that might have been moldy? Cold cereal, hot cereal, bread, crackers, cookies, rice, other grains, fresh fruit, store bought fruit juice, nuts, syrups, pasta, honey? This takes up a large part of any person's diet, even in a single meal. The answer is yes, no doubt you ate moldy food recently.

So you can't catch a cold directly from some sneezy companion, or *E. coli*, or tapeworm stages, or mites. You have to eat moldy food first. This lowers your immunity, allowing any *Adenovirus* to invade your weakest tissues. If that happens to be your respiratory system, you get classic symptoms. (Those same "cold" symptoms can be caused by bacteria, for which I have preliminary evidence of arriving in a similar fashion.)

As fascinating as this whole story is, the bottom line is: how can you stop a cold, in record time?

The Cure

Remember, zapping does not kill your cells. So anything hiding in them will not be harmed by the electric current either. Viruses live inside your cells while they reproduce. You can only kill the outsiders: those stuck in your cell gateways. The rest will be killed by your own cells in time. Not much time. Five or six hours at most. Your cells do it with mucous secretion, inflammation and other unknown ways. So zapping is an imperfect solution.

Using a frequency generator to electrocute *Adenovirus* (393 KHz for three minutes) is not effective either because you are not killing the mites and tapeworm stages at the same time, and the *Adenoviruses* are coming from them.

The best advice to stop a cold is to:

1. **Eat sterile food for 24 hours.** Follow the Mold Free Diet on page 365. Do not eat one questionable item.

2. Take **vitamin C** (10 grams or 2 tsp.), a **B50 complex** (2 tablets), and niacinamide (3 500 mg tablets) to help detoxify the mycotoxins already in you. See *Sources*. It will still take five or six hours for your white blood cells to recover their ability to capture viruses, for the "gag" to wear off.

3. **Zap** for seven minutes, killing all viruses, tapeworm stages and mites together. **Wait** twenty minutes to let viruses and bacteria in the dead larger parasites emerge. **Zap** a second time for seven minutes to kill those viruses and bacteria. **Wait** twenty minutes to let any viruses infecting the killed bacteria emerge. **Zap** a third time for seven minutes to kill the last viruses.

4. Now you need only wait for your tissues to decongest and stop making mucous, etc.

5. Immediately start the Bowel Program (page 546) in case yours is an *E. coli* cold. You can't, and wouldn't want to, kill all the bacteria in your bowel. Zapping kills the escapees, though, to give a bit of relief, and the Bowel Program stops the invasive *E. coli*.

6. Do additional zapping as time permits until the Bowel Program has stemmed the invasion.

In five or six hours your cold could be gone.

Of all these measures, stopping mold consumption is the most important. If you eat peanut butter now, your cold will return with a vengeance. If you eat cheese it will add *Salmonella* to your illness and you may develop a fever. Your own immune system is the most powerful cold killer, so stop handicapping it.

Test yourself for the presence of molds to see if you are accomplishing your goal. The various molds I have tested had these emitting frequencies: 77, 88, 100, 126, 133, 177, 181, 188, 232, 242, 277, 288, 295 KHz.

In about five hours, some relief will be felt. The time it takes depends on how much mold you ate. But if you stop immediately and eat only perfectly safe food, your illness will be over in the shortest time. Shorter than merely zapping.

Mold Free Diet

Stick to this for 24 hours, even if you feel better much sooner.

Before starting to cook sterilize your kitchen sponge (microwave it for three minutes), and wash hands.

Breakfast

- 1 or 2 eggs any style. The egg carton and egg exterior have *Salmonella* on them, so remove the eggs, replace the carton, wash the exterior of the eggs and then your hands again before cracking them. You don't want a *Salmonella* infection added to your cold.
- Hash brown potatoes
- Pancakes or waffles with artificial maple syrup made with brown sugar and vitamin C.
- 1 cup herb tea with vitamin C, cinnamon, or other spice.

- Water with a tsp. of vinegar and honey.

Lunch

- Soup without noodles, without rice or any grain product.
- Homemade biscuits or bakery bread with butter.
- Homemade pudding or custard, all ingredients well cooked.

Supper

- Well cooked fish or seafood (canned O.K., like sardines, salmon and tuna).
- Fresh green vegetables, in perfect condition.
- Cooked vegetables with olive oil and salt (pure, see *Sources*).
- Canned beans, any variety.
- Baked or boiled potato (don't eat skin) with olive oil and salt as described on page 310.
- Hot water with whipping cream and cinnamon.
- A perfectly unblemished banana.
- Water with lemon.

You can "mix and match" these safe foods. If you get a hefty dose of mold at the outset of your cold, the toxicity lasts quite a long time. Repeat the diet the next day and the next until you are well. In animal experiments reported by scientists, toxicity from mold usually lasted three weeks. Sometimes the real damage was only <u>seen</u> after three weeks! Keep up your vigilance. When you decide to take some risks, make sure vitamin C has been added to the new food and mixed with it thoroughly.

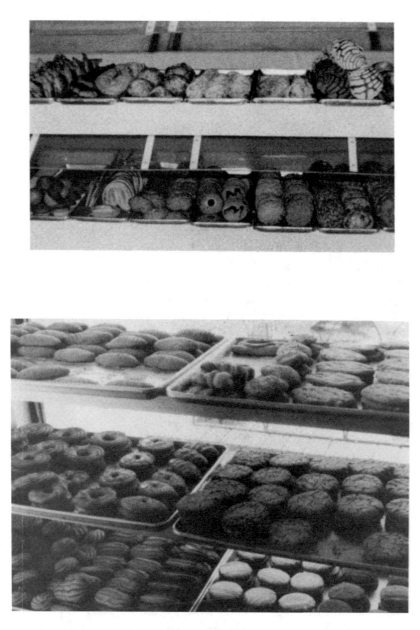

*Fig. 48 Goods baked in a panaderia (Mexican style bakery)
never tested positive to molds.*

Prevention

What is the best way to prevent a cold? Stop eating moldy food. We were never meant to eat rotting, spoiling food. We were meant to be repelled by the bad odor, the bad appearance, the bad taste. Our parents were supposed to teach us in childhood to distinguish between good and bad food. This system no longer works. By mixing spoiled food with good food, by adding flavors and changing the food consistency, parents can't distinguish substandard foods, nor teach their children to.

We rely on government agency assurances, like beef grades, expiration dates, approved food colors and additives. And when they fail? We land in a debacle such as the present one, where large segments of society are ill with uncontrollable behavior (called crime), suffer from hormone imbalances and sexual disturbances, are sidelined by chronic fatigue and new illness. But the greatest social disaster is lowered immunity—AIDS.

We cannot individually control the destiny of our species. But we can get ourselves out of the path of the falling human tide. We can dissent. We can say **NO** to rotten moldy food.

What about exposure to a cold? Won't you catch one if you're in a roomful of coughing, sneezing people? Or you shake hands with a coughing, sneezing person? Or you drink from the same glass as a person with a cold? Or your child plays with the same toys as sick children?

Yes, you will catch the virus, but you won't get sick. If you are tracking *Adenovirus* using the electronic techniques in this book, you will see that it infects you immediately after eating coughed-on food. It stays in you about twenty minutes. Then it disappears, evidently eaten up by your white blood cells, **provided there is no mold toxin in you**. But if you do have a mold toxin in you, the virus spreads, multiplies and gives you a cold! I have only followed *Adenovirus* behavior. There are numerous other "cold bugs" left for you to track. Each illness in your family could provide you with a specimen to research.

This throws light on self infection, too. When we cough into our hands and then eat with them, we self-infect. But it only makes us sicker if we harbor molds.

Curing Symptoms

Cold <u>symptoms</u> alone can be cured much faster than the cold. Taking drugs proves that. Most of the drugs on the market can cure some symptoms in less than one hour. But not without a price, such as a harmful side effect.

Homeopathy can cure cold symptoms too, without side effects. There are three or four favorite homeopathic remedies for colds and eight or nine less common ones. To use them you read the symptoms listed and take the remedy with the closest match.

Homeopathic Remedy	For These Symptoms
Aconitum	early cold with fever, headache, hoarse cough
Allium	clear runny nose with burning of lips or eyes
Arsenicum	sneezing cold, frontal headache, tickling cough
Belladonna	high fever cold with flushed face, throbbing head
Kali bi	thick post nasal drip, colored discharge, sinus headache
Spongia	croupy cough

Fig. 49 Starter set of homeopathic remedies.

There are lots more remedies with fascinating symptoms to try to match with your own. Books suggest that you start with a 6X or a 12X remedy, but success is more certain with 30X. Use three remedies simultaneously. If you get total relief at some point, stop. If the cold has moved or won't budge, try another set of three after an hour. Don't take them within 15 minutes of food or anything else. Homeopathy makes very interesting reading.

Homeopaths say they stimulate the immune system specifically. My results show they do much more. They go right to the gateways of your cells and evict the tiny parasite, bacteria or virus stuck to the latch and trying to get in. Your immune system would be able to gobble them all up if they weren't gagged by the food mold you ate.

Different homeopathic remedies go to different tissues, so you can only clear one tissue at a time. If you plan on trying this for yourself, order the set of cold remedies listed above (see *Sources*). The homeopathic method would be a beautiful cold cure if it weren't for the mold intrusion.

Herbs, too, can cure symptoms rather quickly. **Elderberry tea** mixed with **peppermint** is cited in herbal textbooks and it could probably do a lot if it weren't for the mold immuno-suppression. If you plan on trying these start with a set of **thyme**, **fenugreek**, **sage** (for throat). Since both herbs and homeopathic remedies work on the principle of ejection, they could eject each other. Maybe the last one to arrive takes over. This is an exciting field for you to explore.

Ultimately, the length of time your own white blood cells are bound and gagged decides how soon you are really cured of your cold. Remember taking vitamin C (10 grams or more) helps detoxify the molds. If you find a recipe that works for everybody in less than five hours, be sure to let everybody know.

True Origins Of Viruses

Your body can eliminate any virus in a short time, such as hours or days. It can even keep up with a steady stream that is coming from tapeworm stages!

Let us apply these new insights to several diseases we are familiar with. Let us speculate what could really be happening.

Epstein Barre Virus (EBV) is a mysterious disease because in spite of building up antibodies, it attacks repeatedly. I only see EBV if the person also has *Eurytrema* (pancreatic fluke) in the pancreas. When the fluke is gone, I no longer find EBV in the white blood cells. This suggests that the virus comes from the fluke. As each fluke dies and is finally removed, the body's white blood cells can catch up with the viruses and you begin to feel better again, which can be as quick as one day. But reinfection with an EBV-carrying *Eurytrema* (plus a wood alcohol containing beverage to allow the fluke to go to the pancreas) can spark the next recurrence.

Shingles is a recurrence of chicken pox. I always find *Ascaris* in persons with shingles! Unfortunately, killing the *Ascaris* does not cure shingles. *Herpes Zoster* (the shingles/chicken pox virus) is known to hide in nerve cells. Perhaps *Ascaris* facilitates it's release, or simply suppresses the immune system in a way that allows it to suddenly multiply.

Polio was once a scourge. At that time, we can theorize that a new large parasite was making its appearance. Was a new animal association taking place in the early 1900's? Life was indeed becoming more urban with horse manure on all streets. Owning a dog for a house pet was becoming an acceptable lifestyle. Could the tapeworms of these animals give us a tapeworm stage that hosts polio virus? Many polio sufferers also had migraines. These are caused by *Strongyloides*, a horse threadworm. Does *Strongyloides* host polio virus?

The **HIV** virus infects us during the time the intestinal fluke, *Fasciolopsis buskii*, is being hosted. Persons test negative to HIV shortly after the fluke and its stages are eliminated.

Coxsackie viruses give us some of our encephalitises. I never see *Coxsackie* viruses without the bacteria, *Bacteroides fragilis*, and I never see *Bacteroides fragilis* without *Ascaris* (a roundworm.) I conclude that one lives inside the other!

We may be deriving viruses from all the roundworms, flukes, tapeworms and bacteria that infect us! It would be a fascinating study, simply to examine each of these parasites singly, searching for their viruses with an electron microscope. They could also be searched for using immunological methods.

Fortunately, your health improvement does not need to wait on such studies. Your electronic technique can detect them in your body long before you are made ill by them. You don't need to know their hosts in order to stop hosting them yourself.

It is a time of great change for this planet as pollution spreads from pole to pole. The growth of industrial activity, mining, chemical manufacturing, the food "industry", and personal habits like smoking have spread new chemicals to every corner of the globe. The element *polonium*, which is radioactive and in tobacco smoke, is harmful to human lungs, but <u>may not be harmful</u> to a small lung parasite, like *Pneumocystis carnii*.

Benzene, which is a solvent and extremely harmful to humans, may not be harmful to fluke parasites living within us. Propyl alcohol facilitates the intestinal fluke but is toxic to us.

Parasites are doing abnormal things. Is this because of pollution?

The tables are gradually being turned <u>against</u> us in favor of our parasites and pathogens. Such large changes are called evolutionary. Is the human species doomed, or will some of us "adapt". Will some of us survive to pass on our "better" genes to a new population of cancer-resistant, AIDS-resistant, Alzheimer's-resistant, etc.-resistant humans? How many of us will die trying?

The common cold should not be so common!

Body Wisdom and Why Bad Food Tastes Good

Don't let yourself eat junk food just because your body craves something in it. Try to figure out what it is your body craves. Could it be fat? Could it be salt? Could it be starch?

Salt

If it's salt, you might also love popcorn and other salty food. This implicates the adrenal glands. Maybe they're letting too much salt (sodium chloride) leave the body through the kidneys. Maybe they're letting too much potassium chloride through, too. A diuretic pill could certainly have a similar effect.

Help the adrenal glands do their job of regulating sodium and potassium chloride by cleaning them up. Let salt-hunger be your signal to do a kidney cleanse (page 549). This will clean adrenals too. Even a slight drop in sodium and potassium chloride in the blood (body fluids) can make you too fatigued to tie your own shoelaces.

Remember, when your body craves potato chips, it craves <u>something in</u> the potato chips. If you let yourself eat highly salted food while you're giving the adrenals a clean up, at least add potassium chloride to your diet. Make yourself a mixture of equal parts of sodium chloride and potassium chloride. Part of salt hunger is actually potassium hunger. Let your body (your taste) decide on the amount of potassium chloride to add. Maybe one part potassium chloride to two or three parts sodium chloride is a better mixture for you. After mixing, store it in the original containers (re-label them) to prevent caking. If you put it in an ordinary salt shaker, it will cake soon. Use a shaker with a lid that closes.

Fats

Maybe you like French fries because of the fat. If you deprive yourself of the "good" normal greases that come from plant or animal sources which would ordinarily make up 25% of your calories, of course you'll crave grease. But what a bad trade it is. Now you are getting lab-made (hydrogenated) grease with a non-biological structure, and loaded with the carcinogen nickel.

So if you're body tells you that you need grease, go back to olive oil, butter, cheese (baked only), lard, avocados, nuts and nut butters (homemade only) and seeds. Humankind has been eating these natural fats long before cholesterol was vilified. The key to cholesterol control is not fat avoidance, but a liver cleanse!

Starch

If switching to natural greases doesn't satisfy your "fat-tooth", maybe its the potato in the French fries that your body craves. Plain, pure starch. Do you also love bread and pasta (more pure starch though very inferior to potatoes)? Pure starch is very easy to digest and has a large adsorptive capability for toxins. In fact, if any family member should accidentally eat something poisonous, drinking cornstarch will quickly mop it up and keep it stuck so it can't enter your tissues. (This doesn't work for all poisons.) By craving pure starches, your body could be telling you about a need to improve your digestion (liver disorders) or to eat and breathe less toxic things.

Maybe a stomach-full of baby *Ascaris* is telling you to eat only food that doesn't need a lot of acid: "just potatoes, bread and pasta, please, and skip the sauce." *Ascaris* inhibits acid production by the stomach. This can result in an aversion to meat.

It doesn't take much acid to digest pure starch and get it on its way out of the stomach. And out of the stomach means relief: relief of the pressure on the diaphragm and liver, heartburn, that too-full feeling, and other digestive disturbances.

Sugar

Your body runs on sugar. If you are short on sugar it will turn fat into sugar. If you are short on both, it will turn your muscles into sugar. However eating more sugar doesn't cure the craving. You have to find out why you are so short, in spite of eating it.

The first thing to try is 1 mg chromium (five 200 mcg tablets, see *Sources*) per day. If you still crave sugar after a week the problem is something else. Perhaps you have pancreatic flukes upsetting your sugar regulation. Kill them and go off commercial beverages that may contain wood alcohol. Sugar regulation is very complex, but these two approaches help most of the time.

Dislikes

Respect your body's opinion when it says, "No, I don't want to eat that." Our education about nutritive value of food may be sound but there are other facts to consider. We should take a lesson from nursing babies: when they refuse to nurse, there is something unpalatable in the mother's milk. Usually the mother has eaten onions or members of the cabbage family. The baby tries it once, and learns to reject it immediately. The baby's liver, in its wisdom, does not want the baby to eat what it can't properly digest. The mother may feel: "Now, this breast milk is good for you and drink it you must, or you shall go hungry." Unfortunately, this works for 2-year-olds and up. They are forced to eat carrots, peas, and other vegetables; vegetables that taste terrible, (modern agriculture has ruined the flavor). They alone taste the bitterness of PIT, a cyanide-related chemical, and very difficult for the liver to metabolize. Broccoli and onions may burn the tongue with its sulfur-containing acids. Green beans, onions, garlic, eggplant, all have unique chemicals in them. If you or your child are not ready to eat them, avoid them carefully, so you don't get a surprise dose of the toxic chemical.

The more mold a child eats, inadvertently, in peanut butter, bread, potato chips, syrups, the less capable the liver is of detoxifying foods. This will certainly increase the "pickiness" of a child's appetite. If your child has too many foods on her or his personal "off list", let this signal you to improve liver function. Stop the barrage of chemicals that comes with cold cereals, canned soup, grocery bread, instant cheese dishes, artificially flavored gelatin, canned whipped cream, fancy yogurts and cookies or chips. Move to a simpler diet, cooked cereal with honey, cinnamon and whipping cream (only 4 ingredients), milk (boiled), bakery bread, canned tuna or salmon, plain cooked or fried potatoes with butter, and slices of raw vegetables and fruit without any sauces, except honey or homemade tomato sauce, to dip into.

It is frustrating to cook "a fine meal" for the family and find everybody likes it except Ms. Picky. The good news is that she can usually think of something she would rather eat. If it's nutritious, be thankful. If it's not say No.

Adults should hide their junk food, including everything off limits to children. Don't "hide" your junk food in the refrigerator and lower level cupboards! Treat yourself as well as your child. If a food tastes bad, don't eat it. If you crave it, try to understand the message.

Outwit The Cravings

Here are some examples. Suppose you crave these items:

- **Pickles**. They supply vinegar and are often loved by persons with little acid in their stomachs or a lot of yeast (vinegar is a yeast inhibitor). Start drinking water with lemon juice or vinegar and honey.
- **Bacon**. The fat soothes the stomach and slows down digestion. Switch to butter and cream, with meals.
- **Sugar coated cereals.** Loved by persons with disturbed sugar regulation. Kill parasites, avoid wood alcohol, use chromium tablets and a lot of cinnamon.
- **Crunchy munchies**. Your jaw and teeth want some work to do. Try salads, an apple, raw sunflower seeds (beware of moldy seeds, nuts and dried fruit).
- **Ice cream.** Ice cold food stimulates the thyroid; loved by low thyroid persons. Clean up the thyroid by doing dental work and liver cleanses.
- **Caffeine**-laced beverages. Stimulate many body tissues, raise blood pressure. Loved by low energy people. Do a general body and environment cleanup. (There are people who say coffee puts them to sleep. Insomnia has better solutions than caffeine, though.)
- **Candy.** The more you eat the more you crave because chromium is being used up as you eat it and yet it is necessary to utilize more sugar. Give yourself chromium (GTF) tablets totaling 1 mg. (1,000 mcg.) a day and watch your sugar craving shrink.
- **Pretzels.** You want salt plus crunch.

- **Potato chips.** You want salt, grease, starch and crunch. No wonder they are so popular!

If your body still has its wisdom, or most of it, why can't it detect the mold in peanuts, crackers and bread for us? There is a very sound reason. Our food manufacturers have gone to great lengths to fool our native senses. Salt and sugar, roasting and flavoring, do most of it.

Your body is accustomed, natively, to interpret sugar, salt, and flavors as "good, good, good." Of course, the mold is "bad, bad, bad." But when you mix them, what is your body to read? The "goods" always win; manufacturers don't stop until they do. More flavorings are added. The result is that you can be eating rotten moldy food without knowing it.

Food that is predominantly concocted can't be interpreted by your body wisdom. You must use your second-best ally, your intelligence.

How would you interpret these situations, taken from real life:

- An elderly person can't stand butter, wants and enjoys margarine.
- A child prefers canned spaghetti for the real thing.
- A child wants to eat only sweets, everything else must be coaxed down.
- A young man needs "his" beer to enjoy a cook-out.
- A young man with serious mental illness drinks half a gallon of Mellow Yellow™ a day.
- A child wants ketchup on everything.
- A pregnant woman puts herself on a pickled pigs feet and white bread diet.

Back To Normal

Body wisdom was not meant to substitute for parental teaching. They must both be there. But when there is conflict, trust your wisdom. Will you ever get your primitive body wisdom back and enjoy vegetables, fruit, simple styles of cooking and baking them? Yes, to a considerable extent. You'll hold your nose at all seeds and nuts and most flour (they smell so rancid). You'll back away from cookies and cakes, especially icing (they taste like you imagine shortening tastes). You'll retreat from deep fat fried foods: the dripping grease will just undo the appetite. You'll say "No thanks" to canned food and metal cutlery (you can taste the metal now). You'd have to force yourself to eat grocery bread (it's so doughy and sour smelling). Wheat germ smells terrible (rancidity). Even vitamin tablets may smell awful.

Has life been ruined, now that plain potatoes and butter taste good? Your body wisdom has returned. You are the true gourmet. It is as different as corn on the cob is from the canned variety. Perhaps you are "spoiled" now by eating un-rotten food. Accept the charge with humor and dignity—as long as you're not expected to eat any more spoiled, moldy food.

Toxic Food

Grilled food develops *benzopyrenes* in it that are very toxic.

In an age of lowered immunity, it makes little sense to deliberately poison the food with benzopyrenes. Especially for children, who will be faced with new viruses and parasites in their lifetimes. Will they be able to overcome them or succumb at middle age? Only the strength of their immune system decides this.

Benzopyrenes must be detoxified using the liver's valuable benzene-detoxification system. With so many benzene-polluted items, there is hardly enough detoxification capability to get it all taken care of. NAD enzymes (the N stands for niacin) come into play too. These are essential for alcohol detoxification. If you have consumed alcohol, like a can of beer, NAD enzymes must be shared between the alcohol in the beer and the benzene in the beer. It takes longer to detoxify both the benzene and alcohol. The time delay is a time of lowered immunity and facilitates a growth spurt for parasites and pathogens.

Foods that are raised to very high temperatures, made possible with a microwave oven, produce benzopyrenes. Ordinary bread-toasters can do this too! Old fashioned toasters had a layer of metal separating the bread from the wires. Toasting bread in a frying pan or a stove top surface protects it too. But your stove grill, whether electric or flame, will produce benzopyrenes in your food unless there is a separating wall between them.

It does not matter what kind of fuel is used, the benzopyrenes develop due to lack of shielding between the food and heat source. A metal wall between them absorbs some of the heat.

Do not burn your food in a microwave oven. Since the temperature may go higher than your regular oven, you can produce benzopyrenes. Your regular oven is thermostated so that it cannot go higher than it states. Baking and browning is never done above 425°F. This is your safety feature. If anything in your microwave has turned dark brown or black or has melted plastic, throw it out!

Supplements that help your body to detoxify the benzopyrenes are:

1. Niacin or niacinamide. These are NAD-builders. Take 50 mg with each meal.
2. Vitamin B_2 (riboflavin). Take 50 mg with each meal.

For unpolluted vitamins see *Sources*.

It would be wise to teach children the habits that maximize their immune strength. Avoiding food toxins that are specifically immune-lowering is most important. Besides the benzopyrenes, certain mold toxins and solvents do this and are found in foods.

Moldy Food

Everything that's animal or vegetable can get moldy. While living things are alive, the mold attackers can be held at bay. As soon as they are dead, molding begins. First it molds; then bacterial action sets in. This is what makes things biodegradable. It is a precious phenomenon. It does away with filth—in an exquisite manner. Without mold and decay the streets of New York would still be full of horse manure from the days of the horse and buggy and our lakes too full of dead fish to swim in.

Every grain has its molds; every fruit has its molds; tea and coffee plants have their molds; as do all herbs, and vegetables. Nuts have their molds; nuts grown in the ground (peanuts) are especially moldy because the earth is so full of mold spores. But the wind carries these spores high up into trees, and even up to the stratosphere. Molds are not very choosy. They have their preference for certain plants and conditions. But the same molds can grow on many plants. This is why aflatoxin, for instance, is found not just in your cereal, bread and pasta but in nuts, maple syrup, orange juice, vinegar, wine, etc. Where is it not? It is not in dairy products or fresh fruit and vegetables, provided you wash the outside. It is not in meat, eggs, and fish. It is not in water.

Although I find aflatoxin in commercial bread, I do not find it in carefully screened wheat that has had its discolored, shriveled seeds removed before using it for making bread, cereals

381

and noodles. It is not in baked goods bought at bakeries, left open to air. Evidently the system of wrapping baked goods in plastic keeps moisture trapped and starts the molding process. In spite of adding mold inhibitors, American bread-stuff is far inferior to Mexican baked goods in which I do not find aflatoxin!

Here is some good news for cooks: if you bake it yourself, adding a bit of vitamin C to the dough, your breads will be mold free for an extended period (and rise higher).

Aflatoxin

What is so important about molds? Some of them produce very, very toxic chemicals wherever they grow. They produce some of the most toxic chemicals known to exist. Aflatoxin is one of these. My tests show it is always present in cancer patients; in other words it has built up due to the body's inability to detoxify it in a reasonable time. A great deal of research has been done on aflatoxin. Any library would have more information.

Aflatoxin reaches the liver and simply kills portions of it. After a hefty dose the liver is weakened for a long time— possibly years. Hepatitis and cirrhosis cases always reveal aflatoxin. The liver fights hard to detoxify aflatoxin and manage its own survival. It manages for 2 to 3 weeks; then a portion of it succumbs. So the toxic effects of a dose of aflatoxin aren't even noticeable for several weeks! And without a taste or smell to guide you, how would you know to stop eating the moldy peanut butter or spaghetti? The answer is:

1. make and bake things for yourself
2. test the things you dearly love but can't make
3. treat things that are treatable for molds
4. throw the rest out of your diet

Treatments mentioned in the industrial research journals are hydrogen peroxide, strong alkali such as lime-water, metabisulfite (a common reducing agent) and high heat. I have tried heat and vitamin C, which is also a reducing agent.

Just heating a food to the boiling point does not kill the molds. Boiling for many minutes at a higher temperature or baking does kill them (but not ergot, another mold) and also destroys aflatoxin they produced and left in the food. For foods you can't heat that high, for example nuts that are already roasted, or vinegar, vitamin C comes to the rescue. I suppose it acts a lot like the bisulfite; chemically destroying the mold toxin molecules.

Eradicating Aflatoxin

Simply sprinkling vitamin C over **roasted nuts** is not effective because the molds have penetrated the surface. Rinse the nuts in water first (a lot of mold is removed in this simple way). Cover the nuts with water, add about ¼ tsp. vitamin C powder (for a pint of nuts) and mix. Let stand for 5 minutes. The water penetrates the nuts, taking the vitamin C with it and detoxifies them. Pour off the water and dry the nuts in the oven at low heat. (Don't burn them or you will make benzopyrenes.)

Rice and **pastas** can be demolded partly by cooking and partly by adding vitamin C before or after cooking. There is no need to add so much it affects the flavor. Brown rice is especially moldy.

Vinegars can simply have vitamin C added and placed in the refrigerator.

Honey can be warmed and treated the same way (¼ tsp. per pint).

Bread cannot be salvaged. Switch to bakery breads or homemade. Use it up in a few days, left in its paper bag. Or slice and place in a plastic bag in the freezer.

Since all foods have both their own and others' molds, there must be thousands of molds. Very many have been studied besides aflatoxin producers.

Zearalenone

Zearalenone, an anabolic and uterotrophic metabolite, is frequently found in commercial cereal grains and in processed foods and feeds, and is often reported as causative agent of naturally occurring hyperestrogenism and infertility in swine, poultry and cattle.[18]

What this means is, in animals, "zear" looks likes extra estrogen to the body. Does it affect humans the same way? Are high estrogen levels a problem for us? I find nearly every breast cancer case shows a too-high estrogen level for <u>years before</u> the cancer is found! It starts females maturing too early, too. It could cause PMS, ovarian cysts and infertility. Not everybody gets all of these effects. And what is the effect on men and boys of eating an estrogen-like mycotoxin in their daily diet? This female hormone could have a drastic effect on the maturing process even in small amounts.

Zearalenone ("zear") and aflatoxin both have immune lowering effects. Zearalenone can induce thymic atrophy and macrophage activation.[19] If you have low immunity (low T-

---

[18] Bottalico, A., Lerario, P., and Visconti, A., <u>Production of Zearalenone, Trichothecenes and Moniliformin By *Fusarium* Species From Cereals, In Italy</u>. From *Toxigenic Fungi, Vol 7*, edited by H. Kurata and Y. Ueno, copublished by Kodansha Ltd, Tokyo and Elsevier Science Publishers B. V., Amsterdam, 1984, page 199.

[19] Luster, M.I., Boorman, G.A., Korach, K.S., Dieter, M.P., and Hong, L. 1984. <u>Myelotoxicity toxicity resulting from exogenous estrogens evidence for bimodal mechanism of action</u>. Int. J. Immunopharmacol. 6:287-297.

cells, low white blood cell count, and so forth), immediately go off moldy food suspects.

"Zear" is the mycotoxin that prevents you from detoxifying benzene. Every AIDS sufferer I see has a crippled ability to detoxify benzene; they also have zear!

The main zear sources I have found so far are popcorn, corn chips, and brown rice. But it was absent in fresh corn, canned corn, corn tortillas, and white rice, making me wonder how it gets in our processed corn products.

Sterigmatocystin

Sterigmatocystin ("sterig") is plentiful in **pasta**. Emphasize baked pasta dishes, not boiled. This raises the temperature much higher than boiling. Better yet, make your own pasta with a pasta maker. U.S. bread flour is quite free of mold; the mold in our pastas must come from using inferior quality flour. Always add vitamin C to pasta before or after cooking.

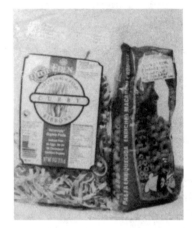

Fig. 50 All U.S. brands of pasta I tested had mold, including health food brands like the one shown here (left). No Mexican brands of pasta, like the one pictured (right), had any molds.

Ergot

A food mold that causes strange feelings and behavior is *ergot*. Although laws regulate the amount of ergot allowed in foods,[20] this is not enough protection. Ergotoxins, for example LSD, are active in extremely minute (less than a microgram, about one thousandth of a fly speck) quantities. They are not destroyed by heat and are especially toxic to children. I found traces in cereals, whole grain breads, wines, and honey. It can be detoxified by adding vitamin C but takes longer; about 10 minutes. Detoxify all your **honey** as soon as it arrives in your house. Warm it slightly and add vitamin C (1/8 tsp. per cup). Stir with wood or plastic.

Ergot toxicity could explain "Jekyll and Hyde" behavior in children, commonly attributed to "allergies". In fact, the mechanism, inability by the liver to keep up with detoxification, fits well into the "allergic" concept. If your child has undesirable behavior, try going off the moldy food suspects for three weeks (cold cereals, nuts and nut butters, store bought breads and baked goods, syrups). Substitute cooked cereals, bakery breads, potatoes, and honeys. Add vitamin C to honey, pasta and cooked cereals. Pancakes and waffles made from scratch would be O.K.

Combining alcohol with ergot is more toxic than either is alone. Alcohol seems to drive the toxin deeper into your tissues. I have found ergot <u>and aflatoxin</u> in beer and wine! Perhaps some of the bizarre behavior and speech of intoxication is really due to the mold-alcohol combination. By delaying alcohol detoxification, the mold could even be responsible for deaths "due to" alcoholism. It would be safer to brew your own alcoholic beverages. Start with pristine fruit. Or at least add vitamin C (1/8 tsp. per cup) to the store bought container you are consuming.

Older children and adults are quite susceptible to ergot too. If bizarre behavior shows up, such as saying mean and cruel things, expressing unusual, irrational thoughts, feeling emo-

---

[20]Canada allows one ergot grain per 300 grains of #3 or #4 wheat.

tionless or unreal, try the same diet changes, but put alcoholic beverages, soy sauces and other sauces, and other grain derived foods on the "off" list. Try this diet on yourself if you have a temper or crying spells or frequent colds! Ergot can make you super religious, hearing voices of command or threat. Ergot also causes seizures!

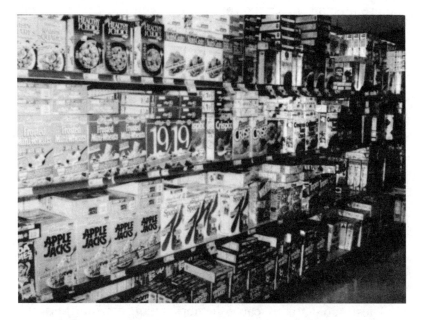

Fig. 51 All cold cereals I tested were full of mold toxins (besides solvents), health food varieties were worst.

Cytochalasin B

Cytochalasin B ("cyto B") is another immune lowering fungus. I find it mostly in pasta. It stops cells from dividing. Dead portions of the liver cannot regenerate as they otherwise would after a toxic encounter!

Kojic Acid

Kojic acid is a mycotoxin that appears to be responsible for wood alcohol build up. In other words, the toxic effect prevents you from detoxifying wood alcohol. This leads to pancreas damage, invites pancreatic fluke infestation, and typically results in diabetes. I find it in potatoes; don't eat potato skins. If you are a potato lover fix your own so you can peel them and remove any gray parts. I have also found it in regular coffee.

T-2 Toxin

T-2 toxin is a mold I have found in all cases of high blood pressure and kidney disease. It is present on dried peas and beans but it can be detoxified in 5 minutes by adding vitamin C to the water they are soaked in. Remember to throw away imperfect ones, first.

Sorghum Molds

Sorghum and millet carry these. Don't buy sorghum syrup. Rinse millet in vitamin C water before cooking, or add vitamin C to the cooking water.

These mold toxins cause hemorrhaging, appetite loss, and inability to swallow. Elderly people are more easily poisoned than others; their hemorrhages show up as strokes and purple blotches on the skin.

Patulin

is <u>the</u> major fruit mold toxin. It is present in most common fruits if they are bruised. It is particularly hazardous since the mold that produces it can actually grow in your intestine in patches. At these locations, bowel bacteria, *E. coli* and *Shigella*, can climb through the colon wall to invade you. These bacteria are then free to spread to regions of injury and tumors.

If you have cancer or bowel disease go off fresh fruit (bananas and lemons are OK) for a few weeks. Then choose your fruit meticulously. Peel everything so you can see and avoid every bruise. Also take a 2 tsp. dose of Black Walnut Hull Tincture Extra Strength. This kills these bowel fungi. But you can reinfect with a single soft grape.

Mold Avoidance

We should be much more critical of our food.

Crackers are notoriously moldy. Never let your child eat crackers. Make crisp things in the oven from left over bakery goods. Just sprinkle with cinnamon.

Dried fruits are very moldy. Soak them in vitamin C water. Rinse and bake to dry again. Then store in the refrigerator or freezer. When fresh fruit gets overripe, don't quickly bake it or preserve it. It's too late.

Peanut butter (store bought) and other nut butters can't be detoxified by adding vitamin C due to the mixing problem, even if you stir it in thoroughly. Make your own. Making your own peanut butter is a great adventure (see *Recipes*). Mix it with home made preserves, honey, marmalade, not very homogeneously so the bright colors and individual flavors stand out in contrast. Having three or four such spreads in the refrigerator will give your children the right perspective on food— homemade is better. Store bought jams are sweeter and brighter in color but strangely low in flavor and often indistinguishable from each other. Let your children eat the polluted foods that friends and restaurants serve (but not rare-cooked meats) so they can experience the difference. Their livers are strong enough to detoxify occasional small amounts.

Tea is quite moldy if purchased in bags. Although I used to recommend single herb teas (tea mixtures have solvents), I can now only recommend single herb teas from fresh sources in bulk (see *Sources*). This also gets you away from the benzalkonium chloride and possibly other antiseptics in the bag itself. When you get them, store them in their original double plastic bag. These herbs are so fresh, you'll only need half as much to make a cup of tea. Use a bamboo strainer (non metal). Bake the strainer occasionally or put through the dishwasher to keep it sterile.

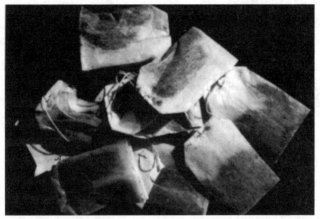

Fig. 52 Packaged herb tea is moldy and polluted with solvents. Get yours in bulk from an herb company.

It comes as a surprise that pure, genuine **maple syrup** has the deadly aflatoxin and other molds. You can often see mold yourself, as a thin scum on the surface or an opaque spot on the inside of the glass after the syrup has stood some time, even in the refrigerator. Some mold spores were in it to begin with. Others flew in. After some time they grew enough to be visible. In my testing, aflatoxin can be cleared with vitamin C but sterig and others need to be treated with a high temperature as well. Fortunately, this is easy to do with a syrup. Heat to near boiling while in the original jar with the lid removed. Keep refrigerated afterwards.

Artificial maple flavor did not have benzene, propyl alcohol or wood alcohol, nor molds. **Turbinado sugar** had none of these contaminants either. **Brown sugar** had sorghum mold. **White sugar** had propyl alcohol pollution. You can make your own syrup, safely, with artificial flavor and turbinado sugar. Of

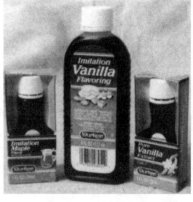

Fig. 53 Three safe flavorings.

course, you'll be missing the taste and nutritional minerals provided by the natural maple product but in a contest between nutritional value and toxicity, always choose the safe product.

The mold in our **hot cereals** can be spotted. Pick out all dark colored, shriveled bits. This represents most of it. Add honey, and salt while it's cooking—this raises the boiling temperature and detoxifies more. At the end, turn off heat and add a sprinkle of vitamin C powder. Rolled oats never showed molds in my testing, although they have their characteristic fungi, too. Don't let grains mold on your shelves simply from aging. Nothing should be more than six months old. Remember you can't see or smell molds when they begin. Molds must have a degree of moisture. As soon as you open a cereal grain, put the whole box in a plastic bag to keep moisture out. This keeps out weevils too, so you won't have to put the box in the freezer later to kill them.

Anything that is put in the refrigerator or freezer and then taken out develops moisture inside. Store cereals in kitchen cupboards or the freezer.

No government agency can test for all of these mycotoxins in all of our foods. Production and storage methods must be better regulated so as to be fail-safe. Simply sending inspectors out to look into the bins at grain elevators is not sufficient. Crusts of mold, sometimes several feet thick, that form on top of grain bins can be simply shoveled away before the inspector arrives. The humidity and temperature of stored grain should be regulated, requiring automated controls. This would soon be cost effective, too, in terms of reduced spoilage losses and higher quality prices earned. I believe that zear, aflatoxin and ergot require special regulations. Products that are imported should be subjected to the same tests as ours. Test results should be on the label.

Getting Away From Grains

In view of the many molds that are grain-related, and because these cannot be seen or smelled in pastas, breads, cold cereals, it would be wise to steer away from grain consumption. Always choose potatoes, because it is a vegetable instead of a grain, if you have a choice. The potato appears on your plate the way it was harvested. Whereas grain was hulled, stored for quite a long time, perhaps degerminated (the bran and germ picks up

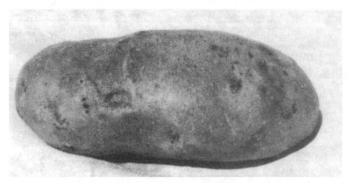

Fig. 54 Don't eat the green on the potato.

mold the fastest). Then it was mixed with assorted chemicals (fumigation, anti oxidants), each polluted in its own way, packaged again and stored again. Grains have a more tortuous history than potatoes that simply get sprayed.

The spray isn't simple, of course. Scrub it off under the tap. If potatoes weren't heavily sprayed they'd be sprouting in the stores. The spray accumulates in the eyes. Cut away all the eyes. By the time you have done this you may as well have peeled them. But no blemish, no cut, no dark spot inside may be left for you to eat. Don't buy potatoes that show a tint of green on them (the green color is due to *scopolamine*; it is toxic). Red potatoes have different chemistry that doesn't produce the green toxin, buy these often. Store potatoes out of the light, to slow down the greening process. They are still a nutritious, vitamin C-rich food—provided you don't fry them in benzene-polluted, hydrogenated grease!

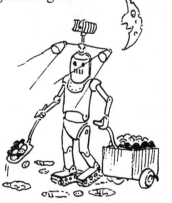

Potatoes have their molds but they are nicely visible. And washing and peeling does away with them. Old literature advises that potatoes should be harvested by moonlight so the green drug isn't produced in the white varieties. With modern mechanized harvesting this should pose no problem. But perhaps this must await the age of robots.

Fig. 55 Potato harvest of the future.

393

Pets Teach Health Lessons

Dogs don't eat hay and cats don't eat fruit. This is not simply due to their inability to digest them. Nor to training. Their body wisdom guides them. But we can trick them into eating corn and soybeans by adding the flavors they like and thereby defeat their wisdom the same way we defeat ours. A concoction is made for them that is called "complete nutrition" and we feed this meal after meal, day after day, a most unnatural situation. The liver is deluged with the same set of pollutants time after time and never gets a rest. Humans still obey their body wisdom about varying their meals. This gives the liver a chance to catch up with detoxifying one pollutant while the new one builds up. If the liver is absolutely unable to handle something, you are informed quite quickly with an allergic reaction to the food.

Cats and dogs with their monolithic diet get no opportunity to reject food (except by vomiting or starvation). It is not surprising they are getting cancer with increasing frequency, a situation where the liver can no longer detoxify isopropyl alcohol, a common pollutant in their food.

Should we go back to the old days and make their food for them? Yes, they deserve pure food, they deserve variety. Table scraps would be much less toxic for them than their commercial feed. But what if they like and prefer their monolithic "scientific", "complete", polluted diet? If our food was doused with sugar for breakfast, lunch and supper, we wouldn't care much about what was under the sugar either. And we'd continue wanting sugar, sugar, sugar the way a pet might want its favorite food and nothing else. Such is the deception of flavorings.

All change should be brought about slowly and with kindness for animals and humans alike. Learn what makes a good pet diet. Cats and dogs are both meat eaters. Cook chicken in a pressure cooker to kill all parasites. Put portions in the freezer. Add table scraps, dressed with a little butter, cheese or lard.

Don't wash the pet dishes with your own—dishwashers don't reach the boiling point. Serve fresh water daily. Standing water picks up bacteria. Don't let food get more than a day old in the dishes. It picks up molds. Don't feed pets at the table, keep them outdoors during mealtime.

After your pets have stopped eating propyl alcohol polluted food and are not getting propyl alcohol in their shampoos, there is no way they can get cancer. Whatever cancer they have will clear up by this change in diet and by giving them the pet parasite program.

Now they are back to a natural state and do not host human flukes. What a relief it is not to worry about reinfection from your pets.

Easy Lifestyle Improvements

None of us likes to change a habit. But once it is changed you are back to an automatic way of doing something. By selecting wise habits your improved lifestyle pays you back for the rest of your life.

Living Hand To Mouth

Hands do everything. They pick up things from the floor. They handle money. They touch other peoples' hands. They clean up bottoms. They touch all kinds of door knobs. And then they pick up food to eat. Some people even lick their fingers when they're sticky or just to turn a page!

What is on the hands that you don't want to eat but can't see? **Bacteria** and **viruses** from coughing and sneezing into your hands! And **cysts**! Cysts are the "eggs" made by parasites. Cysts are so tough not even bleach kills them. They hide under our fingernails when we wash our hands. Then we eat them along with our food. This is called *oral-fecal route*. They hatch in the stomach and go to the intestine to live.

To stop reinfecting yourself the little cysts under the nails need to be killed. Food grade alcohol solution kills them. Buy Everclear™ or Protec (potable) alcohol and make a 5% solution (add ¼ cup of 95% alcohol to a quart of water). Keep it in a small pump bottle at the sink. After using the bathroom and washing your hands, treat your fingernails with alcohol. Pump alcohol into one palm. Put the fingernails of the other hand into it. Scratch a bit. Pour it into the other palm and do the remaining fingernails. Rinse.

- **Don't** eat with your hands! Use a fork.
- **Never** eat food off the floor!
- **Always** wash hands after petting an animal!
- **Never** touch the bottoms of shoes! Keep shoes off couch or bed or chair.
- **Always** cough or sneeze into your clothing or a tissue, not your hands.
- **Keep** your fingers out of your mouth. Don't lick your fingers to turn pages or open plastic bags.

Sick persons need a 50% alcohol solution. Add ½ cup 95% alcohol to ½ cup cold tap water or buy plain vodka, 80 to 100 proof. Pour the vodka into the pump bottle. Be careful that nobody tries drinking it. If there are teenagers in the house, add a hefty dose of cayenne to it.

Lugol's iodine will also sterilize your hands. However most commercial Lugol's is polluted with isopropyl alcohol. Ask your pharmacist to make it from scratch for you (there are only two ingredients and water, see *Recipes*). Then make a solution to wash in (1 tsp. to a quart of water). This can stain some things. Do not use "tincture of iodine."

Better Laundry Habits

Boil your underwear. In long-ago days, all sheets, towels, table cloths, and underwear were <u>separated</u> and boiled.

With the convenience of our electric washing machine, we tend to overlook the fact that underwear is <u>always</u> contaminated by fecal matter and urogenital secretions and excretions. Mixing these with socks and towels and dishcloths is all right if you are going to kill everything anyway. But if you don't kill them, as in cold water washes, you are mixing the yeast, parasite eggs, bacterial spores, and fungus from underwear with all the other clothing you and your family wear. An enlightened system would be to add an antiseptic to the wash or rinse cycle. Lime water (calcium hydroxide) or iodine based antiseptics seem obviously simple methods to accomplish this. In the absence of this protection, use dryer heat to do your sterilizing. Underwear should be dried until too hot to handle.

Bleach can kill a lot, but doesn't kill *Giardia* spores and a lot of types of fungus. Don't rely on bleaching. Besides, your skin absorbs it from clothing, it is quite toxic to you, and can cause mental effects.

Commercial detergents are polluted with PCBs and have cobalt added. Both of these are easily picked up through your skin. Use **washing soda** and **borax** in the wash cycle. They do not clean quite as well as modern detergents, but there is less static cling, eliminating the need to put more chemicals in your dryer. For spot removal use homemade bar soap.

Better Kitchen Habits

Once a day, sterilize the sponge or cloth you use to wipe up the table, counter tops and sink. This little piece of contaminated cloth is the most infectious thing in the house, besides the toilet. It's more dangerous than the toilet because you do not suspect it. Sometimes it has a slight odor at first, which may warn you, but most pathogens do not have an odor! As we wipe up droplets of milk, we give the milk bacteria, *Salmonellas* and *Shigellas*, a new home to multiply and thrive in. We add crumbs, picking up molds this way. We add dust, picking up parasite eggs and stages. They all feed on the milk and food residue.

As the counter and table and stove get wiped "clean" a film of contamination is left everywhere. A few varieties may die but most of them don't. The general moisture in the kitchen is enough for them to survive. The cloth or sponge recolonizes the kitchen and dining room table several times a day.

No doubt, the last thing you do before leaving the kitchen is squeeze it dry <u>with your hands</u>. Now all the pathogens are on your hands!

Where do your fingers go? To your mouth to remove a hull or bit of something from your teeth. Or to eat a last bite of something. Or to turn a page of the telephone directory. You have just eaten a culture sampling from your own kitchen sponge. In two hours they are already multiplying in the greatest culture system of all: your body! You have given yourself your next sore throat, or cold or headache. The worst possible habit is to wipe a child's face and hands with the kitchen cloth. Or to have a handy towel hanging from the refrigerator handle.

To sterilize the sponge: **drop it into a 50% solution of grain alcohol** at the end of each day. Keep a wide mouth glass quart jar handy just for this. Keep the jar tightly closed and out of the reach of children. Dunk your sponge and plop it onto the sink. If you stand it on end in the sink it will partly dry overnight.

Another way to sterilize the sponge or cloth is to **microwave it**, after wetting it, for 3 minutes. Any shorter time simply warms and <u>cultures</u> the pathogens and multiplies them. Or **boil the cloth** like our grandparents did. Drying out the dish cloth helps kill many—but not all—pathogens. It takes three days of drying to kill all! Another strategy is to **use a fresh cloth** or sponge each day, putting the used one to dry until laundry day.

During the day, set the sponge on end to start drying and slow down culturing.

Don't eat food directly off the counter top or table top. You wouldn't slice a tomato or egg directly on the counter top. It would pick up something: some little particle of dust or dirt. Treat bread the same way. Always on a new clean surface, such as a plate. The counter and table top have on them whatever is in the kitchen dust and on the wipe cloth. Dust is always falling! And the sponge is always culturing. Don't eat the dust!

Keep the cutting board sterile like dishes. Wash it the same way and keep it in the cupboard.

Keep food containers closed. Milk or water glasses are picking up dust as soon as you set them out. Dust is everywhere. Every step on the carpet sends up a puff of dust. Vacuuming sends up a hurricane of dust and distributes bathroom dust to the kitchen and kitchen dust to the bedrooms. So if one person has brought in a new infection, the whole family is exposed to it in hours via the dust.

It is very helpful <u>not to eat</u> the new infectious pathogen. Breathing it is not so damaging. Our noses collect such pathogens and we blow them out again. Touching the infected person is not very damaging either; the pathogens can't get through our skins and since we wash hands before eating we are not at great risk of infection this way. But <u>eating</u> the pathogen is 100% effective in infecting us. The new pathogen is in the dust. The newly contaminated dust drops into your ready and waiting glasses on the table and the open foods. Of course, there is no defense if somebody should cough or sneeze at the table.

Teach children to cough and sneeze into a suitable collecting place like a tissue, <u>not their hands</u>. Pathogens live bountifully on hands. Hands not only provide moisture but often food from the last meal. Hands are second only to the dish cloth in contamination level. If you must cough or sneeze and a tissue is not within reach fast enough, <u>use your clothing</u>! That's what clothing is for—to protect you. Cough and sneeze into your own clothing; this protects the cougher and sneezer, as well as everybody else. A sleeve is handy for children. The inside of your T-shirt for T-shirt wearers. The inside of coat for suited persons. The inside of the neck line for dresses. Of course, paper is best, but in emergency use cloth. Never, never your hands unless you are free to immediately dash into the washroom and clean the contamination off your hands.

Teach children this old rearranged verse:

> If you cough or sneeze or sniff
> Grab a tissue, quick-quick-quick!
> And if you're sitting at the table
> Do it in your sleeve if able.

Better Housekeeping

Throw out as much of the wall to wall carpeting as you can bear to part with. It is injurious to everyone's health, even though it's comforting to bare feet and looks pretty.

Carpets clean our shoes. Modern shoes, with their deep treads, bring in huge amounts of outdoor filth which settles deep down into the carpets. In spite of vacuuming every week, the filth accumulates.

Vacuum the carpets when the children, the sick and elderly are out of the house. The dust raised and distributed throughout the house isn't just dirt, it's infectious dirt. It lands on tables and counters. These get wiped with a cloth or sponge and then applied to dishes. The dust in the kitchen falls on open food and into open containers.

Clean carpets with a "steam cleaner". When you see how much filth is in the water and realize how much dirt you were living with, you might be willing to trade in the "beauty" of carpets for the cleaner living of smooth floors. Don't add chemicals (commercial cleaning solutions) to the steam cleaning machine; these chemicals leave a residue in the carpet which dries and flies up into the air to add to the dust. Popular stain resistance treatments contain arsenic. Cobalt, which adds "lustre" to carpets, causes skin and heart disease after it has built up in your organs. Use borax instead of detergent. Use boric acid to leave a residue that kills roaches and fleas (but not ants). Add vinegar that leaves a residue to repel ants. Nothing controls fleas reliably, except getting rid of the carpets and cloth furniture (keep pets out of bedrooms). Removing all the borax is what brings luster to the carpet. Use citric acid in the rinse water for this purpose. Adding lemon peel to the rinse also adds luster and ant deterrence. Just drop the whole lemon in the tank so it can't block the hoses.

Fleas and other vermin in the carpet simply crawl below the wetness level when you wash the carpet. Spraying a grain alcohol solution with lemon peel in it (it needs to extract for a half hour) on the damp carpet will reach and kill a lot of these, together with the residual bacteria. The damp carpet lets it spread evenly and reach all the crevices.

We are trapped in our dwellings. Primitive peoples were mobile. This got them away from accumulations of filth and rubbish in their living space. Much living was done outdoors, the cleanest space of all.

Now, air conditioning has made indoor living more comfortable. But also has added new hazards. The strong currents of air blow the dust about continuously. Molds and bacteria that grow right on the air conditioning unit get blown about for all to inhale. Never, never use fiberglass as a filter or to insulate your air conditioner around the sides. It is a carcinogen. And the danger of freon escaping from a tiny leak is another major health hazard.

Forced air heating systems are undesirable, too. All dirt brought into the house by shoes gets circulated throughout the house by forced air systems of heating or cooling. Old fashioned radiant heat from radiators or a stove did not distribute the dust so effectively. A return to linoleum floor covering for kitchen and bathroom and hardwood for other rooms would be a good step of progress for a health conscious society. Mopping, instead of the vacuum cleaner, keeps dirt to a minimum. Throw rugs at doors and bedside, easy to clean, would "catch the dirt" as was the original intention. Carpets were intended to help keep filth <u>out</u> of the air. These smaller rugs should be laundered weekly.

Furniture should be wood, cane, or plastic, with cushions to soften the impact. These can be washed weekly if the covers are removable. Modern cloth furniture with its foam interior is a repository of filth and fumes and a constant source of infectious dust.

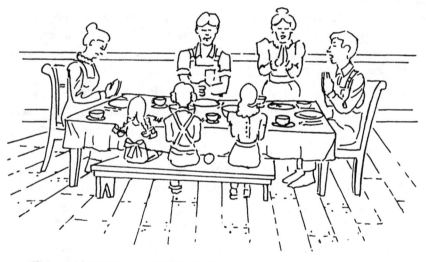

This old fashioned setting is more progressive than our carpeted, modern homes.
Fig. 56 Smooth floors allow every bit of dust to be removed.

Dust your furniture with a damp paper towel. You are picking up and removing highly infectious filth (*Ascaris* and pinworm eggs, pet parasites, "dander" and house mites). Instead of distributing these from room to room, throw the paper towel away after each room is done. Use plain water or vinegar water (50%), not a chemical combination which further pollutes the air.

Clean windows with vinegar water, too. Use a spray bottle.

Keep your dishes in cupboards. This keeps them free of dust. This principle is ancient. It is tempting to leave some of them out. If you must keep the juicer or dishes outside of cupboards, keep them covered or placed upside down so they don't catch dust. Even inside cupboards, store them upside down. When using the "good" dishes or glasses, that haven't been used in a while, wash them first.

Windows Open Or Closed?

In places like Chicago where you can smell the air as you approach the city, it is wiser to keep your windows shut. You can't breath the industrial "soup" all day and night and expect to stay healthy. Of course, it all enters the houses anyway. Central air conditioning and a plain carbon filter at the furnace location (see *Sources*) may be the best solution in spite of blowing dust around the house. Keep the vents to the bedrooms closed to reduce the air turbulence there but leave the cold air return open. Clean the vents in other rooms each week along with floors and carpets by pulling up the grating and reaching down the passage as far as possible.

If you believe the air is free of highway exhaust and industrial smoke open the windows every day. This will let some of the indoor toxins blow away. Asbestos, fiberglass, freon, radon and plain dust can be reduced to a minimum by keeping windows open. If you are ill, sit outdoors (on the porch) as much as you can. Escape to a suitable climate that makes this possible.

Just a few decades ago, many people had summer living quarters that were different from winter living quarters. Gone was all the accumulated infectious dust of half a year of habitation.

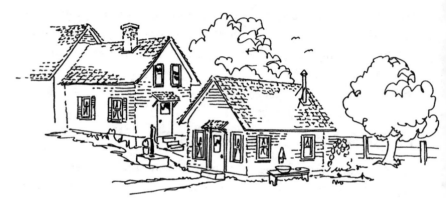

Fig. 57 Moving into the summer kitchen got you away from the accumulation of filth from winter!

Don't have a basement where you stockpile toxic items. Basements invite mold, mice and radon besides toxic things. Fumes travel upward where you live! Keep your toxic things in the attic. If there is no attic, store them in the utility room. Close off the ventilation between utility room and the rest of your house. If you have none of these, perhaps because you live in a senior citizen community or condominium, don't keep any toxic things stored anywhere. Don't save any leftover paints, solvents or cleaners. Buy such small quantities that you can afford to throw it all away when you are done with them.

Live on <u>top</u> of the earth as was intended by nature.

<u>Never</u> have a basement room "finished" for actual living space. Don't buy a house that has a "lower level" built into the

earth. This will be the most polluted and dangerous room in your house. If you are ill, move out of such a room. There is no way that it can be "cleaned up". Move to the other end of the house and furthest away from an attached garage door.

What Kind Of Heat

The worst is coal. The best is none. Breathing coal fumes during the beginning of the industrial age may have brought the new lung diseases: tuberculosis (TB), and pneumonia. It may also have worsened alcohol addiction (beryllium toxicity). Choose electric heat if possible. Even though electricity is based on other fuel consumption, you don't have to breathe those fumes directly.

Wood stoves can be made safe by making sure the chimney works properly. Never use a lighter fluid. Don't fill the house with smoke when stoking.

Minimize your use of fossil fuels in every way you can.

Getting Rid of Mites

We do not tolerate external parasites like bedbugs, lice, ticks, leeches. Bedbugs were once a scourge amongst northern Europeans. I remember our parents spraying for them (kerosene) in the bedroom. This only "controlled" them. What eliminated them was a law against sale of used mattresses. Lice were originally "controlled" by frequent washing, louse combs, and ironing the seams of clothing. What eliminated them was the cutting of long hair as a societal practice. But what about **mites**? They live with us and other animals.

Mites are too tiny to see, tiny enough to ride on a dust particle as if it were a magic carpet. They resemble insects. Chiggers are really mites. Mange in animals is a mite infestation. Dust mites live on our dander (scales of dead skin).

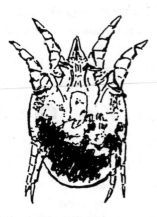

Get rid of their breeding places: beds, cloth covered chairs and soft sofas. Humans leave enough dander behind in these places to

Fig. 58 Mite.

support these ultra small insects. Cover mattresses with plastic covers. Use throws on easy chairs and sofas and wash them often. Never allow a pet into the bedroom or the dust will have tapeworm eggs as well as mites. Throw out rugs that have been pet-beds. Spray the air with a mist of 50% grain alcohol before vacuuming. If you have an illness wear a mask to vacuum. Deep, soft, wall to wall carpets compromise an ancient concept: everything should be washable and cleanable, without throwing the dirt into the air for humans to inhale. Vacuuming a carpet blasts mites and tape eggs into the air. Never shake bedding or rugs where the dust will blow back into the house behind you.

Mites don't bite us but we inhale them as they float in the ever present dust in our homes. The mucus in our lungs traps them and in a few days they die, only to release a drove of *Adenoviruses* (common cold virus) in us.

Four Clean-ups

Chronic health problems are not due to exposures of the past. They are ongoing. Your body is constantly fighting to remove pollutants. In order to stay sick, you must be constantly resupplied! These four clean-ups–dental, diet, body, home–are aimed at removing parasites and pollutants at their source. Only then can your body heal.

Dental Clean-up

(This section on dentistry was contributed by Frank Jerome, DDS)

Dr. Jerome: The philosophy of dental treatment taught in America is that teeth are to be saved by whatever means available, using the strongest, most long lasting materials. Long-term toxic effects are of little concern. The attitude of the majority of dentists is: whatever the American Dental Association (ADA) says is OK, they will do.

A more reasonable philosophy is that <u>there is no tooth worth saving if it damages your</u> immune system. Use this as your guideline.

The reason dentists do not see toxic results is that they do not <u>look</u> or <u>ask</u>. If a patient has three mercury amalgam fillings placed in the mouth and a week later has a kidney problem, will she call the dentist—or the doctor? Will they ever tell the dentist about the kidney problem or tell the doctor about the three fillings? A connection will never be made.

It is common for patients who have had their <u>metal</u> fillings removed to have various symptoms go away but, again, they do not tell the dentist. The patient has to be asked! Once the patient begins to feel well they take it for granted, and don't make the connection, either. If everybody's results were instantaneous, there would be no controversy.

Find an alternative dentist. They have been leading the movement to ban mercury from dental supplies. Not only mercury, but all metal needs to be banned. If your dentist will not follow the necessary procedures, then you must find one that will. The questions to ask when you phone a new dental office are:

1. Do you place mercury fillings? (The correct answer is NO. If they do, they probably don't have enough experience in the use of non-metal composites.)
2. Do you do root canals? (The correct answer is NO. If they do, they do not understand good alternative dentistry.)
3. Do you remove amalgam tattoos? (The correct answer is YES. Tattoos are pieces of mercury left in the gum tissue.)
4. Do you treat cavitations? (The correct answer is YES. By cleaning them.) The complete name of *cavitations* is *alveolar cavitational osteopathosis*. They are holes (cavities) left in the jawbone by an incompletely extracted tooth. A properly cleaned socket which is left after an extraction will heal and fill with bone. Dentists routinely do NOT clean the socket of tissue remnants or infected bone. A dry socket (really an infected socket) is a common result. These sockets never fully heal. Thirty years after an extraction, a cavitation will still be there. It is a form of *osteomyelitis*, which means bone infection.

Ninety percent or more of dental offices will not be able to answer ANY of the above questions correctly. If you allow the work to be done by a dentist who does not understand the importance of the above list, you could end up with new problems. Find the right dentist first even if you must travel hundreds of miles. There are 6,000 to 10,000 dentists who should be able to help. Some can do part of the work and refer you to a specialist for the rest. Five hundred to one thousand of these dentists can do it all.

Normal treatment cost is about $1,000 for replacement of 6 to 8 metal fillings including the examination and X-rays. For people with a metal filling in every tooth, or for the extraction of all teeth (plus dentures), it may be up to $3,000 (or more in some places).

Remember, the simpler the treatment, the better. If the dentist says that he or she can change your metal fillings to plastic but it would be better to <u>crown</u> them, say "NO!"

Guidelines For A Healthy Mouth

If you have	What to do
Metal fillings	change to plastic fillings
Inlays and onlays	change to plastic fillings
Crowns (all types)	change to plastic crowns
Bridges	change to plastic crowns, partials
Metal partials	change to plastic partials(Flexite™)
Pink dentures	change to clear plastic
Porcelain denture teeth	change to plastic denture teeth
Badly damaged teeth	become extractions
Root canals	become extractions
Braces and implants	avoid
Cavitations	need to be surgically cleaned
Temporary crowns	use plastic
Temporary fillings	use Duralon™

Fig. 59 Dental replacements.

The guidelines can be summarized as:

1. Remove all metal from the mouth.
2. Remove all infected teeth and clean cavitations.

Dr. Clark: Removing all metal means removing all root canals, metal fillings and crowns. Take out all bridge work or partials made of metal and never put them back in. But you may feel quite attached to the gold, so ask the dentist to give you everything she or he removes. Look at the underside. You will be glad you switched.

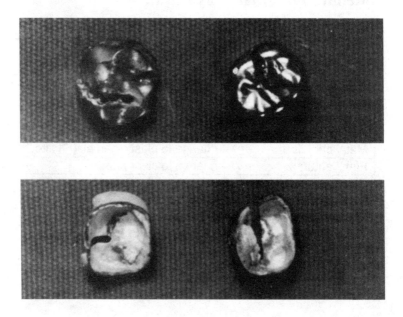

The top surfaces of tooth fillings are kept glossy by brushing (you swallow some of what is removed). Underneath is tarnish and foulness. Ask to see your crowns when they are removed.

Fig. 60 Tops and bottoms of some metal crowns.

The stench of the infection under some teeth may be overwhelming as they are pulled. Bad breath in the morning is due to such hidden tooth infections, not a deficiency of mouthwash!

All metal must come out, no matter how glossy it looks on the surface. Metal does not belong in your body. It is an unnatural chemical. Do this as soon as you have found a dentist able to do it. Find a dentist with experience and knowledge about this subject. It is more than replacing acknowledged culprits like mercury-amalgam fillings. This is metal-free dentistry. Only metal-free plastic should be put back in your mouth.

Dr. Jerome: If your dentist tells you that mercury and other metals will not cause any problems, you will not be able to change his or her mind. Seek treatment elsewhere!

Your dentist should do a complete X-ray examination of your mouth. Ask for the *panoramic* X-ray rather than the usual series of 14 to 16 small X-rays (called full mouth series). The panoramic X-ray shows the whole mouth including the jaws and the sinuses. This lets the dentist see impacted teeth, root fragments, bits of mercury buried in the bone and deep infections. Cavitations are visible in a panoramic X-ray that may not be seen in a full mouth series.

The cost of removing metals should be viewed in the proper light. It took years or decades to get into your present condition. When you do a lot of dental repair in a short time, it can seem to be costly. Unfortunately, many people are in a tight financial position because of the cost of years of ineffective treatment, trying to get well.

Your dentist may recommend crowning teeth to "protect" or strengthen them. Unfortunately, the very concept of crowning teeth is flawed. First, the enamel is removed from a tooth to prepare for the crown. This is permanent and serious damage! Many teeth, up to 20%, may die after being crowned and will need to be extracted. For this reason, you should only get REPLACEMENT crowns and NO NEW crowns. Your metal crowns can be changed to plastic. (Remember, no metal must be left <u>under</u> the crown.)

If you have many crowns, you should have them all removed as quickly as possible. But you should <u>not</u> spend more than two hours in the dentist's chair at any one time. That is too much stress for your body.

Dr. Clark: Don't accept intravenous (IV) treatments during amalgam removal. Both IV bags and the supplements used in them are polluted with propyl alcohol, benzene, and wood alcohol.

Dr. Jerome: It is quite all right to have <u>temporary</u> crowns placed on all teeth that need them in the <u>first visit</u>. You may then go back and complete treatment over the next 6 to 12 months. It is common to find a crowned tooth to be very weak and not worth replacing the crown, particularly if you are already having a partial made and could include this tooth in it.

Dr. Clark: We are accustomed to thinking that plastic is metal-free. This is wrong. The original dental plastic, methyl methacrylate was metal-free. But modern plastic contains metal. The metal is ground up very finely and added to the plastic in order to make it harder, give it sheen, color, etc.

Dr. Jerome: Dentists are not commonly given information on these metals used in plastics. The information that comes with dental supplies does not list them either. Most dentists never look at a dental materials book after they graduate. The ADA, however, has a library full of such information.[21]

Dr. Clark: There are many lanthanide (Rare Earth) metals used in dental plastic. Their effects on the body from dentalware

---

[21] Call the American Dental Association at (800) 621-8099 (Illinois (800) 572-8309, Alaska or Hawaii (800) 621-3291). Members can ask for the Bureau of Library Services, non-members ask for Public Information.

have NOT been studied. Yet their cancer-promoting ability is known in many cases.[22] Only metal-free plastic is safe.

Dr. Jerome: These are the acceptable plastics; they can be procured at any dental lab.

- Plastic for dentures: <u>Methyl Methacrylate</u>. Available in clear and pink. <u>Do not use pink</u>.[23]
- Plastic for partial dentures: <u>Flexite</u>™ Available in clear and pink. <u>Do not use pink</u>.
- Plastic for fillings: <u>Composite Materials</u>. This is the material that has been used in front teeth for 30 years. It has been used in back teeth for 10 years. There are many brands and there are new ones being marketed constantly. The new ones are very much superior to those used 10 years ago and they will continue to improve. They do, however, contain enough barium or zirconium to make them visible on X-rays. There are no alternatives available without these metals.

Dr. Clark: Composites with barium are not good, but I haven't seen enough barium toxicity from fillings at this time to merit advising extraction instead. Hopefully, a barium-free variety will become available soon to remove this health risk.

Dr. Jerome: Many people (and dentists too) believe that porcelain is a good substitute for plastic. Porcelain is aluminum oxide with other metals added to get different colors (shades). The metal DOES come out of the porcelain! It has many technical drawbacks as well. Porcelain is not recommended. Some-

---

[22] Thulium and ytterbium have been studied for their tumor-seeking ability. See page 321 in the book *METAL IONS In BIOLOGICAL SYSTEMS, Vol. 10, Carcinogenicity and Metal Ions*. Editor Helmut Sigel 1980.

[23] The pink color is from mercury or cadmium which is added to the plastic.

times the white composite fillings are called porcelain fillings but they are not. They also require more tooth structure to be removed.

If you have a large bridge, it cannot be replaced with a plastic bridge because it isn't strong enough. A large bridge must be replaced with a removable partial (Flexite™).

The methods used to remove metals and infections are technical and complicated. See dental information in *Sources*.

Dr. Clark: *I'd like to thank Dr. Jerome for his contributions to this section, and his pioneering work in metal-free dentistry. I hope more dentists acquire his techniques.*

Horrors Of Metal Dentistry

Why are highly toxic metals put in materials for our mouths? Because not everyone agrees on what is toxic at what level. Just decades ago lead was commonly found in paint, and until recently in gasoline. Lead was not less toxic then, we were just less informed! The government sets standards of toxicity, but those "standards" change as more research is done (and more people speak out). You can do better than the government by dropping your standard for toxic metals to zero! Simply remove them.

The debate still rages over mercury amalgam fillings. No one disputes the extreme toxicity of mercury compounds and mercury vapor. 'The ADA feels that mercury amalgam fillings are safe because they do not vaporize or form toxic compounds to a significant degree. Opponents cite scientific studies that implicate mercury amalgams as disease causing. Many dentists advocate mercury amalgam fillings simply because they are accepted by the ADA, which they believe protects them from malpractice litigation. Why risk your health and life on their opinions? Remember everything corrodes and everything seeps, so amalgams must too.

Cadmium is used to make the pink color in dentures! Cadmium is five times as toxic as lead, and is strongly linked to high blood pressure.

Occasionally, thallium and germanium are found together in mercury amalgam tooth fillings. Thallium causes leg pain, leg weakness, and paraplegia. <u>If you are in a wheelchair without a very reliable diagnosis, have all the metal removed from your mouth.</u> Ask the dentist to give you the grindings. Try to have them analyzed for thallium using the most sensitive methods available, possibly at a research institute or university.

I was astonished to find thallium in mercury amalgams! It couldn't be put there intentionally, look how toxic it is:

TEJ500   **HR: 3**
THALLIUM COMPOUNDS
Thallium and its compounds are on the Community Right To Know List.

THR: Extremely toxic. The lethal dose for a man by ingestion is 0.5-1.0 gram. Effects are cumulative and with continuous exposure toxicity occurs at much lower levels. Major effects are on the nervous system, skin and cardiovascular tract. The peripheral nervous system can be severely affected with dying-back of the longest sensory and motor fibers. Reproductive organs and the fetus are highly susceptible. Acute poisoning has followed the ingestion of toxic quantities of a thallium-bearing depilatory and accidental or suicidal ingestion of rat poison. Acute poisoning results in swelling of the feet and legs, arthralgia, vomiting, insomnia, hyperesthesia and paresthesia [numbness] of the hands and feet, mental confusion, polyneuritis with severe pains in the legs and loins, partial paralysis of the legs with reaction of degeneration, angina-like pains, nephritis, wasting and weakness, and lymphocytosis and eosinophilia. About the 18th day, complete loss of the hair on the body and head may occur. Fatal poisoning has been known to occur. Recovery requires months and may be incomplete. Industrial poisoning is reported to have caused discoloration of the hair (which later falls out), joint pain, loss of appetite, fatigue, severe pain in the calves of the legs, albuminuria, eosinophilia, lymphocytosis and optic neuritis followed by atrophy. Cases of industrial poisoning are rare, however. Thallium is an experimental teratogen [used to induce birth defects for study]. When heated to decomposition they [sic] emit highly toxic fumes of Tl [thallium]. See also THALLIUM and specific compounds.[24]

Fig. 61 Thallium excerpt.

Thallium pollution frightens me more than lead, cadmium and mercury combined, because it is completely unsuspected. Its last major use, rat poison, was banned in the 1970s. Every <u>wheelchair</u> patient I tested was positive for thallium! One current use for thallium is in Arctic/Antarctic thermostats. When added to mercury the mercury will stay liquid at lower temperatures. Are mercury suppliers then providing the dental industry with tainted amalgam?

The cancer causing or carcinogenic action of metals has been studied for a long time, although it doesn't get attention by our regulatory agencies. A scientific book on this subject was published in 1980.[25] One table from this book is shown on page 431. We can see that chromium and nickel compounds are the <u>most</u> carcinogenic metals. Nickel is used in gold crowns, braces, and children's crowns!

Note that the form of the metal is very important. For instance chromium is an essential element of *glucose tolerance*

[24] *Dangerous Properties of Industrial Materials,* 7th ed. by N. Irving Sax and Richard J. Lewis Sr., Van NOSTRAND, Reinhold N.Y. 1989.

[25] The title is *Carcinogenicity and Metal Ions.* It is volume 10 of a series called *Metal Ions in Biological Systems,* edited by Helmut Sigel. A university chemistry library should have this book. It has a fascinating chapter on the leukemias by two scientists from the Academy of Sciences of the USSR, E. L. Andronikashvili and L. Mosulishvili. Their brilliant work and discussion was largely responsible for my pursuit of the whole subject of cancer.

factor, but most of its other compounds are extremely toxic. In general, xenobiotic compounds (foreign) are to be avoided! Metal doesn't belong in our foods or in our bodies.

Dental Rewards

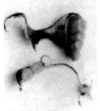

Fig. 62 More dental metal.

After your mouth is metal and infection-free, notice whether your sinus condition, ear-ringing, enlarged neck glands, headache, enlarged spleen, bloated condition, knee pain, foot pain, hip pain, dizziness, aching bones and joints improve.

Keep a small notebook to write down these improvements. It will show you which symptoms came originally from your teeth. Symptoms often come back! So go back to your dentist, to search for a hidden infection under one or more of your teeth, or <u>where your teeth once were</u>! That infection can be the cause of tinnitus, TMJ, arthritis, neck pain, loss of balance, and heart attacks!

Dentures can be beautiful. Of course, plastic isn't natural, but it is the best compromise that can be made to restore your mouth. At least it isn't positively charged like metals; it can't set up an electric current nor a magnetic field in your mouth, all of which may be harmful.

Do not be swayed by arguments that plastic is not as strong as metal. You see dentures everywhere and they seem strong enough to eat with. You will be told that "noble" metals like gold and platinum

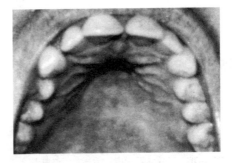

Fig. 63 Beautiful plastic mouth.

and silver are OK, that they are "inert" and do not corrode or seep. Nothing could be more untrue. You may be keeping them glossy by the constant polishing action of your toothpaste. But if you look at the underside, the view is frightful. **Everything tarnishes and everything seeps.** You wouldn't expect even a gold or silver coin that was dropped in a fountain 50 years ago to be intact. As metal corrodes your body absorbs it!

In breast cancer, especially, you find that metals from dentalware have dissolved and accumulated in the breast. <u>They will leave the breast</u> if you clear them out of your mouth (and diet, body, home). **The cysts shrink and are simply gone.** No need to do surgery!

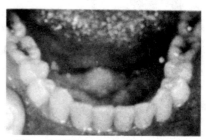

Fig. 64 Ugly metal in mouth.

Diet Clean-up

Breakfast

Cook your cereal from scratch. Don't eat cold cereal; it has numerous solvents and molds. Buy hot cereals that say "no salt added," like cream of wheat, steel cut oats or old fashioned oats,[26] millet, corn meal, cream of rice, or Wheatena. Cook it

---

[26] Rolled oats have 235 mcg <u>nickel</u> per serving of 4 ounces, picked up from the rollers, according to *Food Values* 14th ed. by Pennington and Church, 1985. I have only found nickel in the "one-minute" or "instant" variety of oats, however.

with milk to add nutritive value. Add your own (non-aluminum) salt and a pinch of vitamin C before cooking. Make granola from a recipe (see *Recipes*). Use honey, or brown sugar. Add raisins that were soaked for 5 minutes in vitamin C water. Use whipping cream or butter (both boiled) if you need to gain weight. Isn't this a delicious way to start your day! Add cinnamon to flavor, or frozen fruit and honey.

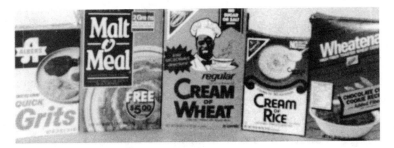

Fig. 65 Unpolluted breakfast cereals.

Or start your day with fried potatoes, an egg, and glass of milk. Don't worry about cholesterol since you will be doing liver cleanses anyway. (We have been told that eggs carry *Salmonella* bacteria. I found *Salmonellas* only on the <u>outside</u> shell and the egg carton—never inside! Could the researchers have accidentally transferred the bacteria from the shell to the inside while they were testing?)

The milk should be 2% or more butterfat because the calcium in milk cannot be absorbed without at least this much fat. Eat homemade yogurt and add honey or homemade preserves yourself. You need 3 cups of a milk product each day. Homemade buttermilk is fine. If you don't tolerate milk, and get diarrhea from it, try a milk digestant tablet to go with it. Start with only ¼ cup at a time. Do not choose chocolate milk. There is no substitute for milk; calcium tablets are not satisfactory. Vegetable matter, although high in calcium, does not give you *available* calcium either, unless you buy a juicer and make vegetable juice out of it. Eating fish can give you a lot of calcium, but it is in the tiny bones hidden in the fish. Don't try to remove them. Canned salmon has a lot of calcium; tuna does not. On a day that you eat fish, you would not need milk. Goat milk is probably better than cows' milk, but more difficult to get used to.

Lunch

Cook your food from scratch. Don't start with cans or packages or frozen items to make some recipe. In fact, don't bother with <u>any</u> fancy recipes. Just cook two or three vegetables for lunch and eat them with butter and salt or homemade sauces. Bread and milk rounds it out, plus fruit (not canned or frozen). Soup is a nice change. Cook it with all the vegetables you can find. Don't start with a can or packet or cube. Use a bit of onion and genuine herbs to give it zest. Thyme and fenugreek, together, make a flavorful combination you can purchase in capsules. Just pull apart and season.

If all this is too much work, make fresh vegetable juice once a week and freeze enough so that you can have a daily nutritious meal just by pouring a glass of it, together with bread and yogurt or milk.

Never diet during illness

This is a rule based on common sense. A weight-loss diet must wait at least two years.

Bake your own bread! I found aflatoxin in commercial bread after just four days in my bread box, but none in homemade bread even after two weeks! Aflatoxin is a most potent carcinogen and immunosuppressant. Aflatoxin is the toxin in your diet that keeps you from clearing propyl alcohol from your body (see 382)! Aflatoxin is a substance made by mold; bread starts to mold on the grocery store shelf. Don't buy plastic-wrapped bread. Don't <u>ever</u> salvage moldy food, whether it is fruit, breads or leftovers in the refrigerator. Throw them out. <u>Buy a bread maker</u>. It can do everything, including baking the bread. Use unbleached (unbrominated) flour and add ½ tsp. vitamin C powder per loaf to help retard mold further (it also makes the bread rise higher).

Supper

Cook your supper from scratch. Emphasize fish for animal food, not beef, pork, turkey or chicken. Don't buy bread crumbs, use your own. Don't buy batter, make your own. Use genuine eggs, not substitutes. Wash your hands after handling raw meat or eggs.

Make your own salad and salad dressing out of olive oil, fresh lemon juice or white distilled vinegar (apple cider vinegar has aflatoxins), honey, salt and herbs to flavor. If your digestion isn't strong enough for raw vegetables or fruit, make juice. Get a sturdy juicer and make your juice about half carrot juice and half from vegetables like celery, squash, lettuce, and broccoli. Make your own tomato sauce with pure herb seasoning, not from a jar or can (home canned foods are fine, of course, as long as they are not made in a big aluminum pot with aluminum-containing salt).

Cook real potatoes, not instant varieties. Peel them to get rid of Kojic acid (mycotoxin) and scopolamine (the green part). Make mashed potatoes from scratch, with milk, not box potatoes, nor chips nor French fries. Chips and fries were made in chemical grease called "hydrogenated." There is a large amount of nickel in hydrogenated fats.[27] Fry your potatoes in butter, lard or olive oil. Find butter that is not wrapped in foil and is not salted. Salt your own butter, using aluminum-free salt.[28] Don't wrap potatoes in foil to bake, coat with butter or olive oil. Don't eat the peels.

Eat no meat that hasn't been cooked as thoroughly as if it were pork.

Other animals are as parasitized as we, full of flukes and worms and *Schistosomes* in every imaginable stage, and if the blood carries these, would we not be eating live parasites if we eat animals in the raw state? We have been taught to cook thoroughly any pork, fish or seafood. Now we must cook thoroughly any beef, chicken or turkey. It must be at cooking temperature (212°F or 100°C) for 20 minutes. Freezing is not adequate. Canned meats are safe from living parasites, but are not recommended due to added chemicals.

Beverages

Drink 6 kinds of beverages:

- milk
- water
- fruit juices
- vegetable juices
- herb teas
- homemade (see *Recipes*)

---

[27] 114 mcg/100 g. Taken from *Food Values* 14th ed. by Pennington and Church, 1985.

[28] Salt has aluminum in it to keep it from caking. Buy salt that has magnesium carbonate as its anti-caking agent. Sea salt must be baked for 5 minutes at 400°F to destroy molds. Or buy chemically pure salt (see *Sources*).

This means getting off caffeine. And if you are already fatigued, this means you might be even more fatigued for a short time. You might have headaches from withdrawal, too. But they will only last 10 days. Mark your calendar and count off the days. Take headache medicine, if necessary, but make sure it does not contain caffeine. For energy, to replace caffeine, take one arginine (500 mg, see *Sources*) upon rising in the morning and before lunch. Soon you won't need it.

Cutting down on coffee, decaf, soda pop and powdered drinks won't do. You must be completely off. They contain very toxic solvents due to careless, unregulated production methods. Much is imported and can't be sufficiently regulated.

Even though grain (drinking) alcohol is the recommended substitute for propyl alcohol, that doesn't mean you may safely drink it. It is inadvisable to drink any form of alcohol at least until you are fully recovered.

1. Milk: 2% or higher, drink three 8 oz. glasses a day. Alternate brands. Buttermilk will do. Homemade yogurt is fine. Goat milk is also fine. Start with ¼ cup and increase gradually, if you are not used to it. If you do not drink milk because it gives you more mucous, try to drink milk anyway. If you have other reactions, like diarrhea, try milk digestant tablets (available at health food stores). Milk is too valuable to avoid: there are many unwanted chemicals in most brands of milk, but it is solvent-free, mold-free and very nutritious. The only exception should be for serious symptoms, like swelling, colitis, flu, or chronic diarrhea.

But all milk, whether goat or cow, is contaminated with *Salmonella* and *Shigella* bacteria as well as fluke parasite stages. Cattle are immunized against *Salmonella* but it does not prevent its persistence in the bowel. All these are <u>very harmful</u>. Pasteurization does not kill all of them. Only heating to a rolling boil makes milk safe. To do this in the easiest way, pour 1 or 2 quarts milk into an enamel double boiler or microwavable glass jar. Stay in the kitchen while the heat is on. When the bubbles have risen to indicate boiling, turn off the heat. You may throw away the "skin". Pour into glass jar and refrigerate. Another easy way is to use a pressure cooker that holds several pint jars of milk. All dairy products that have only been pasteurized are still contaminated. Ultrapasteurization does not improve matters. Dairy products that cannot be sterilized should not be consumed. It may be possible to find sterilized milk in paper containers on the store shelf—not in the refrigerator; if it wasn't sterile it would go foul in a day! Canned milk has solvent pollution. Powdered milk has both solvent and bacterial pollution.

2. Water: 2 pints. Drink one pint upon rising in the morning, the other pint in the afternoon sometime. The cold water faucet may be bringing you cadmium, copper or lead, but it is safer than purchased water, which inevitably has solvents in it. Let it run before using it. Filters are rather useless because water pollution comes in surges. A single surge of PCB contaminates your filter. All the water you use after this surge is now polluted, so you will be getting it chronically, whereas the unfiltered water cleans up again after the surge passes. Until you can test your own water for solvents, PCBs and metals, no expensive filter is worth the investment. An inexpensive pure carbon filter that is replaced <u>every</u> <u>month</u> may improve your tap water. Inflexible plastic pitchers fitted with a carbon filter pack are available (see *Sources*). <u>Never</u> buy filters with silver or other chemicals, even if they are just added to the carbon. Keep the filter sterile by soaking in diluted grain alcohol weekly.

3. Fruit juice: fresh squeezed only. Some stores make it while you wait. If they freeze some of it, you could purchase the frozen containers. Bottled fruit juices have traces of numerous solvents, as do the frozen concentrates, as do the refrigerated ones, <u>don't buy them</u>. You have to <u>see it being made</u>, but watch carefully: I recently went to a juice bar where they made everything fresh, before your very eyes. And I saw them take the fruit right from the refrigerator and spray it with a special wash "to get rid of any pesticides," then put a special detergent on it to clean off the wash! So instead of getting traces of pesticide, I got traces of propyl alcohol![29] Another grocery store had a machine that squeezed the oranges while you watched. But if you did not watch them filling the jugs, you missed seeing them add a tablespoon of concentrate, from a bottle out of sight, to give it better flavor. It still qualifies as "Fresh squeezed 100% orange juice," but thanks to that concentrate it now has toluene and xylene in it! Best of all, buy a juicer, select completely unbruised fruit, wash with plain water, and make your own juice (enough for a week—freeze it in half pint plastic bottles). For stronger flavor, leave some of the peel in the juice.

4. Vegetable juice: fresh or frozen only. If you or a friend would be willing to make fresh juice, this would be much better than purchased juice. Start with carrot juice. Peel carrots (don't scrape them, it's too easy to miss small dirt spots) and remove all blemishes carefully, then rinse. Drink ½ glass a day. After you are accustomed to this, add other vegetables and greens to the juice to make up half of it. Use celery, lettuce, cabbage, cucumber, beet, squash, tomato, everything raw that you normally have in your refrigerator. Then drink one glass a day.

5. Herb tea: fresh or bulk packaged. Tea bag varieties are moldy. Buy a non-metal (bamboo is common) tea strainer. Sweeten with honey or brown sugar with vitamin C added.

6. Homemade beverage. If you will miss your coffee or decaf, try just plain hot water with boiled whipping cream. Sweeten with honey. Please see *Recipes* for many more suggestions.

---

[29] Yes, I took a sample of the wash to test.

Horrors In Commercial Beverages

Commercial beverages are especially toxic due to traces of solvents left over from the manufacturing process. There are solvents in decaffeinated beverages, herb tea blends (not single herb teas), carbonated drinks, beverages with Nutrasweet™, fla-vored coffee, diet and health mixes, and fruit juices, even when the label states "not from concentrate" or "fresh from the or-chard," or "100% pure."

It is allowable to use solvents to clean machinery used in bottling (please look again at page 347)! It is also allowable to use solvents to make spice oleoresins, which are used as fla-voring.

21 CFR 173.240 (4-1-94 Edition) Isopropyl Alcohol.
Isopropyl alcohol may be present in the following foods un-der the conditions specified:
- (a) In spice oleoresins as a residue from the extraction of spice, at a level not to exceed 50 parts per million.
- (b) In lemon oil as a residue in production of the oil, at a level not to exceed 6 parts per million.
- (c) [Discusses its use in hops extract.]

Here is a summary of other solvents mentioned:

Solvent	Allowable residue in spice oleoresins	Paragraph in 21 CFR
Acetone	30 PPM	173.210
Ethylene dichloride	30 PPM	173.230
Methyl alcohol	50 PPM	173.250
Methylene chloride	30 PPM	173.255
Hexane	25 PPM	173.270
Trichloroethylene	30 PPM	173.290

Fig. 66 Lawful uses of solvents in food.

I have found all these solvents and others in commercial beverages! Some of the solvents I have found are just too toxic to be believed! Yet you can build the test apparatus yourself (page 457), buy foods at your grocery store, and tabulate your own results. I hope you do, and I hope you find that the food in your area is cleaner than mine! Remember that the Syncrometer can only determine the presence or absence of something, not the concentration. There may only be a few parts per billion, but a sick person trying to get well cannot afford <u>any</u> solvent intake. For that matter, <u>none</u> of us should tolerate any of these:

- **Acetone** in carbonated drinks
- **Benzene** in store-bought drinking water (including distilled), store-bought fruit juice (including health varieties)
- **Carbon tetrachloride** in store-bought drinking water
- **Decane** in health foods and beverages
- **Hexanes** in decafs
- **Hexanedione** in flavored foods
- **Isophorone** in flavored foods
- **Methyl butyl ketone** and **Methyl ethyl ketone** in flavored foods
- **Methylene chloride** in fruit juice
- **Pentane** in decafs
- **Propyl alcohol** in bottled water, commercial fruit juices, commercial beverages.
- **Toluene** and **xylene** in carbonated drinks
- **Trichloroethane**(TCE), **TC Ethylene** in flavored foods
- **Wood alcohol** (methanol) in carbonated drinks, diet drinks, herb tea blends, store-bought water, infant formula

If you allowed a tiny drop of kerosene or carpet cleaning fluid to get into your pet's food every day, wouldn't you expect your pet to get sick? Why would <u>you</u> not expect to be sick with these solvents in your daily food? I imagine these solvents are just tiny amounts, introduced by sterilizing equipment, the manufacturing process, and adding flavor or color. Flavors and colors for food must be extracted somehow from the leaves or bark or beans from which they come. But until safe methods are invented, such food should be considered unsafe for human consumption (or pets or livestock!).

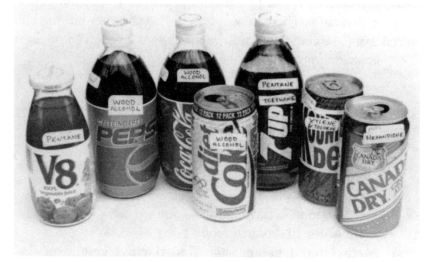

Fig. 67 Some unsafe beverages.

Food Preparation

Cook your food in glass, enamel, ceramic or microwavable pots and pans. Throw away all metal ware, foil wrap, and metal-capped salt shakers since you will never use them again. If you don't plan to fry much (only once a week), you might keep the Teflon™ or Silverstone™ coated fry-pan, otherwise get an enamel coated metal pan. Stir and serve food with wood or plastic, not metal utensils. If you have recurring urinary tract infections, you should reduce your metal contact even further; eat with plastic cutlery. Sturdy decorative plastic ware can be found in hardware and camping stores. Don't drink out of styrofoam cups (styrene is toxic). Don't eat toast (many toasters spit tungsten all over your bread and make benzopyrenes besides). Don't buy things made with baking powder (it has aluminum) or baked in aluminum pans. Choose goods made with baking soda and sold in paper or microwavable pans. Don't run your drinking water through the freezer or fountain or refrigerator. Don't heat your water in a coffee maker or tea kettle. Don't use a plastic thermos jug (the plastic liner has lanthanides) the inside must be glass. Don't drink from a personal water bottle (it begins to breed bacteria) unless you sterilize it daily.

Why are we still using stainless steel cookware when it contains 18% chromium and 8% nickel? Because it is rustproof and shiny and we can't <u>see</u> any deterioration. **But all metal seeps!** Throw those metal pots away. Get your essential minerals from foods, not cookware.

Never, never drink or cook with the water from your hot water faucet. If you have an electric hot water heater the heating element releases metal. Even if you have a gas hot water heater, the heated water leaches metals or glues from your pipes. If your kitchen tap is the single lever type, make sure it is fully on cold for cooking. Teach children this rule.

Food Guidelines

It is impossible to remember everything about every food, but in general do not buy foods that are highly processed. Here are a few foods; see if you can guess whether they should be in your diet or not.

breads	Yes, but only from a bakery, and <u>never</u> wrapped in plastic.
toast	No. It has benzopyrene and tungsten. Yes, if made on a cookie sheet or in a frying pan.
cheese	Yes, if used in baked dishes.
chicken	Only if cooked for 20 minutes at boiling point, as in soup, or canned (never prepare raw chicken yourself).
wine with dinner	No.

431

peanut butter	Yes if you grind it yourself and add ¼ tsp. vitamin C powder as you grind.
cottage cheese	No, it can't be sterilized easily.
desserts	Yes, but again, only if flavored with safe extracts.
rice	Yes, if vitamin C is added before cooking. Use white only, brown is too moldy.
pasta	Yes, with homemade sauce and vitamin C.
Jell-O™	No, it has artificial flavor and color.
egg dishes	Yes, but not "imitation", cholesterol-free or cholesterol-reduced varieties.
fish, seafood	Yes!
soy foods (tofu)	No. It's the extensive processing that taints it.
soup	Yes, if seasoned only with herbs (no bouillon cube).
sugar	Yes, turbinado or brown if treated with vitamin C.
herb tea	Yes, if not in a bag and not in a mixture of herbs.
cheesecake	Yes.

Fig. 68 Some good foods.

Choose brands with the shortest list of ingredients. Alternate brands every time you shop.

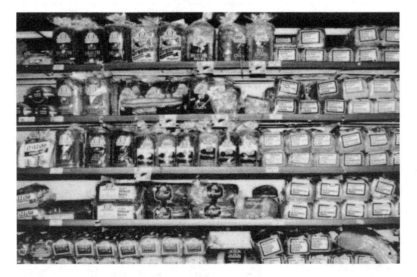

Fig. 69 All breads I tested had mold if they were in plastic.

Dining Out

Restaurants (excluding fast food) are generally quite safe to eat at. Here are some do's and don'ts:

Do carry your own aluminum-free salt and vitamin C powder with you.

Do ask for plastic cutlery.

Do drink the water if from the tap.

Do ask for boiled, not just steamed, milk.

Don't eat or drink from styrofoam. If getting food "to go," get it in clear plastic containers, or ask them to line the styrofoam container with paper or plastic wrap, and line the styrofoam cup with a plastic baggy.

Don't use their ketchup and condiments (they have been standing out too long).

Here is a list of things that are generally safe to order:

pancakes, French toast, waffles	Don't use their imitation syrup (has benzoate), use honey instead.
eggs	Any style except soft boiled and scrambled. The white should be solid.
hash browns	If lightly fried, not deep fried.
soup	Only if nothing else is available. (It probably came in a can and was cooked in an aluminum pot and is full of aluminized salt.)
vegetarian sand-wiches	But no soy products (too processed).
baked or boiled po-tatoes	Use only cheese sauce, bring your own salt, don't eat the skin.
cooked vegetables	Broccoli, Brussels sprouts, beets, corn, squash, and so forth.
vegetable salads	Don't eat the croutons, bacon bits, and anything that doesn't look fresh.
vegetarian dishes	But no soy ingredients and or sauces. Fresh ketchup OK.
bread and biscuits	White only, not toasted, not "cholesterol-free" varieties.
fish and seafood	Anything but deep fried (the oil may have benzene) is fine: baked, steamed, fish cakes, seafood cock-tails, etc.
Mexican food	Any of the numerous baked dishes.
Chinese food	Except dishes with tofu or MSG.
fruit cup	With honey and cinnamon.
fruit pies, cobblers	But not with ice cream (every flavor has benzene).
lemon or lime me-ringue pie	Indulge yourself.

Fig. 70 Good restaurant foods.

As you see your symptoms disappear, one after another, you will feel the magic of healing. Many sick persons have 50 or more symptoms to start out! They could fill two sheets of paper, one symptom to each line. It can be quite shocking to see a list of all your symptoms.

Sometimes a new symptom appears as fast as an old one disappears. The coincidence makes it tempting to believe that one symptom turns into a different one. But it is not so. If a new symptom appears, it is because another pathogen has become activated due to a new toxin. Try to identify the new item. Stop using any new food, supplement, or body product, even if it is a health variety, and see if it goes away.

Body Clean-up

We are living in a very fortunate time. We are not expected to all look alike! The 60's brought us this wonderful freedom. Freedom to dress in a variety of styles, use make-up or no make-up, jewelry or no jewelry, any kind of hair style, any kind of shoes.

You will need to go off <u>every</u> cosmetic and body product that you are <u>now</u> using. Not a single one can be continued. They are full of titanium, zirconium, benzalkonium, bismuth, anti-mony[30], barium[31], strontium[32], aluminum, tin, chromium, not to mention pollution solvents such as benzene and PCBs.

Do not use any commercial salves, ointments, lotions, colognes, perfumes, massage oils, deodorant, mouthwash, toothpaste, even when touted as "herbal" and health-food-type. See *Recipes* for homemade substitutes.

---

[30] Breast cancer cases show titanium, zirconium, benzalkonium, bismuth and antimony accumulation in the breast.

[31] Barium is described in the *Merck Index* as "Caution: All water or acid soluble barium compounds are POISONOUS." 10th ed. p. 139 1983.

[32] This element goes to bones.

People are trying desperately to use less toxic products. They seek health for themselves. So they reach for products that just list herbs and other natural ingredients. Unfortunately, the buyers are being duped. The Food and Drug Administration (FDA) requires all body products to have sufficient antiseptic in them. Some of these antiseptics are substances <u>you must avoid</u>! But you won't see them on the label because manufacturers prefer to use quantities below the levels they must disclose. And by using a variety of antiseptics in these small amounts they can still meet sterility requirements. The only ingredient you might see is "grapefruit seed" or similar healthy-sounding natural antiseptic. This is sad for the consumer of health food varieties.

- I have seen rocks sold as "Aluminum-Free Natural Deodorant". You rub the rock under your arms. It works because the rock is made of magnesium-<u>aluminum</u>-silicate.
- Men's hair color has lead in it.
- Lipstick has barium, aluminum, titanium.
- Eye pencil and shadow have chromium.
- Toothpaste has benzene, tin, and strontium.
- Hair spray has propyl alcohol and PCBs. BEWARE! Stop using it <u>today</u>.
- Shampoo, even health varieties, has propyl alcohol! BEWARE! Stop using it <u>today</u>.
- Cigarettes have lead, mercury, nickel and *Tobacco Mosaic virus.*
- Chewing tobacco has ytterbium

Some of the unnatural chemicals listed are present because of residues in the manufacturing process, but others you will actually see listed on the label!

Propyl alcohol and wood alcohol are present because the tubing used to fill the bottles is sterilized and cleaned with them. Ice cream machines are "oiled" with a gel containing petroleum products. This could explain why I always find benzene in ice cream.

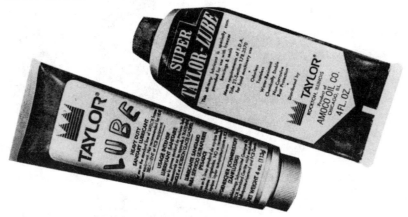

Fig. 71 Examples of commercial "food lube."

How can propyl alcohol in shampoo get into your body in significant amounts? The skin is more absorbent than we realize, and time and time again I see cancer victims who have gone off every body product <u>except</u> their favorite shampoo. They harbor propyl alcohol until they make that final sacrifice. It is better to switch shampoos than to not need any due to radiation and chemotherapy!

See *Recipes* for easy-to-make, natural cosmetics. But you might consider just stopping them all. Especially if you're going on vacation.

Use nothing that you wouldn't use on a new-born baby. This is a permissive age. You will be the only one feeling "naked." Others won't even notice. Don't forget advertising is aimed at you, even if other people's eyes are not!

Don't even use soap unless it is homemade soap (see *Recipes*) or borax straight from the box. Borax was the traditional pioneer soap. It is antibacterial and can be made into a solution. It is also a water softener and is the main ingredient in non-chlorine bleach. Borax can remove grease, too, and some stains.

But even borax is not natural to your body and it is therefore wise to use as little as necessary. See *Recipes* for anti-bacterial borax soap.

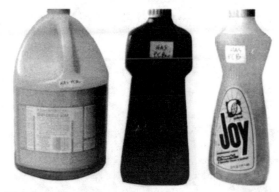

Dishes and clothing are primary source of PCBs.
Fig. 72 Detergents with PCBs.

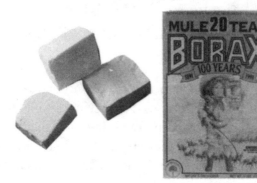

homemade soap   pure borax
Fig. 73 Safe soaps.

Don't use toothpaste, not even health-food varieties. To clean teeth, use plain water or chemically pure baking soda (see *Sources*)—but dissolve it in water first, otherwise it is too abrasive. Or brush with hydrogen peroxide <u>food grade</u>, not the regular variety (see *Sources*). Don't use floss; use 2 or 4-pound monofilament fish line. Floss has mercury antiseptics (with thallium pollution!). Throw away your old toothbrush—solvents don't wash away.

Don't use mouthwash. Use saltwater (aluminum-free salt) or food grade hydrogen peroxide (a few drops in water).

Don't use hair spray.

Don't use massage oils of any kind. Use olive oil.

Don't use bath oil. Take showers, not baths, if you are strong enough to stand. Showers are cleaner.

Don't use perfumes or colognes.

Don't use commercial lotions or personal lubricants.

Stop Using Supplements

Stop using your vitamin supplements. They, too, are heavily polluted. This is the saddest, most tragic part of your instructions. I have found solvents, heavy metals and lanthanides in 90% or more of the popular vitamin and mineral capsules and

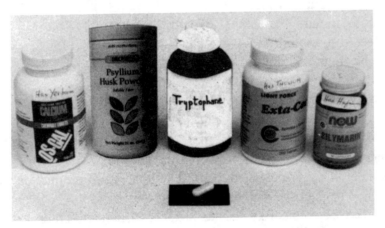

The capsule in the foreground is a notorious tryptophane capsule. It had the following pollutants: PCBs, mercury, ruthenium, thulium, strontium, praseodymium, aluminum, benzalkonium.

Fig. 74 Some polluted supplements.

tablets I test. These substances will do more harm in the long run than the supplement can make up for in benefits.

<u>Most</u> of the varieties of vitamin C that I have tested are polluted with thulium! Until all vitamins and minerals and other food supplements have been analyzed for pollutants, <u>after they are encapsulated or tableted</u>, they are not safe. We need more disclosure on our products. No manufactured product is pure. We can't expect that. But at least we should be able to tell what impurities we are getting, and how much.

It <u>is</u> possible to do detailed analysis of foods or products at a reasonable price. Look at the bottle of common table salt, sodium chloride, that is used by beginning chemistry students to do experiments. It must be thoroughly analyzed for them because minute impurities affect their results. (Those minute impurities, like lead, affect <u>you</u>, too.) Look at the label on the bottle in the picture. Even after all these tests, the cost of laboratory salt is only $2.80 per pound.[33]

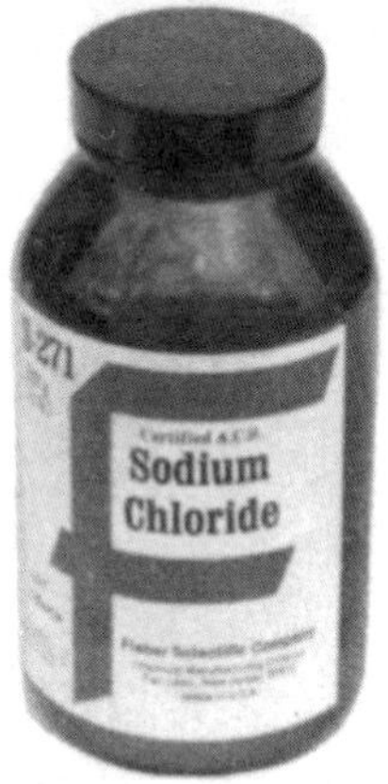

Fig. 75 Pure salt.

It is most important not to be fooled by ingredient claims, like "made from organically grown vegetables". Sure that's great, but the analysis *I* trust would be done on the final, cleaned, cooked and packaged product on the shelf. The package is a major <u>unlisted</u> ingredient.

Toxic solvents like decane, hexane, carbon tetrachloride and benzene will get more flavor or fat or cholesterol out of things than metabolizable grain alcohol. Of course, the extraction process calls for washing out the solvent later. But it can't all be washed out, and a detailed analysis <u>on the final product</u> would

---

[33] You will pay about $8.00 per pound (Spectrum Chemical Co.) for USP (United States Pharmaceutical) grade. But the same analysis is done on the cheaper grades, and my point is that the analysis is cost effective enough that it should be done on our daily foods.

give the public the information they need to make informed choices.

> ## All supplements must be tested for purity by yourself. If this cannot be done, don't take them.
>
> Polluted supplements do much more harm than good. Get your super-nutrition by juicing vegetables of all kinds and making herbal teas.

Safe Supplements

There are, no doubt, lots of safe supplements to be had. The problem is knowing which they are. The nature of pollution is such that one bottle might be safe, while another of the same brand is not. In view of this, as I found a polluted bottle, I stopped using any more of that brand. That is why I am reduced to recommending only the ones in the *Sources* at this time.

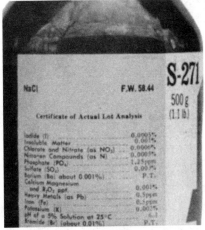

Common salt for student use is thoroughly analyzed for pollution. The label gives you the final "Actual Lot Analysis" of the product. It is not expensive.

Fig. 76 Laboratory salt label.

Vitamin C, in crystal form, is a must in your lifestyle. It helps the liver, and possibly other organs, detoxify things. It also helps retard mold, and perhaps even <u>destroys</u> aflatoxins! Keep some next to your refrigerator so it is handy when you put away groceries. Add 1/8 tsp. to maple syrup, vinegar, cooked cereal, fruit juice, leftovers. Have ¼ tsp. (1 gram) with each meal.

Vitamin B₂, 100 mg. This is the vitamin that helps detoxify benzene! Take one to three a day. While recovering from AIDS you need 3 tablets three times a day.

Vitamin B₆, 250 mg, and B-complex, 50 mg. Undoubtedly these help the liver and kidneys in many ways. One a day.

Magnesium oxide, 300 mg., is another must. Take one or two a day. It is a major mineral; all of our cells need lots of it. Only leafy vegetables provide it.

Hydrogen peroxide, food grade. It is advantageous to kill bacteria and viruses to some extent every day. Hydrogen peroxide lets you do this. It should never come in contact with metal, including its container or metal tooth fillings. If you get a few drops on your skin it may turn white and sting, but does no harm, so simply wash it off. Instructions for its use come with the product.

Herbs. These are excellent supplements, both in bulk and capsules, but not extracts, concentrates, or concoctions. There are many books that describe their uses.

Thioctic acid or lipoic acid. Presumably this chelates (traps and prepares for elimination) heavy metals, and helps the liver in detoxifying obscure and deadly poisons. Everyone would benefit from 100 mg. per day. I find it outstanding, and give it to many ill persons, even when not mentioned in the case histories. It comes as a 100 mg. capsule (see *Sources*). I use it at doses from one capsule, 3 times a day, to 2 capsules, 5 times a day. I have seen no side effects at these dosages, even in very sick persons.

Lugol's Iodine Solution (see *Recipes*) is old-fashioned "iodine." Iodine has a distinctive trait: it hangs up on anything and everything. In fact, it attaches itself so quickly we consider everything it touches as "stained." This is just the property we want to make it safe for use. The amount you use is immediately hung up, or attached, to your mucous and can not be quickly absorbed into the blood or other organs. It stays in the stomach. And for this reason it is so useful for killing vicious bacteria like *Salmonella*.

Do not take Lugol's iodine if you know you are allergic to iodine. It could be fatal.

Six drops of Lugol's solution can end it all for *Salmonella*. If you have gas and bloating, pour yourself ½ glass of water. Add 6 drops of Lugol's (not more, not less), stir with wood or plastic, and drink all at once. The action is noticeable in an hour. Take this dose 4 times a day, after meals and at bedtime, for 3 days in a row, then as needed. This eradicates even a stubborn case of *Salmonella*.

Notice how calming 6 drops of Lugol's can be, soothing a manic stage and bringing a peaceful state where anxiety ruled before.

Lugol's is perfectly safe (if not allergic) to take day after day, when needed, because of its peculiar attaching property. It arrives in the stomach, reattaches to everything in proximity. Doomed are all *Salmonellas*; doomed also are eggs of parasites that might be in the stomach (cysts).

Naturally, one would not leave such medicine within the reach of children. Also, one would not use anything medicinal, including Lugol's unless there were a need, like cancer, AIDS, or bowel disease. When the gas and bloating problem has stopped, stop using Lugol's. If one or two doses of Lugol's cures the problem, stop. Store it in a perfectly secure place. In the past, 2/3 of a teaspoon (60 drops) of Lugol's was the standard dose of iodine given to persons with thyroid disease. Six drops is small by comparison.

Turmeric and **fennel** are herbs also used as cooking spices. They can eradicate invasive *E. coli* and *Shigella* bacteria! They are completely harmless, and are part of the Bowel Program.

Other supplements. The concept of supplementing the diet is excellent, but the pollution problem makes it prohibitive. Use only supplements and brands recommended in *Sources*, although the best approach is to test them yourself with your Syncrometer. I can't guarantee the brands in *Sources* will stay pure. If in doubt, leave it out.

Home Clean-up

This is the easiest task because it mostly involves throwing things out. Hopefully your family and friends will jump to your assistance.

- The basement gets cleaned.
- The garage gets cleaned.
- Every room in the house gets cleaned.

Your Basement

To clean your basement, remove all paint, varnish, thinners, brush cleaners, and related supplies. Remove all cleaners such as carpet cleaner, leather cleaner, rust remover. Remove all chemicals that are in cans, bottles or buckets.

You may keep your laundry supplies: borax, washing soda, white distilled vinegar, bleach and homemade soap. You may keep canned goods, tools, items that are not chemicals. You may move your chemicals into your garage. Also move any car tires and automotive supplies like waxes, oil, transmission fluid, and the spare gas can (even if it is empty) into your garage or discard them.

Seal cracks in the basement and around pipes where they come through the wall with black plastic roofing cement. In a few days it will be hard enough to caulk with a prettier color. Spread a sheet of plastic over the sewer or sump pump.

Your Garage

Do you have a garage that is a separate building from your home? This is the best arrangement. You can move all the basement chemicals into this garage. Things that will freeze, such as latex paint, you may as well discard. But if your garage is attached, you have a problem. <u>Never, never use your door between the garage and house</u>. Walk around the outside. Don't allow this door to be used. Tack a sheet of plastic over it to slow down the rate of fume entrance into the house. Your house acts like a chimney for the garage. Your house is taller and warmer than the garage so garage-air is pulled in and up as the warm air in the house rises. See the drawing.

In medieval days, the barn for the animals was attached to the house. We think such an arrangement with its penetrating odors is unsavory. But what of the gasoline and motor fumes we are getting now due to parked vehicles? These are toxic besides! This is even more medieval.

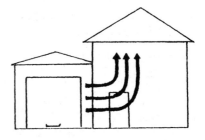

Fig. 77 Garage fumes.

If your garage is under your house, you cannot keep the pollution from entering your home. In this case, leave the cars and lawnmower <u>outside</u>. Remove cans of gasoline, solvents, etc. Put up a separate shed for these items.

445

Special Clean-up for Freon (CFCs)

Because I consider Freon to be the top health hazard in our home, I recommend turning in your refrigerator for a non-CFC variety. Dispose of all spare units. Remove window air conditioners or test the dust in your home (page 485) for Freon. Have your car's air conditioning system checked. Dispose of old pressurized cans. Even one whiff is too much. It never leaves the body because the body has no detoxification methods for it!

Only one useful reaction with Freon comes to mind. Freon is thought to be responsible for the ozone "hole" at the South Pole. Would Freon react with ozone supplied to your body and thereby become biodegradable? Indeed, it does! But only if you drink it as ozonated water. Other ozone routes, as intravenous or rectal, have not been observed to be as effective.

If you are following your progress with the Syncrometer, you will see that Freon now appears in the liver for the first time. (Before this, it was marooned in the parathyroids, thymus, and other organs.) You may also detect a feeling like indigestion. You must come to the assistance of your liver. Even ozonated Freon is extremely burdensome to the liver.

A combination of herbs (Liver Herb Drink in *Recipes*, page 552) rescues the liver from its plight, and prevents the indigestion. After drinking liver herbs you will see that the Freon now appears in the kidneys. Yet it is marooned there unless you assist them. Take the kidney cleanse to assist the kidneys so they can finally excrete the Freon into the urine.

It's an elaborate detoxifying program and usually takes six to eight weeks to get most of the Freon out. Afterward, continue the programs at one fourth dosage for half a year.

Forane is one of the new refrigerants. Although toxic, at least I observe it in the liver directly, suggesting that your body is capable of handling it. Remember your new refrigerator will still be using a toxic coolant, and it would be best to keep it outside or at least vented to the outside.

Special Clean-up for Fiberglass

Fiberglass insulation has microscopically small bits of glass that are free to blow into the air. When house drafts pull it into the air you will inhale them. They cut their way through your lungs and organs like millions of tiny knives, spreading through your body, since there is no way out for them. You smell nothing and feel nothing. This makes it a very sinister poison. Your body, though, recognizes these sharp, pointed bits and tries to stop their spread by sequestering them in cysts.

Most solid malignant tumors contain fiberglass or asbestos, another glass-like particle. In nearly all cases a hole can be found in the ceiling or walls, leading to fiberglass insulated parts of the house. When these holes are sealed in an air-tight manner the house air no longer is positive for fiberglass. Covering with paneling is not sufficient. Check your dwelling for uncovered fiberglass. Repair immediately. Search for small screw holes intended for pictures, or electric outlet plates that are missing.

Also remove fiberglass jackets from water heater and fiberglass filter from furnace. Replace with foam or carbon. Best of all, hire a crew to remove it all from your home, and replace insulation with blown-in shredded paper or other innocuous substance.

Never build a new house using fiberglass for any purpose.

Special Clean-up for Asbestos

The biggest source of asbestos is not building materials! It is the clothes dryer belt and hair dryer! To be safe, remove the belt from your dryer and check to see if it says "Made in USA" on the belt itself. If so, it is OK. If not, it is imported, and probably contains asbestos. Exchange it for a USA belt (see *Sources*).

Hair dryers, too, may be imported and shed asbestos. It is especially hazardous to be aiming a stream of hot asbestos right at your face! If you can't find a safe model (see *Sources*), or are unsure, don't use any. If you have cancer or are ill, <u>no one in the house</u> should use an unsafe hair dryer.

Turn off radiators and electric heaters and cover them with big plastic garbage bags, or paint them, or remove them. They give off asbestos if their paint is old.

Your House

To clean the house, start with the bedroom. Remove everything that has any smell to it whatever: candles, potpourri, soaps, mending glue, cleaners, repair chemicals, felt markers, colognes, perfumes, and especially plug-in air "fresheners". Store them in the garage, not the basement. Since all vapor rises, they would come back up if you put them in a downstairs garage or basement.

Do not sleep in a bedroom that is paneled or has wallpaper. They give off arsenic and formaldehyde. Either remove them or move your bed to a different room. Leave the house while this is being done. If other rooms have paneling or wallpaper, close their doors and spend no time in them.

Next clean the kitchen. Take all cans and bottles of chemicals out from under the sink or in a closet. Remove them to the garage. Keep only the borax, washing soda, white distilled vinegar and homemade soap. Use these for all purposes. For exact amounts to use for dishwasher, dishes, windows, dusting, see *Recipes*. Remove all cans, bottles, roach and ant killer, moth balls, and chemicals that kill insects or mice. These should not be stored anywhere. They should be thrown out. Remember to check the crawl space, attic and closets for hidden poisons also.

To keep out mice, walk all around your house, stuffing holes and cracks with steel wool. Use old-fashioned mouse traps. For cockroaches and other insects (except ants) sprinkle handfuls of boric acid[34] (not borax) under your shelf paper, behind sink, stove, refrigerator, under carpets, etc. Use vinegar on your kitchen wipe-up cloth to leave a residue that keeps out ants. Do this regularly. To wax the floor, get the wax from the garage and put it back there. A sick person should not be in the house while house cleaning or floor waxing is being done.

Remove all cans and bottles of "stuff" from the bathroom. The chlorine bleach is stored in the garage. Someone else can bring it in to clean the toilet (only). Leave only the borax soap, homemade soap, and grain alcohol antiseptic. Toilet paper and tissues should be <u>unfragranced</u>, <u>uncolored</u>. All colognes, after shave, anything you can smell must be removed. Family members should buy unfragranced products. They should smoke outdoors, blow-dry their hair outdoors or in the garage, use nail polish and polish remover outdoors or in the garage.

Do not keep new foam furniture in the house. If it is less than one year old, move it into the garage until you are well. It gives off formaldehyde. So does new clothing; it is in the sizing. Wash all new clothes before wearing. If you have a respiratory illness, move <u>all</u> the clothes in the clothes closet out of your bedroom to a different closet.

Do not use the hot water from an electric hot water heater for cooking or drinking. It has tungsten. Do not drink water that sits in glazed crock ware (the glaze seeps toxic elements like cadmium) like some water dispensers have. Do not buy water from your health food store that runs through a long plastic hose from their bulk tank (I always see cesium picked up from flexi-

---

[34] Boric acid is available by the pound from farm supply stores and from Now Foods. Because it looks like sugar keep it in the garage to prevent accidental poisoning.

ble clear plastic). Also ask them how and when they clean their tank. Best is to observe that it is done with non-toxic methods.

If your house is more than 10 years old, change all the galvanized pipe to PVC plastic. Although PVC is a toxic substance, amazingly, the water is free of PVC in three weeks! If your house has copper pipes don't wait for cancer or schizophrenia to claim a family member. Change all the copper pipe to PVC plastic immediately. If the pipes are not accessible, ask a plumber to lay an extra line, outside the walls. This is less expensive, too.

If you have a water softener, by-pass it immediately and replace the metal pipe on the user side of the softener tank. Softener salts are polluted with strontium and chromate; they are also full of aluminum. The salts corrode the pipes so the pipes begin to seep cadmium into the water. After changing your pipes to plastic, there will be so little iron and hardness left, you may not need a softener. If the water comes from a well, consider changing the well-pipe to PVC to get rid of iron. While the well is open, have the pump checked for PCBs. Call the Health Department to arrange the testing. If you must have softening after all this, check into the new magnetic varieties of water softener (although they only work well when used with plastic plumbing).

The cleanest heat is electric. Go total electric if possible. If you must stay with gas, have a furnace repair person check your furnace and look for gas leaks before the heating season starts. Don't call the gas company even though it is free. The gas company misses 4 out of 5 leaks! The Health Department does not miss any; call them! House builders and contractors are also reliable in their gas leak detection.

Unnatural Chemicals

And where I found them...

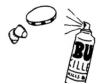

ARSENIC

in ant & roach hives,
grains of pesticide

in carpet & furniture"treated"
for stain resistance

in wallpaper

BARIUM

MOLYBDENUM

in lipstick

in bus exhaust

in "molys"

COBALT

in laundry
detergent

in dishwasher
detergent

in skin bracer

in mouthwash

ANTIMONY

CADMIUM and COPPER

TITANIUM

in eye liner

in water running
through old metal pipes

in face powder &
other powders, and
in metal dental ware

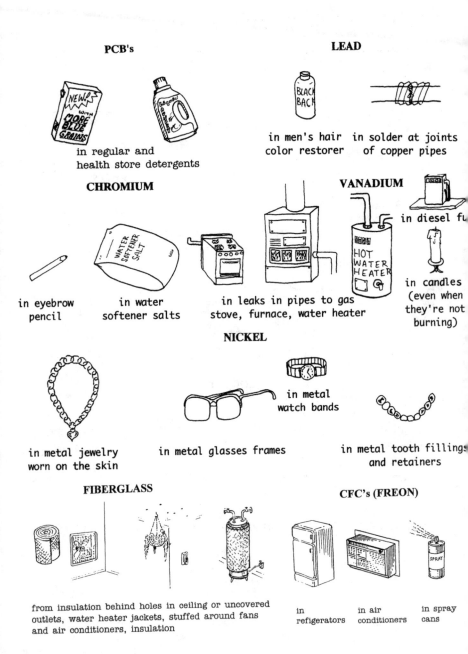

PCB's

in regular and
health store detergents

LEAD

in men's hair
color restorer

in solder at joints
of copper pipes

CHROMIUM

in eyebrow
pencil

in water
softener salts

in leaks in pipes to gas
stove, furnace, water heater

VANADIUM

in diesel fu

in candles
(even when
they're not
burning)

NICKEL

in metal
watch bands

in metal jewelry
worn on the skin

in metal glasses frames

in metal tooth fillings
and retainers

FIBERGLASS

from insulation behind holes in ceiling or uncovered
outlets, water heater jackets, stuffed around fans
and air conditioners, insulation

CFC's (FREON)

in
refrigerators

in air
conditioners

in spray
cans

MERCURY and THALLIUM

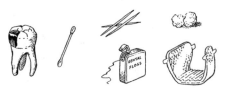

in tooth fillings, sanitary napkins, cotton balls
dental floss, toothpicks, cotton swabs

THULIUM

in most brands of
vitamin C I tested

DYSPROSIUM and LUTETIUM

in paint, varnish,
shellac

HOLMIUM

in hand cleaners

HAFNIUM

in nail polish
& hair spray

RHENIUM

in spray starch

BISMUTH

in cologne and
stomache aids

CESIUM

in clear-as-glass
plastic

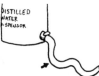

after running through
long plastic hose

TIN and STRONTIUM

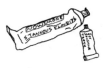

in toothpaste

YTTERBIUM, ERBIUM TERBIUM

PRASEODYMIUM, NIOBIUM, NEODYMIUM, YTTRIUM

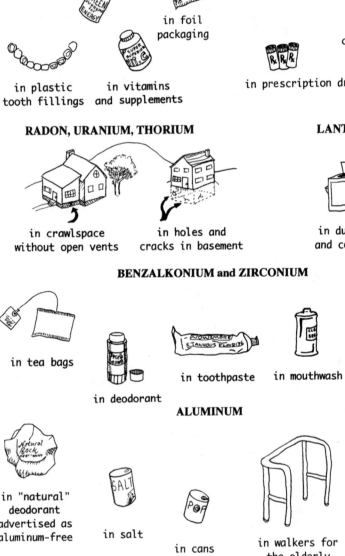

in foil packaging

in over the counter drugs

in prescription drugs

in plastic tooth fillings

in vitamins and supplements

RADON, URANIUM, THORIUM

LANTHANUM

in crawlspace without open vents

in holes and cracks in basement

in duplicator and copier ink

BENZALKONIUM and ZIRCONIUM

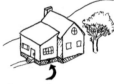

in tea bags

in deodorant

in toothpaste

in mouthwash

in cosmetics

ALUMINUM

in "natural" deodorant advertised as aluminum-free

in salt

in cans

in walkers for the elderly

in lotions

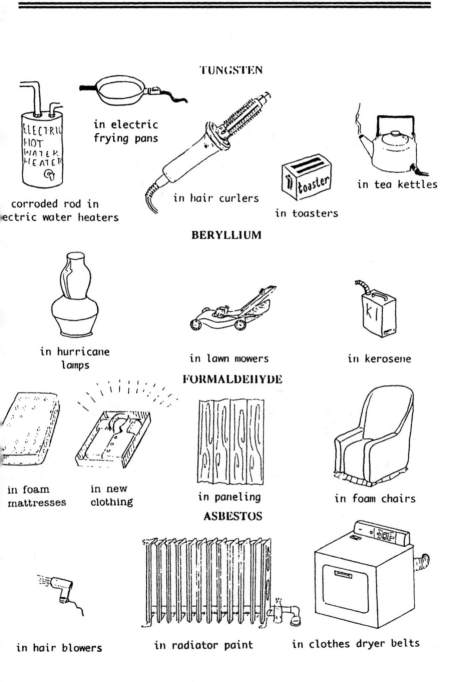

TUNGSTEN

corroded rod in electric water heaters

in electric frying pans

in hair curlers

in toasters

in tea kettles

BERYLLIUM

in hurricane lamps

in lawn mowers

in kerosene

FORMALDEHYDE

in foam mattresses

in new clothing

in paneling

in foam chairs

ASBESTOS

in hair blowers

in radiator paint

in clothes dryer belts

455

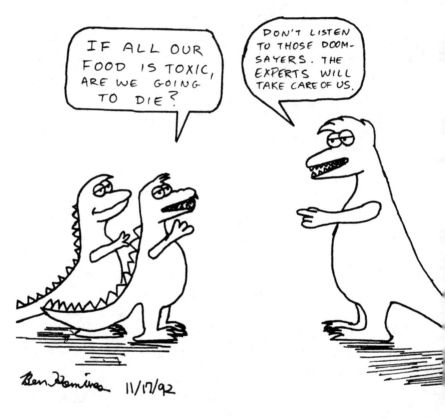

Fig. 78 Our future, unless we act.

Bioelectronics

The most important electronic device to make or buy is a **zapper**—a compact pulse generator operating from a common 9 volt battery whose output is about 30 KHz. It kills all parasites, bacteria, viruses, molds, and fungi even though their individual resonant frequencies are either higher or lower (50 KHz to 900 KHz). Building a zapper is described in an earlier chapter.

The next most useful device to have is a **Syncrometer.™** It lets you diagnose yourself and monitor your progress until you are cured. It consists of an audio oscillator circuit with your body as part of the circuit. Utilizing samples of parasites or pollutants, it lets you test for them in any product or body tissue. I include a design that you can make yourself.

A third very useful device is a **frequency generator.** You can use it to electrocute individual organisms, or together with the Syncrometer™ to find an organism's particular frequency. You need one that operates in the parasite, bacteria and virus ranges, from 50 KHz to 900 KHz. It must also be able to select a particular frequency, like 434 KHz, quickly and accurately. Frequency generators are available for as little as $300.00, but it is worth paying a little more to get a digital display of the frequency.

Making A Syncrometer

This is an *audio oscillator circuit* in which you include yourself by means of a handhold. You listen to the current in your circuit with a loudspeaker. Other oscillator circuits will work, too. A lot of fascinating opportunities present themselves with this concept.

I have previously published three ways to build the Syncrometer circuit.[35] Here is the circuit diagram:

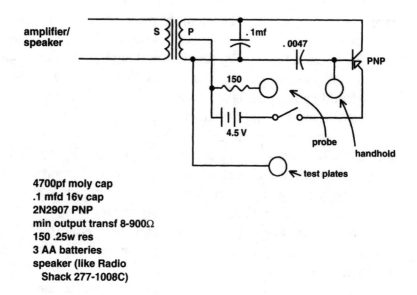

Fig. 79 Syncrometer schematic.

If you are not an electronics enthusiast, you can still assemble a Syncrometer using a hobby kit. No soldering is required. Here is what you need:

Making a Hobby Kit Syncrometer

Item	Radio Shack Cat. No.
200 in One Electronic Project Lab by Science Fair	28-262
3 AA 1½ volt batteries	

[35]In *The Cure for all Cancers* and *The Cure for HIV/AIDS*.

Alligator clip test jumpers	You need 2.
Handhold. A four inch length of ¾ inch copper pipe, like for plumbing. These dimensions are critical to assure maximum skin contact.	
Probe. A banana plug.	Precision Mini-Hook Test Lead Set (contains two, you only need one) 278-1160A
Pencil, new.	

Fig. 80 Syncrometer parts list.

Build <u>The Electrosonic Human</u> in the *200 in One Electronic Project Lab*. It takes about 10 minutes.

Later, when you use the probe to press against your knuckle you may find getting the right sound is painful. In this case try substituting the .005 microfarad capacitor for the .01 microfarad capacitor in the circuit.

Attach the Probe. The Archer Precision Mini-Hook Test Lead Set has a banana plug for the probe on one end and a mini-hook on the other end for easy attachment to the circuit. Tape a long, new pencil to the probe to make it easier to hold. Connect the Probe to middle post of the primary side of the transformer (it also connects to the negative battery post). <u>You will not be using the two connections the instuctions tell you to hold</u>.

Attach the Handhold. Clip the Handhold to one end of an alligator clip test jumper, and clip the other end to the base (B) of the transistor used in the circuit.

Attach an alligator clip to the post of the transformer that connects to the two capacitors. This will go to the **test plates**.

Final test. Turn the control knob on and keep turning the potentiometer to nearly the maximum. (This reduces the resistance. The schematic has a 150 ohm fixed resistor in place of the potentiometer.) Make sure you have good batteries installed. Test the circuit by briefly touching the Probe to the Handhold. The speaker should produce a sound like popping corn. If it does not, check that your alligator clips are not bending the spring terminals so much that other wires attached there are loose. Finally, turn switches OFF.

Making Test Plates

This is the box you attach to the basic Syncrometer circuit. It has test plates to put your test substances and tissue samples on. The wiring in it is arranged so that you can test for a toxin in a product, as well as search in yourself. This means you can search for *Salmonella* in the milk or cheese you just ate, not just for *Salmonella* in your stomach.

Only if the resonant frequency of an item on one plate is equal to the resonant frequency of an item on the other plate will the entire circuit oscillate or resonate! This implies the two plates have something in common. By putting a known pure sample on one plate you can reliably conclude the other sample contains it if the circuit resonates.

You may build a test plate box into a cardboard box (such as a facial tissue box) or a plastic box. Here are the instructions for the cardboard box model.

Test Plates Parts List

- Stiff paper.
- Aluminum foil.
- A facial tissue box is easiest. A plastic project box, about 7" x 4" x 1½," makes a more durable product, but requires a drill, and you should discard any metal lid it comes with.

- 3 bolts (tapered heads) about 1 inch long, 1/8 inch diameter and 6 washers and nuts to fit.
- toggle switch with OFF-ON positions.
- Alligator clip test leads.

Test Plates Assembly

Cut two 3-1/2 inch squares out of stiff paper such as a milk carton. Cover them with 4½ inch squares of aluminum foil, smoothed evenly and tucked snugly under the edges. You have just made yourself a set of open capacitors. Turn the box upside down and draw squares where you will mount them at the ends of the box. Don't actually mount them, to save wear and tear on them, until the rest of the box is complete.

Mount the ON OFF switch on the front of the box, underneath the right hand plate. Line it up so ON is downward and OFF is up. (An electronics shop can determine this for you at the time of purchase.) Label the box with ON and OFF signs.

Two bolts will be reserved for the plates. The third bolt is used as a terminal where the current from the oscillator circuit will arrive. Make a hole on the side of the box, near the left hand plate and mount the bolt so it sticks half way inside and halfway outside the box. It does not matter whether the head is inside or outside. Tighten it there with a nut on each side of the box. Label it TERMINAL. It merely means connecting place.

Mark the center of each square that you drew and each capacitor you built. Pierce first with a pin; follow with a pencil until a round hole is made at the center. Mount each plate with a bolt, fastening it below with a nut. Washers are optional.

The left side connection (terminal) gets attached to the left plate (bolt) with an alligator clip. Use another clip to attach the same left plate (bolt) to the ON OFF switch (there are two connections, use either one). Finally attach the ON OFF switch connection you didn't use to the right plate (bolt). Make sure the connections at the switch are not touching each other; you might tape them to guard against this.

All these connections should be checked carefully to make sure they are not touching others accidentally. But if you leave the box open so you can see any problems and use clear tape around connections to prevent accidental touching to the wrong connection, it should work OK.

Finally, trace your current. It comes in from the Syncrometer at the main terminal on the left. It is brought to the left plate. When the switch is ON it is simultaneously brought to the right plate. Notice that the plates are not connected to anything else. They are simply capacitors, letting current in and out momentarily and at a rate that is set by the frequency of the oscillator circuit, about 1,000 hertz. This frequency goes up as the resistance (of the circuit or your body) goes down.

The probe and handhold allow you to include yourself in the Syncrometer circuit. You grasp these when testing. This makes you part of the circuit.

The speaker lets you "listen" to the current. As resistance drops, current goes higher and frequency goes up. As frequencies go higher in the circuit, pitch goes higher. You will be comparing the sound of a standard "control" current with a test current.

Using The Syncrometer

Fill a saucer with cold filtered tap water. Fold a paper towel four times and place it in this dish. It should be entirely wet.

Cut paper strips about 1 inch wide from a piece of white, unfragranced, paper towel. Dampen a paper strip on the towel and wind it around the copper pipe handhold to completely cover it. The wetness improves conductivity and the paper towel keeps the metal off your skin.

- Start with the test plate switch at OFF.
- Turn the control knob (potentiometer) on, and to near maximum.
- Touch each plate with the probe, while holding the copper pipe with one hand. Only the left plate should give you a sound from the speaker. Turn the test plate switch ON. Now both plates should give you a sound when the probe touches them.
- Turn the test plate switch OFF again.
- Pick up the handhold, squeeze it free of excess water.
- Pick up the probe in the same hand, holding it like a pen, between thumb and forefinger.

Dampen your other hand by making a fist and dunking your knuckles into the wet paper towel in the saucer. You will be using the area on top of the first knuckle of the middle finger or forefinger to learn the technique. Become proficient with both. Immediately after dunking your knuckles dry them on a paper towel folded in quarters and placed beside the saucer. The degree of dampness of your skin affects the resistance in the circuit and is a very important variable that you must learn to keep constant. Make your probe as soon as your knuckles have been dried (within two seconds) since they begin to air dry further immediately.

With the handhold and probe both in one hand press the probe against the knuckle of the other hand, keeping the knuckles bent. Press lightly at first, then harder, taking one half second. Repeat a half second later, with the second half of the probe at the same location. There is an additive effect and you get two chances to listen to the current. All of this takes less than two seconds. Don't linger because your body will change and your next probe will be affected.

463

Subsequent probes are made in exactly the same way. As you develop skill, your probes will become identical. Plan to practice for one or two hours each day. It takes most people at least twelve hours of practice in order to be so consistent with their probes that they can hear the slight difference when the circuit is resonant.

For reference you may wish to use a piano. The starting sound when you touch down on the skin should be F, an octave and a half above middle C. The sound rises to a C as you press to the knuckle bone, then slips back to B, then back up to C-sharp as you complete the second half of your first probe. If you have a multitester you can connect it in series with the handhold or probe: the current should rise to about 50 microamps. If you have a frequency counter the frequency should reach 1000 Hz. You should arrive at C-sharp just before the probe becomes painful.

Two things change the sound of the probes even when your technique doesn't change.

1. The patch of skin chosen for probing will change its properties. The more it is used, the redder it gets and the higher the sound goes when you probe. Move to a nearby location, such as the edge of the patch, when the sound is too high to begin with, rather than adjusting the potentiometer.

2. Your body has cycles which make the sound go noticeably higher and lower. If you are getting strangely higher sounds for identical probes, stop and only probe every five minutes until you think the sound has gone down to standard. This could take five to twenty minutes. <u>Learn this higher sound</u> so you can avoid testing during this period.

You may also find times when it is impossible to reach the necessary sound without pressing so hard it causes pain. You may adjust the potentiometer if that helps.

464

All tests are momentary.

This means less than one second. It is tempting to hold the probe to your skin and just listen to the sound go up and down, but if you prolong the test you must let your body rest ten minutes, each time, before resuming probe practice!

For our purposes, it is not necessary to locate acupuncture points.

Resonance

The information you are seeking is whether or not there is *resonance*, or *feedback oscillation,* in the circuit. If there is the test is **YES** (positive). You hear resonance by comparing the second probe to the first. You can never hear resonance on the first probe, for reasons that are technical and beyond the scope of this book. You are not merely comparing pitch in the two probes. During resonance a higher pitch is reached faster; it seems to want to go infinitely high.

Remember that more electricity flows, and the pitch gets higher, as your skin reddens or your body changes cycle. These effects are not resonance.

Resonance is a small extra hum at the high end of the probe. As soon as you hear it, stop probing. Your body needs a short recovery time (10 to 20 seconds) after every resonant probe. The longer the resonant probe, the longer the recovery time to reach the standard level again.

Using musical notes, here is a NO (negative result): F-C-B-C# (first probe) F-C-B-C# (compare, it is the same sound). Here is a YES (positive) result: F-C-B-C# (first probe) F-D (stop quickly because you heard resonance). In between the first and second probe a test substance will be switched in as described in lessons below.

465

It is not possible to produce a resonant sound by pressing harder on the skin, although you can make the pitch go higher. To avoid confusion it is important to practice making probes of the same pressure. (Practice getting the F-C-B-C# tune.)

Making Pure Water for Testing Purposes

Since the water you purchase is likely to have solvents in it and since your tap water may be polluted with heavy metals and since your (or a store's) filtration system may be clogged, it is important to make your own pure water.

Purchase a "filter pitcher" made of hard, opaque plastic, not the clear or flexible variety (see *Sources*). Fill the pitcher with cold tap water, only, not reverse osmosis, distilled, or any other water, since solvents do not filter out as easily as heavy metals. The filter should be made of carbon only. To make test substances, use fresh water in the pitcher and pour.

If your water has lead, copper or cadmium from corroded plumbing, the filter will clog in five days of normal use. So use this pitcher sparingly, just for making test substances and for operating the Syncrometer.

Lesson One

Purpose: To identify the sound of resonance in the circuit.

Materials: Potentized (homeopathic) solutions. Prepare these as follows: find three medium-sized vitamin bottles, glass or plastic, with non-metal lids. Remove any shreds of paper sticking to the rim. Rinse well with cold tap water. Then rinse again with filtered water.

Pour filtered water into the first bottle to a depth of about ½ inch. Add about 50 little grains of table salt using the tip of a plastic knife. This is a "pinch." Replace the lid. Make sure the outside is clean. If not, rinse and dry. Now shake hard, holding it snugly in your hand. Count your shakes; shake 120 to 150 times. Use elbow motion so each shake covers about an eight inch distance. Shaken samples <u>are different</u> from unshaken ones, that's why this is so important. When done label the bottle on its side and lid: SALT #1. Wash your hands (without soap).

Next, pour about the same amount of filtered water into the second and third bottles. Open SALT #1 and pour a small amount, like 1/4 to 1/2 of a teaspoon (do not use a spoon) into the second and third bottles. Close all bottles. Now shake the second bottle the same as the first. Clean it and label it SALT #2. Do the same for the third bottle. Label it SALT #2 also and set aside for Lesson Four.

These two solutions have unique properties. SALT # 1 <u>always</u> resonates. Use #1 to train your ear. SALT #2 <u>shouldn't</u> resonate. Use #2 to hear when you (your body's internal resistance) have returned to the standard level.

1. Turn the Syncrometer ON.
2. Place the SALT #2 bottle on the right test plate.
3. Start with the plate switch OFF.
4. Make your first probe (F-C-B-C#).
5. Flip the plate switch ON, taking only one half second. Brace your hand when switching so it is a fast, smooth, operation.
6. Make the second probe (F-C-B-C#). Total probe time is 2½ seconds. Count it out, "a thousand and one (done with first probe) a thou. (done with switching) a thousand and one (done with second probe)."
7. The result should be a NO (negative). If the second probe sounds even a little higher you are <u>not at the standard level</u>. Wait a few more seconds and go back to step 3.
8. If the first result was NO, remove SALT #2 and put SALT #1 on. Put the test plate switch back to OFF and repeat the test. This time the circuit was resonating. Learn to hear the

difference between the last two probes so that a resonant probe can be terminated early (reducing rest time).

9. The skin must now be rested. When SALT #1 is placed in the circuit there is <u>always</u> resonance whether you hear it or not. Therefore, always take the time to rest the skin.

10. How can you be sure that the skin is rested enough? Any time you want to know whether you have returned to the standard level, you may simply test yourself to SALT #2 (just do steps 3 through 6). While you are learning, let your piano also help you to learn the standard level (starts exactly at F). If you do not rest and you resonate the circuit before returning to the standard level, the results will become aberrant and useless. The briefer you keep the resonant probe, the faster you return to the standard level. Don't exceed one half second when probing SALT #1. Hopefully you will soon hear resonance within that time.

This lesson teaches you to first listen to the empty plate, then to SALT #2, to check for standard state. Then to compare the empty plate to SALT #1 to check for resonance. In later lessons we assume you checked for your standard level or are quite sure of it.

Practice hearing resonance in your circuit every day.

White Blood Cells

Checking for resonance between your white blood cells and a toxin is the single most important test you can make.

Your white blood cells are your immune system's first line of defense. In addition to making antibodies, interferon, interleukins, and other attack chemicals, they also "eat" foreign substances in your body and eliminate them. By simply checking your white blood cells for toxins or intruders you save having to check every other tissue in your body. Because no matter where the foreign substance is, chances are some white blood cells are working to remove it.

It took me two years to find this ideal indicator, but it is not perfect. **Tapeworms are a notable exception.** They can be encysted in a particular tissue which will test positive, while the white blood cells continue to test negative. Also, when bacteria and viruses are in their latent form, they do not show up in the white blood cells. Fortunately, in their active form they show up quite nicely. **Freon** is an example of a toxin that is seldom found in the white blood cells; but typically, the white blood cells are excellent indicators of toxins.

Making a White Blood Cell Specimen

Obtain an empty vitamin bottle with a flat plastic lid and a roll of clear tape. The white blood cells are not going into the bottle, they are going on the bottle. The bottle simply makes them easy to handle. Rinse and dry the bottle. Make a second specimen on a clean glass slide if available. Squeeze an oil gland on your face or body to obtain a ribbon of whitish matter (not mixed with blood). Pick this up with the back of your thumb nail. Spread it in a single, small streak across the lid of the bottle or the center of the glass slide. Stick a strip of clear tape over the streak on the bottle cap so that the ends hang over the edge and you can easily see where the specimen was put (see photo). Wipe the lid beside the tape to make sure all white blood cells are covered. For the slide, apply a drop of balsam and a cover slip (see *Sources*). Both types of preparation will give you identical results. The bottle type of white blood cell specimen is used by standing it on its lid (upside down) so that the specimen is next to the plate. The lid is used because it is flat, whereas the bottom of most bottles is not.

Lesson Two

Purpose: To add a white blood cell specimen to the circuit and compare sound.
Method:
1. Turn the Syncrometer ON.
2. Start with test plate switch OFF.
3. Place the white blood cell specimen on the left plate. Place some junk food in a plastic baggy on the right plate.
4. Eat some of the junk food.
5. After ½ minute listen to the current. Flip the plate switch ON and listen again.
6. If the circuit is now resonating, the junk food is already in your white blood cells. It is toxic.

Take vitamin C and a B-50 complex to clear it rapidly; it may have had propyl alcohol or benzene in it. Test every 5 minutes afterward to see how long it takes to clear out.

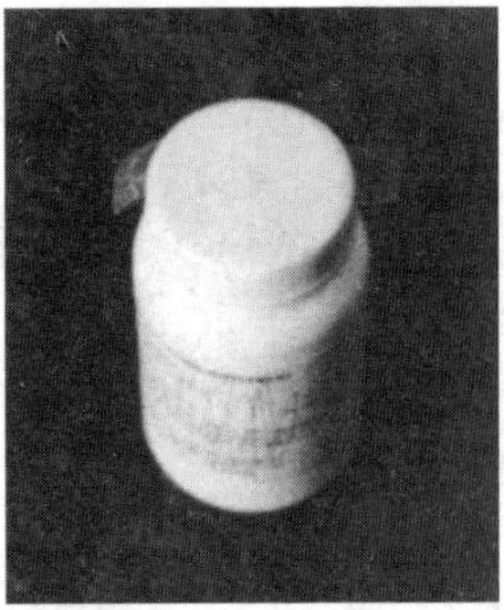

Fig. 81 Bottle with white blood cells taped to top.

Lesson Three

Purpose: To determine the purity of the filtered water you are making.

Method: Pour a few tsp. of filtered water into a bottle or plastic bag. Place your white blood cell specimen on one plate and the water sample on the other. Listen to your circuit. Taste your filtered water. After ½ minute, listen to your circuit again, just as in Lesson Two. If it appears in your white blood cells at any time you can conclude the water is not pure. You must have pure water available to you before continuing.

Lesson Four

Purpose: To determine your percent accuracy in listening for resonance.

Materials: The SALT #1 and SALT #2 solutions you made for Lesson One.

Method: Move the SALT #1 and SALT #2 labels to the bottom of the bottles so you can not tell which bottle is which.

1. Turn the Syncrometer ON.
2. Start with the test switch OFF.
3. Mix the bottles up, select one at random, and place it on the right plate.
4. Listen to the current.
5. Flip the plate switch ON and make your second probe.
6. Resonance indicates a SALT #1, no resonance indicates SALT #2. Check the bottom. Remember to rest after the SALT #1, whether or not you heard resonance.
7. Repeat steps 3 through 5 a number of times. Work toward getting three out of three correct. Practice every day.

Trouble shooting:

a) If you repeat this experiment and you keep getting the same bottles "wrong", start over. You may have accidentally contaminated or mislabeled the outside of the bottle, or switched bottle caps.

b) If you get different bottles wrong each time, the plates may be contaminated. Wash the outside of the bottles and rinse with filtered water and dry. Wipe the plates very gently too, with filtered water and dry. Or replace the plates.

c) If all the bottles read the same, your filtered water is polluted. Change the filter.

Preparing Test Substances

It is possible to prepare dry substances for testing such as a piece of lead or grains of pesticide. They can simply be put in a plastic bag and placed on the test plate. However, I prefer to place a small amount (the size of a pea) of the substance into a ½ ounce bottle of filtered water. There will be many chemical reactions between the substance and the water to produce a number of test substances all contained in one bottle. This simulates the situation in the body.

Within the body, where salt and water are abundant, similar reactions may occur between elements and water. For example, a strip of pure (99.9% pure) copper placed in filtered water might yield copper hydroxide, cuprous oxide, cupric oxide, copper dioxide, and so forth. These may be similar to some of the reaction products one might expect in the body, coming from a copper IUD, copper bracelet or the copper from metal tooth fillings. Since the electronic properties of elemental copper are not the same as for copper compounds, we would miss many test results if we used only dry elemental copper as a test substance.

Impure Test Substances

It is not necessary to have pure test substances. For instance, a tire balancer made of lead can be easily obtained at an auto service station. Leaded gasoline and lead fishing weights also make good test substances for lead. There is a disadvantage, though, to using impure test substances. You are including the extra impurities in your test. If your lead object also has tin in it, you are also testing for tin. Usually, you can infer the truth by some careful maneuvering. If you have searched your kidneys for leaded gasoline, fishing weights and tire balancers and all 3 are resonant with your kidneys, you may infer that you have lead in your kidneys, since the common element in all 3 items is lead. (You will learn how to specify a tissue, such as your kidneys, later.)

Using pure chemicals gives you certainty in your results. You can purchase pure chemicals from chemical supply companies (see *Sources*). Your pharmacy, a child's chemistry set, a paint store, or biological supply company can also supply some.

> The biggest repository of all toxic substances is the grocery store and your own home.

You can make test substances out of your hand soap, water softener salt, and laundry detergent by putting a small amount (1/16 tsp.) in a ½ ounce glass bottle and adding about 2 tsp. filtered water. (Or for quick testing just put them dry or wet in a sealed plastic baggy.) Always use a plastic spoon.

Here are some suggestions for finding sources of toxic products to make your own toxic element test. If the product is a solid, place a small amount in a plastic bag and add a tablespoon of filtered water to get a temporary test product. For permanent use put it in a small amber glass bottle. If the product is a liquid, pour a few drops into a glass bottle and add about 2 tsp. filtered water. Keep all toxic substances in glass bottles for your own safety. Small amber glass dropper bottles can be purchased by the dozen at drug stores (also see *Sources*). Seal your test bottles with tape for safety and to prevent evaporation.

Aflatoxin: scrape the mold off an orange or piece of bread; wash hands afterward.
Acetone: paint supply store or pharmacy.
Arsenic: 1/16 tsp. of arsenate pesticide from a garden shop. A snippet of flypaper.
Aluminum: a piece of aluminum foil (not tin foil) or an aluminum measuring spoon.

Aluminum silicate: a bit of salt that has this free running agent in it.

Asbestos: a small piece of asbestos sheeting, an old furnace gasket, 1/4 inch of a clothes dryer belt that does not say "Made in USA", or a crumb of building material being removed due to its asbestos content (ask a contractor).

Barium: save a few drops from the beverage given clients scheduled for an X-ray. Lipstick that has barium listed in the ingredients.

Benzene: an <u>old</u> can of rubber cement (new supplies do not have it). A tsp. of asphalt crumbs from a driveway.

Beryllium: a piece of coal; a few drops of "coal oil" or lamp oil.

Bismuth: use a few drops of antacid with bismuth in it.

Bromine: bleached "brominated" flour.

Cadmium: scrape a bit off a galvanized nail, paint from a hobby store.

Cesium: scrape the surface of a clear plastic beverage bottle.

CFCs (freon): ask an electronics expert for a squirt from an old aerosol can that used freon as a cleaner. (Squirt into water, outdoors, put the water in a sample bottle.)

Chromate: scrape an old car bumper.

Cobalt: pick out the blue and green crumbs from detergent. A sample of cobalt containing paint should also suffice.

Chlorine: a few drops of pure, old fashioned Clorox.™

Copper: ask your hardware clerk to cut a small fragment off a copper pipe of the purest variety or a ¼ inch of pure copper wire.

Ergot: a teaspoon of rye grains, or rye bread. Add grain alcohol to preserve.

Ether: automotive supply store (engine starting fluid).

Ethyl alcohol (grain alcohol): the purest "drinking" alcohol available. Everclear™ in the United States, Protec™ (potable) in Mexico.

Fiberglass: snip a fragment from insulation.

Fluoride: ask a dentist for a small sample.

Formaldehyde: purchase 37% at a pharmacy. Use a few drops only for your sample.

Gasoline: gas station (leaded and unleaded).

Gold: ask a jeweler for a crumb of the purest gold available or use a wedding ring.

Kerosene: gas station.

Lead: wheel balancers from a gas station, weights used on fishing lines, lead solder from electronics shop.

Mercury: a mercury thermometer (there is no need to break it), piece of amalgam tooth filling.

Methanol: paint supply store (wood alcohol).

Nickel: a nickel plated paper clip, a washed coin.

Patulin (apple mold): cut a sliver of washed, bruised apple.

PCB: water from a quarry known to be polluted with it (a builder or electrical worker may know a source).

Platinum: ask a jeweler for a small specimen.

Propyl alcohol: rubbing alcohol from pharmacy (same as propanol or isopropanol). Use a few drops only, discard the rest. Do not save it.

PVC: glue that lists it in the ingredients (polyvinyl chloride).

Radon: leave a glass jar with an inch of filtered water in it standing open in a basement that tested positive to radon using a kit. After 3 days, close the jar. Pour about 2 tsp. of this water into your specimen bottle.

Silicon: a dab of silicon caulk.

Silver: ask a jeweler for a crumb of very pure silver. Silver solder can be found in electronics shops. Snip the edge of a very old silver coin.

Sorghum mold: 1/8 tsp. sorghum syrup.

Styrene: a chip of styrofoam.

Tantalum: purchase a tantalum drill bit from hardware store.

Tin: scrape a tin bucket at a farm supply. Tin solder. Ask a dentist for a piece of pure tin (used to make braces).

Titanium: purchase a titanium drill bit from a hardware store.

Toluene: a tube of glue that lists toluene as an ingredient.

Tungsten: the filament in a burned out light bulb.

Vanadium: hold a piece of dampened paper towel over a gas stove burner as it is turned on. Cut a bit of this paper into your specimen bottle and add 2 tsp. filtered water.

Xylene: paint store or pharmacy.

Zearalenone: combine leftover crumbs of three kinds of corn chips and three kinds of popcorn.

This list gets you off to a good start. Since few of these specimens are pure, there is a degree of logic that you must apply in most cases. If you are testing for barium in your breast, a positive result would mean that a barium-containing lipstick tests positive and a barium-free lipstick is negative.

A chemistry set for hobbyists is a wonderful addition to your collection of test specimens. Remember, however, the assumptions and errors in such a system. A test for silver using silver chloride might be negative. This does not mean there is no silver present in your body; it only means there is no silver chloride present in the tissue you tested.

You are bound to miss some toxins; don't let this discourage you. There is more than enough that you <u>can</u> find.

The most fruitful kind of testing is, probably, the use of household products themselves as test substances. The soaps, colognes, mouthwash, toothpaste, shampoo, cosmetics, breads, dairy products, juices and cereals can all be made into test specimens. Put about 1/8 tsp. of the product in a small glass bottle, add 2 tsp. filtered water and ¼ tsp. grain alcohol to preserve it. For temporary purposes use a plastic baggy and water only. If you test positive to your household products in your white blood cells you shouldn't use them, even if you can not identify the exact toxin.

For a list of toxins and solvents I use, see page 571. To order pure substances see *Sources* for "chemicals for testing."

Making Organ Specimens

To test for toxic elements or parasites in a particular organ such as the liver or skin, you will need either a fresh or frozen sample of the organ or a prepared microscope slide of this organ. Meat purchased from a grocery store, fresh or frozen, provides you with a variety of organ specimens. Chicken, turkey, beef or pork organs all give the same results. You may purchase chicken gizzards for a sample of stomach, beef liver for liver, pork brains for brain, beef steak for muscle, throat sweet breads for thymus, tripe for stomach lining. Other organs may be ordered from a meat packing plant.

Trim the marrow out of a bone slice to get bone marrow. Scrub the bone slice with hot water to free it of marrow to get a bone specimen. Choose a single piece of meat sample, rinse it and place it in a plastic bag. You may freeze it. To make a durable unfrozen sample, cut a small piece, the size of a pea, and place it in an amber glass bottle (½ oz.). Cover with two tsp. filtered water and ¼ tsp. of grain alcohol (pure vodka will do) to preserve it. These need not be refrigerated but if decay starts, make a fresh specimen.

Pork brains from the grocery store may be dissected to give you the different parts of the brain. Chicken livers often have an attached gallbladder or piece of bile duct, giving you that extra organ. Grocery store "lites" provides you with lung tissue. For kidney, snip a piece off pork or beef kidney. Beef liver may supply you with a blood sample, too. Always wash hands and rinse with grain alcohol after handling raw meat.

I use ½ oz amber glass bottles with bakelite caps (see *Sources*) to hold specimens. However, plastic bags or other containers would suffice. After closing, each bottle is sealed with a Parafilm™ strip to avoid accidental loosening of the cap. You may use masking tape.

To make a specimen of skin, use hangnail bits and skin peeled from a callous, <u>not a wart</u>. A few shreds will do. Remember, they must be very close to the test plate when in use; add 2 tsp. filtered water and ¼ tsp. grain alcohol.

Making a Complete Set of Tissue Samples

My original complete set was made from a frozen fish. As it thawed, different organs were cut away and small pieces placed in bottles for preserving in filtered water and grain alcohol. In this way, organs not available from the grocery store could be obtained. The piece of intestine closest to the anus corresponds to our colon, the part closest to the stomach corresponds to our duodenum. The 2 layers of the stomach and different layers of the eye, the optic nerve and spinal cord were obtained this way.

Another complete set of tissue samples were obtained from a freshly killed steer at a slaughter house. In this way the 4 chambers of the heart were obtained, the lung, trachea, aorta, vein, pancreas, and so forth.

Purchasing a Complete Set of Tissue Samples

Slides of tissues, unstained or stained in a variety of ways for microscope study give identical results to the preparations made by yourself in the ways already described. This fact opens the entire catalog of tissue types for your further study. See *Sources* for places that supply them.

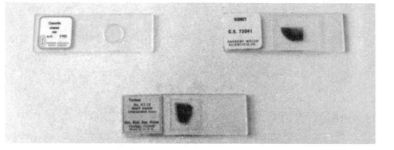

Fig. 82 Some purchased parasite and tissue slides.

You now have a set of organ samples, either fresh, frozen, preserved or on slides. You also have a set of test substances, whether chemical compounds, or elements, or products. Your goal is to search in your own organs and body tissues for the substances that may be robbing you of health.

Keeping yourself healthy will soon be an easy, daily routine.

Body Fluid Specimens

Each of these fluids should be prepared by putting about ¼ tsp. in a ½ oz amber glass bottle. Add about 2 tsp. filtered water and ¼ tsp. grain alcohol for preservation. Undiluted specimens do not work for reasons that are technical and beyond the scope of this book. It is important *not* to shake the specimen, but to mix gently.

Urine. It is desired to have a pure, uninfected urine sample as a tissue specimen. Since this cannot be proved with certainty, obtain several urine samples from different persons whom you believe to be healthy and make several test specimens in order to compare results. Label your specimens Urine A (child), Urine B (woman), Urine C (mine), and so forth.

Semen. A sample from a condom is adequate. Aged specimens (sent by mail, unpreserved and unrefrigerated) work well also. Use one to ten drops or scrape a small amount with a plastic knife.

Blood. One to ten drops of blood should be used. Clotted or chemically treated blood is satisfactory. A blood smear on a slide is very convenient.

Milk. Cow's milk is too polluted with parasites to be useful. Electronically, a dead specimen is equivalent to a live specimen, so that pasteurization of the milk does not help. A human milk specimen is preferred.

Saliva. Use your own, if you have deparasitized yourself and test negative to various fluke stages. Otherwise find a well friend or child.

Specifying a tissue is the most powerful investigative technique in your arsenal. Any of your tissue samples can be tested for any of your toxic substances.

You Can Now Test **Three** Different Ways!

When you test with a substance on one plate and nothing on the other, you are searching your entire body for that substance. Such a test is not very sensitive.

By putting a tissue sample on the other plate you are testing for the substance specifically in that tissue, and this is much more sensitive. The tissue need not be the white blood cells. To find mercury in your kidneys you would use a mercury sample on one plate, and a kidney sample on the other. The technique is the same as when you use white blood cells.

If you put a substance on each plate, a resonating circuit means the two samples have something in common. For example, if you have mercury on one plate and some dental floss on the other, a positive result indicates mercury in the floss.

Lesson Five

Purpose: To watch substances travel through your body.

Materials: Prepare a pint of brown sugar solution (white sugar has propyl alcohol pollution) using filtered water. Use about 1 tsp. brown sugar, 1/8 tsp. vitamin C (to detoxify sorghum mold), and a pint of filtered water. Do not shake it; gently mix. Make a sample bottle by pouring about ½ inch into a clean used vitamin bottle. Rinse and dry the outside of the sample bottle. Finally wash your hands with plain water.

Method:

1. Test your skin for the presence of brown sugar, using the newly made sample bottle and your skin specimen. It should not be there (resonate) yet.
2. Prepare a paper applicator by tearing the corner from a white unfragranced paper towel. Fold it to make a wick.
3. Dip the paper wick in the pint of sugar water and apply it to the skin of your inner arm where you can rub freely.

Rub it in vigorously for about 10 seconds (otherwise it takes minutes to absorb). Leave the shredded wick on the skin and tape it down with a piece of clear tape about 4 inches long (this increases the time you have to work). Quickly wash your fingers.

4. Place your skin tissue specimen on one plate and the sugar specimen bottle on the other plate.

5. Probe for resonance every 5 seconds. As soon as you hear resonance, implying that the skin has absorbed the sugar solution (which may take a full minute), replace the skin specimen with one of liver and listen for resonance again. There should be none, yet.

6. Alternate between the skin and liver. Soon the skin will be clear and the liver will resonate. Also check the pancreas and muscles to see how quickly sugar arrives there.

7. Check white blood cells and kidneys. It should <u>not</u> appear here (unless it is polluted with a toxin).

8. After five to ten minutes the sugar will be gone from all of these tissues and your experiment is ended. Wash your arm with plain water.

Notice that you have only a few minutes to get all your testing done after the skin has absorbed the test substances.

Lesson Six

Purpose: To verify the propyl alcohol and benzene lists.

Method: We will use the Syncrometer to test for a toxin in a product. Assemble the products named in the propyl alcohol list (page 335) and benzene list (page 382)...as many as you can find. Also make sample bottles of benzene and propyl alcohol.

1. Place the propyl alcohol test substance on one plate and your products, in turn, on the other.

2. Listen to the current with only one of the plates in the circuit. Then listen with both plates in (the test plate switch ON). This method can detect one part per quadrillion in concentration. It is not as sensitive as the skin test (Lesson Five).

3. Repeat, with the benzene test substance.

Even tiny amounts of solvents are toxic! They must not be consumed or be left in our environment.

I have found that too many unsuspected products test positive to <u>benzene</u>. This is such a global tragedy that people must protect themselves by using their own tests. Rather than assurances, regulatory agencies should provide the consumer with cheap and simple tests (dip sticks and papers so we need not lug our Syncrometers around). Even if some test should fail, not all tests would fail to find an important pollutant like benzene. It would come to public attention much faster than the present debacle has.

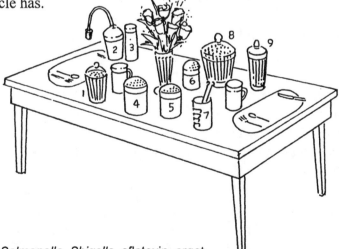

1) *Salmonella*, *Shigella*, aflatoxin, ergot, zearalenone, patulin test sticks; 2) ozonizer; 3) Lugol's; 4) vitamin C powder; 5) sodium/potassium salt; 6) fresh powdered herb spices; 7) food zapper; 8) benzene, propyl alcohol, wood alcohol test sticks; 9) heavy metals and lanthanides test sticks.

Fig. 83 Table of the future.

Lesson Seven

Purpose: To test for the presence of aluminum in your brain and your foods.

Materials: An aluminum measuring spoon, a tsp. of free flowing aluminized salt, a square inch of aluminum foil, a package of pork brain from the grocery store, kept frozen. (Other animal sources will do). Or a stained slide of cerebrum, cerebellum or other brain tissue.

Method:

1. Cut a piece of brain tissue (about 1 tsp.) and place in a plastic bag.
2. Place the aluminum samples in separate plastic bags. Add filtered water to each, about 1 tbs. Keep all surfaces and your hands meticulously clean (do not use soap).
3. Place the aluminum sample on one plate and the brain sample on the other plate.
4. Probe for resonance. If the circuit resonates <u>you</u> have aluminum in <u>your</u> brain.
5. If your aluminum specimen actually has cadmium or copper in it, you are <u>also</u> testing for these in your brain. Repeat the aluminum test with other aluminum objects. If they <u>all</u> resonate, you <u>very, very</u> <u>likely</u> have aluminum in your brain. If you can, test yourself to cadmium and copper, separately. If you don't have these in your brain, the aluminum test result is even more likely to be correct.
6. Of course, it would be desirable to have absolute certainty about this. To achieve this, purchase pure aluminum or an Atomic Absorption Standard. These are available from chemical supply companies.

If you do have aluminum in your brain, where is it coming from?

7. Leave your purest aluminum test substance on one plate, and replace the brain sample with these items, testing them one at a time. Remember to rest after each positive result.
   - a teaspoon of cottage cheese or yogurt taken from the top of a container of a foil-capped variety
   - a piece of cream cheese or butter that was wrapped in foil
   - a chip of bar soap or a bit of hand lotion
   - a piece of cake or rolls baked in an aluminum pan
   - a piece of turkey skin or hot dish that was covered with aluminum foil
   - anything baked with baking powder
   - a carbonated beverage from an aluminum can

Alternative Lesson:

To test for dental metal in your tissues. Use a piece of amalgam from an old tooth filling. This tests for the rest of the alloys in amalgam fillings as well as mercury. If you can't get a piece of mercury amalgam, use a mercury thermometer (don't break it, just put the bulb on the plate). Choose tissues like kidney, nerves, brain, liver, in addition to white blood cells.

I have never dissected human tissues and subjected them to confirmatory laboratory tests. It seems reasonable that because skin and tongue are directly provable, that other tissues work similarly.

Testing the Air

Fine particles and gas molecules that are in the air stick to the dust and eventually fall down onto the table, kitchen counter, and other places. Every night a film of dust accumulates, even though you can't see it. To test for air pollutants, gather some dust. Wipe the kitchen table and counter with a dampened piece of paper towel, two inches by two inches square. Place it in a resealable baggie. Do not get old dust, like from the top of the refrigerator or back shelves, because it does not represent the current air quality.

Testing Someone Else

Seat the person comfortably with their hand resting near you. Choose the first knuckle from the middle or first finger just like you do for yourself. Since you are touching this person, you are putting yourself in the circuit with the subject.

To exclude yourself, you need to add inductance to yourself. A coil of about 10 microhenrys, worn next to the skin, works well and is easily made. Obtain insulated wire and wrap 24 turns around a ball point pen (or something about that size), closely spaced. Cut the ends and tape them down securely. Keep it in a plastic bag, even when in your pocket. A commercial inductance of 4.7 microhenrys, worn touching your skin also works well. It can be worn on a string necklace. (Remember to remove the necklace when testing yourself.) The inductance acts as an RF (radio frequency) choke, limiting the alternating current that can flow through you while testing another person.

Test your inductor in this way. Repeat Lesson One with the coil next to your body. No resonance, even to SALT #1, should occur. If it does, make the coil bigger. Remove the inductor when you are not testing others.

Lesson Eight

Purpose: To detect aluminum in the brain of another person.

Materials: same as previous lesson, you wear the inductor.

Method:

1. Place the aluminum sample on one plate and the brain sample on the other plate.
2. Give the other person the handhold. You use the probe. Hold their finger steady in yours.
3. Probe the other person for resonance. The first probe is with only one plate in the circuit. The second is with both plates in the circuit. Resonance implies there is aluminum in the person's brain.

Saliva Testing

This may become your most useful test. The saliva has in it a bit of almost everything toxic that is in you. But it is not the first tissue to carry the HIV virus or a bit of a tapeworm stage. Nevertheless, *Salmonella* in your liver, mercury in your kidneys, aluminum in the brain all show up in the saliva, too. And saliva can be sent by mail or stored in the refrigerator. It should be frozen for long storage to prevent mold invasion. Or it may have grain alcohol added to preserve it. This test is not as sensitive as having the person present in the circuit, though.

To make a saliva specimen, place a two inch square piece of white, unfragranced paper towel (tear, don't cut) in a lightweight resealable baggy. Hold the open baggy near your mouth. Don't touch the paper towel with your fingers. Drool or spit onto the paper towel until half of it is damp. Zip it shut. Before testing, add enough filtered water to dampen the whole piece of paper.

Lesson Nine

Purpose: To search for shingles or *Herpes*.

Materials: A saliva specimen from the person being tested; they may be thousands of miles away. Also a specimen of the virus. This can be obtained from someone else's lesions—one droplet is enough, picked up on a bit of paper towel. The whole thing, towel and all, can be pushed into a glass bottle for preserving. Water and alcohol should be added. It can also be put on a slide, *Herpes, homemade.* A homeopathic preparation of the virus does not give accurate results for this kind of testing, due to the additional frequency imposed on it by potentizing. (However, homeopathic preparations can be used if the potency matches the tissue frequency where it resides. Hopefully, some way of using homeopathic sources will soon be found.)

Method: Place the saliva specimen in its unopened baggy on one plate. You may wish to open it briefly, though, to add enough filtered water to wet all the paper and add ¼ tsp. grain alcohol to sterilize or preserve it.

Place the virus specimen on the other plate and test as usual (like Lesson Six). A positive result means the person has active *Herpes.*

The main disadvantage of saliva testing is that you do not know which tissue has the pathogen or the toxin. You can only conclude that it is present. Usually this is enough information to carry out a corrective program.

Surrogate Testing

Although saliva testing is so easy, it is also possible to use an adult as a surrogate when testing a baby or pet. The pet or baby is held on the lap of the surrogate. A large pet may sit in front of the person. The handhold is held by the surrogate and pressed firmly against the body of the baby or pet. It can be laid flat against the arm, body or leg of a baby and held in place firmly by the whole hand of the adult. The paper covering should be wet. For a pet, the end is held firmly pressed against the skin, such as between the front legs or on the belly. The other hand of the adult is used for testing in the usual way. The adult <u>must</u> wear an inductor for surrogate testing as well as you, the tester.

An ill or bedridden person may be tested without inconvenience or stress. He or she rests their whole hand on the skin of your leg, just above the knee. A wet piece of paper towel, about 4 inches by 4 inches is placed on your leg, to make better contact. You <u>must</u> use an inductor for yourself with this method. You may now proceed to probe on <u>your</u> hand instead of the ill person's.

Lesson Ten

Purpose: To test for cancer.

Materials: Ortho-phospho-tyrosine. Here are four ways to obtain some:

1. Order a pure sample from a chemical company (see *Sources*). Place a few milligrams (it need not be weighed) in a small glass bottle, add 2 tsp. filtered water and ¼ tsp. grain alcohol.

2. All persons with cancer have ortho-phospho-tyrosine in their urine as well as in the cancerous tissue. It is seldom found in other body fluids. Obtain a urine specimen from a friend who has active cancer. Freeze it if you can't prepare it immediately. Keep such specimens well marked in an additional sealed plastic bag. Persons who have recently been treated clinically for cancer are much less likely to have ortho-phospho-tyrosine in the urine.

   Urine cannot be considered a chemical in the same way as a sugar or salt solution. Urine is a <u>tissue</u> and has its own resonant frequency as do our other tissues. If combined with another tissue on the test plates, it will <u>not</u> resonate as if a solution of pure ortho-phospho-tyrosine were used. To use urine as an ortho-phospho-tyrosine specimen, you must:

a) Pour a few drops of urine into your specimen bottle
b) Add about 2 tsp. of filtered water
c) Add a few drops of grain alcohol
Gently mix, <u>do not shake</u>. Rinse and dry the outside of the bottle. Label it "urine/cancer".

3. Cancer victims also have other growth factors being produced in their bodies. These are the same as can be found in mother's milk—for example, epidermal growth factor and insulin-like growth factor. Obtain a sample of mother's milk and use it to make another test substance for cancer. A few drops is enough.

4. There is still another way to prepare an ortho-phospho-tyrosine test sample. Common snails from a fish tank or outdoor snails are the natural hosts for *Fasciolopsis buskii* (human intestinal fluke) stages. The stages will produce ortho-phospho-tyrosine when the snails are fed fish food polluted with propyl alcohol. Over half the fish food cans I purchased had propyl alcohol pollution. Buy several brands of fish food. Test them for propyl alcohol and benzene. Obtain some snails, put them in a tank, feed them propyl alcohol polluted fish food. (Feed a separate group of snails benzene polluted fish food to obtain samples of HIV.) After two days put each snail in a zipped plastic bag, and test them individually against someone diagnosed with cancer or their saliva. The snails that the person tests positive to have ortho-phospho-tyrosine. Put these snails in the freezer to kill them humanely, then crush them and place in a specimen bottle with 50% grain alcohol to preserve. The bottles can be kept sealed and at room temperature.

Similarly, your benzene snails can be tested against someone known to be HIV positive. Any snails that test positive can be used to prepare an HIV test specimen in the same way. <u>The fish food must be tested for both benzene</u>

490

and propyl alcohol pollution, and separated appropriately, or you run the risk of making specimens that have both ortho-phospho-tyrosine and HIV.

Method:
1. Test for cancer by placing the test sample you just made (any of the four) on one plate and a white blood cell sample on the other plate.
2. If you resonate with both samples in the circuit you have cancer. Immediately, search for your cancer in your breast, prostate, skin, lungs, colon, and so forth.
3. To be more certain, test yourself to the other kinds of test samples. You should not resonate.

As you know by now, you can confirm the cancer by testing yourself to propyl alcohol and the human intestinal fluke in the liver. You should eliminate propyl alcohol from use, and zap all parasites. Keep testing yourself for cancer until it is gone. It should take less than one hour. Also continue to test yourself for propyl alcohol and the intestinal fluke in the white blood cells; make sure they are gone. Also test yourself for aflatoxin and freon.

Lesson Eleven

Purpose: To test for HIV.

Materials: Purchase a few milligrams of Protein 24 antigen (a piece of the HIV virus core) or the complete HIV virus on a slide (see *Sources*). You may use the vial unopened if only one test specimen is needed. To make more specimens, use about 1 milligram per ½ ounce bottle. Add 2 tsp. filtered water and ¼ tsp. grain alcohol. Or prepare an HIV specimen from snails as described in the previous Lesson.

Method: Search in the thymus (throat sweet breads), vagina and penis for the virus because that is where it will reside almost exclusively for the first year or two. If you don't have those tissue specimens, you could search in urine, blood, saliva, or white blood cells, but only a positive result can be trusted. Also search for the human intestinal fluke and benzene in the thymus. Of course, a positive test in these tissues is very significant. If you are positive, zap parasites immediately. You should test negative in less than an hour. Remove benzene polluted items from your lifestyle. Also test yourself to several varieties of popcorn, brown rice, and corn chips as an indication of zearalenone, which must be eliminated in order to get well. Follow up on yourself every few days to be sure your new found health is continuing. Test yourself for freon.

Lesson Twelve

Purpose: To test for diseases of all kinds.

Materials: Use slides and cultures of disease organisms. Homemade preparations of strep throat, acute mononucleosis, thrush (*Candida*), chicken pox, *Herpes* 1 and 2, eczema, shingles, warts, measles, yeast, fungus, rashes, colds, sore throats, sinus problems, tobacco virus, and so forth can all be made by swabbing or scraping the affected part. A plastic spoon or bit of paper towel works well. Put a small bit on a slide. Add a drop of balsam and a cover slip. Or put the towel in a bottle, add water and alcohol as described previously. Microscope slides can greatly expand your test set (see *Sources*).

Method: Test yourself for a variety of diseases, using your white blood cell specimen first. Then search in organs like the liver, pancreas, spleen. Notice how many of these common illnesses don't "go away" at all. They are alive and well in some organ. They are merely not making you sick!

Lesson Thirteen

To test for AIDS.

Materials: Benzene sample, slides of tissue samples like thymus, liver, pancreas, penis, and vagina. Also a collection of disease specimens such as the ones used in the previous lesson.

Method: Search in the thymus for benzene. If it is positive throughout the day, <u>you are at risk</u> for developing AIDS, although you may not be ill. Search other tissues for benzene. The more tissues with benzene in them the more serious the situation. Immediately search all your body products and foods for benzene.

Stay off benzene polluted items forever.

Tally up the diseases you tested positive for in Lesson Twelve. Test at least ten. If you had more than half positive you already have AIDS. (50% is my standard, you may set your own; an ideal standard for defining a healthy person should be 0% positive.)

Lesson Fourteen

Purpose: To test for aflatoxin.

Materials: Do not try to purchase a pure sample of aflatoxin; it is one of the most potent carcinogens known. Having it on hand would constitute unnecessary hazard, even though the bottle would never need to be opened. Simply make specimens of beer, moldy bread, apple cider vinegar, and any kind of peanuts using a very small amount and adding filtered water and grain alcohol as usual.

Method: Test yourself for these. If you have all of them in your white blood cells and the liver then you very, very probably have aflatoxin built up. Next, test your daily foods for their presence in your white blood cells. Those that test positive must be further tested for aflatoxin. Notice the effect of vitamin C on aflatoxin in your liver. Find a time when your liver is positive to aflatoxin (eat a few roasted peanuts from a health food store and wait ten minutes). Take 1 gram vitamin C in a glass of water. Check yourself for aflatoxin every five minutes. Does it clear? If not, take 5 or 10 grams vitamin C. How long does it take?

Lesson Fifteen

Purpose: To test for parasites.

Method: If you test positive to your pet's saliva, you have something in common—a parasite, no doubt. You must search your muscles and liver for these, not saliva or white blood cells, because they are seldom seen in these. Zap yourself for parasites until you no longer test positive to your pets' saliva.

Tapeworms and tapeworm stages can not (and <u>should not</u>) be killed with a regular frequency generator. Each segment, and probably each scolex in a cysticercus has its own frequency and might disperse if your generator misses it. Only <u>zapping</u> kills all and is safe for tapeworms.

Be sure to treat your pet on a daily basis with the pet parasite program.

Lesson Sixteen

Purpose: To test for fluke disease.

A small number of intestinal flukes resident in the intestine may not give you any noticeable symptoms. Similarly, sheep liver flukes resident in the liver and pancreatic flukes in the pancreas may not cause noticeable symptoms. Their eggs are shed through the organ ducts to the intestine and out with the bowel movement. They hatch and go through various stages of development outdoors and in other animals. But if you become the total host so that various stages are developing in your organs, you have what I term *fluke disease*. I have found that cancer, HIV, diabetes, endometriosis, Hodgkin's disease, Alzheimer's disease, lupus, MS and "universal allergy syndrome" are examples of fluke disease.

You can test for fluke disease in two ways: electronically and by microscope observation.

Materials: Cultures or slides of flukes and fluke stages from a biological supply company (see *Sources*) including eggs, miracidia, redia, cercaria, metacercaria. Body fluid specimens to help you locate them for observation under a microscope.

Method: Test for fluke stages in your white blood cells first. If you have any fluke stages in your white blood cells you may wish to see them with your own eyes. To do this, you must first locate them. Place your body fluid samples on one plate, your parasite stages on the other plate, and test for as many as you were able to procure, besides adults. After finding a stage electronically, you stand a better chance of finding it physically with a microscope.

Lesson Seventeen

Purpose: To see how sensitive your measurements can be. (How much of a substance must be present for you to get a positive result?)

Materials: filtered water, salt, glass cup measure, 13 new glass bottles that hold at least ¼ cup, 14 new plastic teaspoons, your skin tissue sample, paper towel.

Method: Some of the best measurement systems available today are immunological (such as an ELISA assay) and can detect as little as 100 fg/ml (femtograms per milliliter). A milliliter is about as big as a pea, and a femtogram is $1/1,000,000,000,000,000$th (10^{-15}) of a gram!

1. Rinse the glass cup measure with filtered water and put one half teaspoon of table salt in it. Fill to one cup, stirring with a plastic spoon. What concentration is this? A teaspoon is about 5 grams, a cup is about 230 ml (milliliters), therefore the starting concentration is about 2½ (2.5) gm per 230 ml, or .01 gm/ml (we will discuss the amount of error later).

2. Label one clean plastic spoon "water" and use it to put nine spoonfuls of filtered water in a clean glass bottle. Use another plastic spoon to transfer one spoonful of the .01 gm/ml salt solution in the cup measure to the glass bottle, stir, then discard the spoon. The glass bottle now has a 1 in 10 dilution, and its concentration is one tenth the original, or .001 gm/ml.

3. Use the "water" spoon to put nine spoonfuls of filtered water in bottle #2. Use a new spoon to transfer a spoonful of salt solution from bottle #1 to bottle #2 and stir briefly (never shake). Label bottle #2 ".0001 gm/ml".

4. Repeat with remaining bottles. Bottle #13 would therefore be labeled ".000000000000001 gm/ml." This is 10^{-15} gm/ml, or 1 femtogram/ml.

5. Do the skin test with water from bottle #13 as in Lesson Five. If you can detect this, you are one hundred times as sensitive as an ELISA assay (and you should make a bottle #14 and continue if you are curious how good your sensitivity can get). If you can not, try to detect water from bottle #12 (ten times as sensitive as ELISA). Continue until you reach a bottle you can detect.

Calculate the error for your experiment by assuming you could be off by as much as 10% when measuring the salt and water adding up to 20% error in each of the 13 dilutions. This is a total error in bottle #13 of 280%, or at most a factor of 3. So bottle #13 could be anywhere from 0.33 to 3 femtogram/ml. If you can detect water from bottle #13, you are <u>definitely</u> more sensitive then an ELISA, in spite of your crude utensils and inexpensive equipment! Note that the starting error of using 2.5 gm instead of 2.3 gm only adds another 10% error.

If you want to calculate how many salt <u>molecules</u> you can detect, select the concentration at the limit of your detection, and put 2 drops on a square inch of paper towel and rub into your skin. Assume one drop can be absorbed. If you can detect water from bottle #13, you have detected 510,000 molecules (10^{-15} fg/ml divided by 58.5 gm/M multiplied by 6.02×10^{23} molecules/M divided by 20 drops/ml). Water in bottle #12 would therefore have 10 times as many molecules in one drop, and so forth. Even if your error is as much as a factor of 2 (100%), you can still get a good idea of what you can measure.

Atomic absorption standards start at exact concentrations; it is easy to make a more exact dilution series with them. When testing for iridium chloride by this skin test method, I was able to detect 3025 molecules!

Troubleshooting:

Always extend your set until you get a negative result (this should happen by at least bottle #18). If you always "detect" salt, then you <u>shook</u> the bottle!

Never try to reuse a bottle if you spill when pouring into it. Get another new bottle.

Sensitivity of Pollutant-In-Product Testing

Get some slides of *Salmonellas* and *Shigellas* and find some milk that tests positive to at least one. Make a dilution series of the milk up to bottle #14, being careful not to shake the bottles. Start with 2 drops of milk in bottle #1. Use an eye dropper to deliver 2 drops to subsequent bottles. Begin testing at bottle #14, using the slide that tested positive. You will learn to search by frequency later. My sensitivity was routinely around bottle #12, for a variety of pathogens. It was the same for toxic elements starting with standard solutions, about 1000 µg/ml, showing this method is less sensitive than skin testing.

Microscopy Lesson

Purpose: To *observe* fluke stages in saliva and urine with a microscope.

Materials:

a. A low power microscope. High power is not needed. A total of 100x magnification is satisfactory for the four common flukes, *Fasciolopsis, sheep liver fluke, human liver fluke* and *pancreatic fluke.*

b. Glass slides and coverslips.

c. A disposable eye dropper.

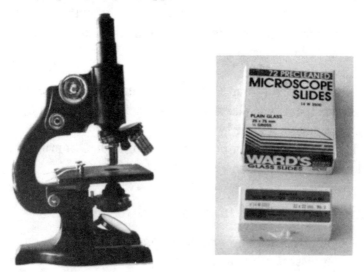

Fig. 84 Microscope, slides and coverslips.

d. For sanitation purposes (wiping table tops, slides, microscope and your hands) a 50% to 70% alcohol solution (not rubbing alcohol!) is best. Dilute 95% grain alcohol 7 parts alcohol plus 3 parts water. Vodka or 76% grain alcohol can be used undiluted.

e. Formaldehyde, 20%. Formaldehyde 37% is commonly available at pharmacies. Dilute this with equal parts of filtered water to get 18½%, which is close enough to 20%, for the purpose of "fixing" (killing) the specimens. Store in a glass bottle in the garage, away from sunlight. Label. Specimens that are fixed properly do not lose their life-like appearance.

f. Iodine solution. This is only useful for the urine specimens. Lugol's iodine and tincture of iodine are both useful. Ask a pharmacist to prepare *Lugol's Iodine Solution* for you, as follows:
   - 44 grams (1½ oz) iodine crystals
   - 88 grams (3 oz) potassium iodide crystals

Dissolve both in 1 liter (quart) filtered water. This may take a day of frequent shaking.

Method for saliva:
1. Pour the 20% formaldehyde into a small amber bottle or other receptacle to a depth of about 1/8 inch. Keep tightly closed.
2. The person to be tested is asked to salivate into the bottle so the organisms are immediately "fixed" without undergoing cooling first. The total volume should be about double the original amount of formaldehyde used. Make a mark on the container so the subject knows how much to produce. The resultant concentration of formaldehyde will be about 10%.
3. Shake the bottle a few times. Set it aside for 24 hours to settle (less if testing is urgent).

4. With a dropper, draw up some of the bottom settlings. Put one drop on a slide and apply a coverslip.

5. View under low power of microscope. Compare objects you observe with specimens obtained on slides from biological supply companies.

Note: Persons with HIV and moderate AIDS will show about one to ten parasite stages per slide. It requires several hours of searching. Persons with HIV and severe AIDS show 10 or more fluke stages per slide; this makes the task of finding them much easier. Persons with terminal untreated cancer have many more fluke stages than relatively well persons.

Method for urine:

1. Prepare bottles of formaldehyde fixative ahead of time. Put about ¼ to ½ inch of 20% formaldehyde in each. Keep tightly closed.

2. Add freshly voided[36] urine from cancer or HIV sufferers to the formaldehyde in approximately equal amounts, resulting in a 10% formaldehyde solution. Shake immediately. Let settle several hours. The sediment has a higher number of fluke stages. Cancer victims with cervical or prostate cancer will show higher numbers of stages in urine than other cancer types.

3. Staining the slide is optional. It helps to outline fluke stages slightly. Prepare Lugol's solution as described above.

   Slides may be stained in either of these two ways:
   - Put a drop of "fixed" urine on a slide. Add a drop of 50% Lugol's (dilute 1:1 with filtered water). Apply coverslip.

---

[36] Urine that has cooled even slightly below body temperature does not show *miracidia* and *redia* in their original shapes.

- Put a drop of "fixed" urine on a slide. Apply coverslip. Add 1 to 3 drops of 50% Lugol's to edge of coverslip and allow it to seep in.

Note: persons who have been treated for cancer or HIV using any of the known drugs may show only 1 to 2 fluke parasite stages per drop of saliva or urine. For this reason, you may need to search through 20 or more slides to find flukes. Very ill persons may show up to 10 parasites per drop (slide).

Taking Pictures Of What You See

You may be unsure of what you see even if you have the microscope slides of labeled flukes and their stages to study and compare. In real life, they vary so much in shape and size that absolute identification is difficult without experience. Unfortunately in a few hours, just as you are getting proficient, your magnificent specimens will be drying out and unfit for observation. To preserve them longer you can seal the edges by painting around the coverslip with fingernail clear enamel. Or dribble hot sealing wax along the edges and then place them in sealed plastic bags (one per bag). Melt sealing wax in a metal jar lid. Make an applicator from a piece of coat hanger wire bent in the shape of a small square to fit around the coverslip and a handle.

Or take photographs. To take pictures of what you see under the microscope you will need a photomicrographic camera, which costs $200.00 and up (see *Sources*). It is easy to use. Remember to label your pictures so you know which slide they came from.

Even photographs do not scientifically prove identity of parasite stages, but it is very good evidence. Proof would require that the saliva or urine sample could be cultured and seen to produce the known parasite stages.

Using A Frequency Generator

Frequency generators come in all sizes and costs and capabilities. If you can purchase one that reads out the frequency for you in numbers (digital type) and lets you produce a fraction of a kilohertz by turning a dial, it meets your most elementary needs. It should also be possible to set it on positive offset (100% positive) and still give you 5 volts. Then it can be used as a zapper. You should also be able to select a sine wave or square wave.

The advantages of having a frequency generator are that you can do your own diagnosing. You can find, in a few minutes:

1. Which invaders you have by dialing in to their frequencies.
2. At what frequencies you are broadcasting to the world.
3. What frequencies are used by other living things.

The Theory

Every living animal and every cell type produces its own frequencies and responds to these frequencies as well. We may speak of frequencies but we really mean waves, waves of energy. All waves have a frequency associated with them, so it's not really misleading to say frequencies when we really mean waves.

When the animal is alive it produces them, when it is dead it still responds to some of them. It is like the opera singer and the glass goblet. The opera singer produces frequencies in the air. The goblet responds to them because of its structure, not because it's alive. The goblet "picks up" on that particular frequency of sound because its own "resonant" frequency is exactly the same. If the singer sings loud enough the goblet shatters from the vibrations set up in it. An identical goblet, made of plastic, would not have the same resonant frequency.

There is not merely a structural and chemical difference between the living and non living. Living things are transmitting energy of some unique kind. And with your simple device, you will be able to trap this energy. And measure its exact frequency. This is not the same as understanding its makeup and source. We must leave that to others. But we can observe and use our observations to track down bacteria and other parasites. We can track down pollutants. We can measure our health quantitatively and perhaps in the future predict life expectancy.

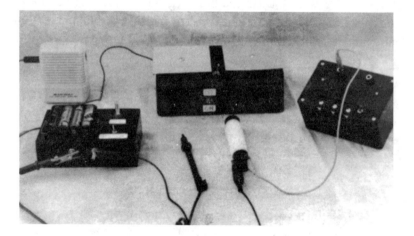

The Syncrometer at left is attached to the handhold. The frequency generator at right is also clipped to the handhold.
Fig. 85 Setup for finding resonant frequencies.

The Syncrometer traps the frequencies that match the ones in the material on the test plates and delivers them to an audio speaker in a range that you are able to hear. **Instead of test tissues or pathogens, we are now going to use pure test frequencies!** Remarkably, few things have overlapping frequencies, making this technique extremely useful for identification, <u>even without a specimen</u>!

Lesson Eighteen

Purpose: To search for the intestinal fluke in your body by listening to its broadcast frequency at 434 KHz.

Method: Turn on the frequency generator, select a frequency a short distance above the one you are interested in, like 438 KHz, turn the voltage (amplitude) down to less than one volt. Select sine waves. The lead coming from the frequency generator will have two connections, usually red and black (ground). We will not use the black (ground), just tape it out of the way. Pick up the handhold and probe in the usual way. Attach the red lead coming from the generator to your handhold. <u>This makes two wires attached to your handhold.</u> Although there is nothing on the test plates, they must be connected as usual with the switch at OFF (one plate is still ON).

Turn the Syncrometer ON. Probe yourself as usual. Your body's waves are being sent to the capacitor (plate) in the test plate box. The frequency from the Syncrometer is sent there, too. And now the 438 KHz waves from the generator are being sent there as well. Three different frequencies are mingling on the plate! If the two from your body and the generator are the same, the circuit will oscillate, and you will hear resonance. Turn the generator to 437 and probe again. Next, 436.

Sometimes, you can hear the resonance start to build. Continue on.

Next try 435. Then 434.

If your body is emitting a frequency of 434 KHz (coming from a live intestinal fluke inside you) it will be reinforced by the generator's 434 KHz. The reinforcement will put oscillations or resonance in the circuit, the same as you are accustomed to hearing with the Syncrometer. If there was none, you don't have the intestinal fluke anywhere in your body. Confirm this by starting at 430 KHz and working your way up.

If you hear resonance, you do have it. You may wish to verify this independently using a prepared slide of the fluke. Kill your flukes immediately as described in the next lesson.

Lesson Nineteen

Purpose: Killing the intestinal fluke with a frequency generator.

Materials: A frequency generator, two handholds with alligator clip leads for them.

Method: Wrap a single layer of paper towel over each of the two handholds. Wet them under the tap; squeeze out excess water. Clip them to the red and black wires of the frequency generator. (We use both wires for this purpose.) Dial up 434 KHz. Set the amplitude (voltage) at 10 volts. Grasp the handholds in each hand and hold on for three minutes. That is all. You have killed whatever tiny invader has a resonant frequency the same as the setting on the generator. Remember to zap all the stages, too; see *Pathogen Frequencies*.

If your frequency generator has a **positive offset** capability, you can use it like a zapper, and a single session will kill all pathogens, provided it is 100% offset and can give at least 5 volts at this setting. When using this technique, the generator can be set to any frequency from 2 KHz to 800 KHz, and you should go for 7 minutes. But even a small percentage of negative voltage will ruin this effect and do more harm than good! To be certain your generator is set correctly it would be best to observe the output on an oscilloscope.

Experiment with other voltage settings. Notice that less than one volt is also effective.

Lesson Twenty

Purpose: To find the bandwidth of a small living animal.

Materials: A fly, beetle or other insect, Syncrometer, frequency generator.

Discussion: Persons using a Syncrometer might have already tried putting a small insect on one of the plates. The circuit <u>always</u> resonates when you join the circuit at the handhold and probe. Even the tiniest ant placed in a glass bottle or plastic baggy will resonate the circuit. Unless it is too far away from the plate. If it has climbed up the side you will lose the resonance. At least one foot must be touching the bottom of the bottle. If the animal is dead this ceases. Obviously the living thing is affecting the circuit differently before and after death. Is it some kind of a wave form energy? To find its frequency you must add another frequency that will reinforce or interfere with the frequency already on the plate. Adding the generator frequency does just that.

Method: Use the same method as described in the last Lesson; however for an ant or fly, start at 1,000 KHz and proceed upward in big steps like 10 KHz. Use the right test plate which is controlled by the ON-OFF switch. Always listen to the current with the switch OFF, first, then ON. Move the frequency up and repeat. Continue until you hear resonance. Stop immediately. Rest your skin and go back down to the nonresonant frequency region. Move up in smaller steps this time. Repeat and repeat until you feel sure you know just where the resonance begins. But where does it end?

Start testing well above the suspected range taking big steps downward until you reach a resonant frequency. Rest and repeat until you find the upper limit of resonant frequencies. Record the bandwidth, for example, 1009-1112 KHz.

Lesson Twenty One

Purpose: To see if similar living things interfere with each other when put on the plate together.

Materials: Two identical living insects or very small living things.

Method: Find the broadcast range of each one separately and then together on the plate.

Note: Identical living things do not interfere with each others' frequencies.

Lesson Twenty Two

Purpose: To see if different living things interfere with each other when put on the plate together.

Method: Find the lower and upper end of the broadcast range of two different living things, such as a fly and a beetle or 2 kinds of flies or beetles. Then put them on the plate together. Notice there is no resonance in the accustomed range for either of them. They are interfering with each other on the plate.

Now add the 2 lower ends, then the two upper ends. Also subtract the 2 lower ends, then the two upper ends. For example imagine two insects, one with a spectrum of 1000 to 1090 KHz, the other with a range of 1050 to 1190 KHz. Adding the lower ends gives us 2050 KHz. Subtracting the lower ends gives us 50 KHz. Adding the upper ends gives 2280. Subtracting the upper ends gives 100. Now search for resonance at 50, 100, 2050, 2280 KHz. (These last two may be outside the range of your frequency generator. Choose more primitive life forms which have lower frequency bandwidths to stay within your limit.)

Notice that you hear resonance at exactly these frequencies and not above or below them. This is evidence for modulation of the frequencies: namely fusing them together.

Lesson Twenty Three

Purpose: To find your own bandwidth of emitted frequencies.

Materials: A frequency generator that goes up to 10 MHz. If yours only goes to 2 MHz you can still investigate the lower end of your band.

Method: You do not need to put yourself on the plate, since you are already there by being in the circuit at the handhold. However, if you are measuring someone else, they can simply touch the plate with a finger. Attach the frequency generator to the circuit at the handhold.

Since human adults begin to emit at about 1560 KHz, start searching at 1550, going upward in 1 KHz steps until you hear resonance.

Younger or healthier humans start emitting at a lower frequency and sometimes end at a higher frequency. In other words, they broadcast on a wider band.

Very young infants begin their band at about 1520 KHz. Could you ever regain this ability?

Most adults terminate at 9375 KHz

By eliminating molds from my diet, killing as many parasites and removing as many toxins as I became aware of, I have been able to expand my bandwidth from an initial 1562-9457 KHz in 1990 to 1520-9580 KHz in 1994! I hope this challenges you to accomplish a health improvement reflected in an even broader bandwidth for yourself.

Lesson Twenty Four

Purpose: To find the effect of a variety of things on the lower end of your spectrum, such as body temperature, eating, time of day, rainy weather, feeling sick. Notice that you may not change for weeks at a time, then suddenly see a shrinking of your bandwidth. You may assume you have eaten a mold.

Search for mold frequencies from 75 KHz to 295 KHz. Or test in your liver with mold samples. If this is positive go on a mold free diet—watching carefully for mold in your white blood cells. Even after removing the mold from your diet, so that no molds appear in your white blood cells, notice that your bandwidth does not recover. It regularly takes 2-3 weeks for mine to recover.

Surely, this sheds light on the poisonous effect of eating bad food.

Lesson Twenty Five

Purpose: To find an emission spectrum using a saliva sample.

Materials: A regular frequency generator.

Method: Search for the bottom of the resonant frequency band as in the previous lesson.

You may store it in the refrigerator for a few weeks without seeing a change. After that the band begins to shrink.

Lesson Twenty Six

Purpose: To observe the effect of dying on the bandwidth.

Method: Freeze the insect you tested in Lesson Twenty to kill it humanely. Repeat the search for its bandwidth. Note the bandwidth has become very narrow.

Note the bandwidth also depends on the accuracy of your particular frequency generator.

Lesson Twenty Seven

Purpose: To find unknown invaders of your body.

Method: Start at 900 KHz and proceed down to 77 KHz in 1 KHz steps, to search for all pathogens. If you find a resonating frequency, go to the Pathogen Frequency Chart (page 561) to identify likely candidates for it. <u>Verify the identity of the invader by using a slide or culture specimen</u>. If your pathogen remains unidentified, add it to the chart. This lets you determine whether the next illness is new or a recurrence of this one. Or just kill it.

Use the frequency generator at one pathogen's frequency. Wait <u>ten minutes</u> and retest all of the ones you found. Only <u>that</u> one will be gone. Now **zap**, wait ten minutes, and test again for all of the ones you found. Notice they are <u>all</u> gone. After one hour, search yet again for the pathogens you had. Any that are back must have come from an internal source not reached by the zapper current, like from the bowel or an abscess.

Lesson Twenty Eight

Purpose: To observe the action of a positive offset frequency on a very small animal. Does the animal die or is it just incapacitated?

Materials: A slug or small earthworm.

Method: Place the small animal in a plastic container like a cottage cheese carton. Add a few tsp. of water to wet the bottom. Attach a metal teaspoon to each of the generator clips. Place them on opposite sides in the carton and fasten with tape. Set the generator to positive offset at a frequency of about 30 KHz and 5 to 10 volts. Experiment with different voltages and compare effectiveness. Measure the time it takes for the animal to seem lifeless. You may try to revive it by keeping it for some time in the presence of food. Retest its emission band.

Lesson Twenty Nine

Purpose: To kill the bacteria in dairy products.

Materials: A glass of regular pasteurized milk, a carton of cottage cheese. A zapper.

Method: Search for *Salmonellas* and *Shigellas* first in the milk and cottage cheese. Search by frequency, using the chart, or with slides of these bacteria. If you don't find any, search different dairy foods until you find some bacteria. Attach metal teaspoons to the red and black leads of the generator. Place them inside the milk glass or cottage cheese carton, across from each other. Secure with masking tape. Attach the zapper. Zap them for 7 minutes. Remove the electrodes and wait 5 minutes. Test again for the same bacteria. They should be gone (but the food is not safe to eat due to the metal released from the teaspoons).

These experiments point to some exciting possibilities. Perhaps water supplies as well as foods and medicines could be sterilized this way. Perhaps sewage could be treated more efficiently, electrically. Best of all, maybe you could protect yourself from unsanitary products. If you do decide to explore this possibility, remember not to put metals in your mouth or food. Nor to use currents greater than 10 milliamps, or for longer than 10 minutes.

There are many commercially available function generators that can meet your needs. Two are shown here.

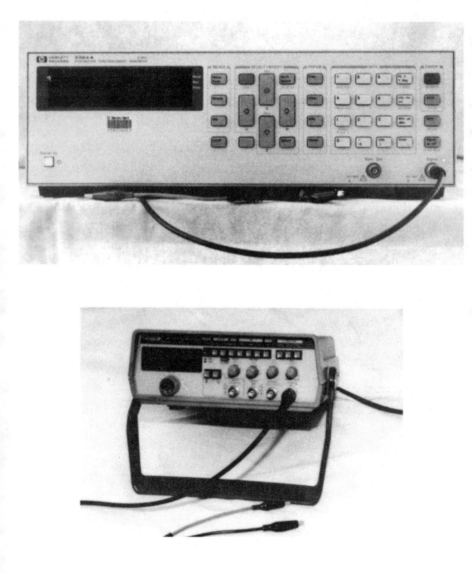

Fig. 86 Function generators.

Recipes

Read old recipe books for the fun and savings of making your own nutritious food. Change the recipes to avoid processed ingredients. Here are some I found:

Beverage Recipes

Anything made in your own juicer is fine. Experiment with new combinations to create different flavorful fruit and vegetable juices. Consider the luxury of preparing gourmet juices which satisfy your own individual palate instead of the mass-produced, polluted varieties sold at grocery stores. Remember to wash all fruit, including citrus before juicing. This removes the ever-present pesticides and common fruit mold.

Lemonade

1 cup fresh lemon juice, 1 cup honey, 1½ quarts water. Bring honey and water to a boil if you plan to keep it several days. Then add lemon juice and store in the refrigerator.

> All honey and maple syrup should have vitamin C added to it as soon as it arrives from the supermarket. Warm it first; then stir in ¼ tsp. per pint.

Fresh Tomato Juice

Simmer for ½ hour: 12 medium-sized raw, ripe tomatoes, ½ cup water, 1 slice onion, 2 ribs celery with leaves, ½ bay leaf, 3 sprigs parsley. Strain these ingredients. Season with: 1 tsp. salt (aluminum-free), ¼ tsp. paprika, ½ tsp. honey. Serve thoroughly chilled. Makes about 4 servings.

Fresh Pineapple Juice

Peel a pineapple. Remove all soft spots. Cut it into cubes. Extract the juice by putting the pineapple through a food grinder or a blender. There will be very little pulp. Strain the juice and serve it on ice with sprigs of mint. Makes about 1½ cups of juice. Mix the pulp with an equal amount of clover honey and use as topping (kept in freezer) for homemade ice cream (below), pancakes, or yogurt.

Maple Milk Shake

For each milk shake, blend or shake together: 1 glass of milk and 2 tablespoons maple syrup.

Remember, all milk gets boiled.

Yankee Drink

Mix together 1 gal. water, 3 cups honey, ½ cup fresh lemon juice or distilled white vinegar, and 1 tsp. ginger.

Hot Vanilla Milk

Add one inch of vanilla bean and one tsp. honey to a glass of milk and bring to a near boil. You may add a pinch of cinnamon or other pure spice. You may even use vanilla extract (see *Sources*).

Red Milk

Equal parts fresh carrot juice (use a juicer) and sterilized milk. Save the carrot pulp for salads and soups.

C-Milk

Milk can absorb a surprising amount of vitamin C powder without curdling or changing its flavor. Try ½ tsp. in a glass of cold milk.

My Own Soda Pop

Excellent for stomach distress. Put 1 tsp. citric acid, 2 tbs. vegetable glycerin (see *Sources*), 2 tbs. honey, and 1 lemon, juiced by hand, into a quart jar and fill with cold water. Refrigerate until ready to use. Then add 1 tsp. baking soda (chemically pure only, see *Sources*) and shake a few times, keeping the lid tight. Pour over a few ice cubes. Many variations are possible: other fruit concentrates, made in the blender, can be used along with some lemon juice; for example, 2 blended whole apples (peeled), blended pineapple, orange or grapefruit. Always add a bit of lemon to give it zip. You may add a pinch of ginger or other pure spice.

Note: The amount of sodium in ½ tsp. baking soda is .476 grams. If you have heart disease, high blood pressure, or edema, use potassium bicarbonate instead. Ask your doctor what an acceptable amount of sodium or potassium bicarbonate is. I would suggest limiting yourself to one glass of soda pop a day, even if you do not have heart disease.

Another Note: the citric acid kills bacteria, while the carbonation brings relief.

My Own Super C-Pop

An excellent way to get lots of vitamin C into a child and relieve stomach distress at the same time. Squeeze 1 slice of lemon and 1 whole orange into an 8 ounce bottle that has a tight lid. Add 1 tsp. vitamin C powder (ascorbic acid), ¼ tsp. citric acid, and 2 tbs. vegetable glycerin (you may also experiment with honey for sweetness). Fill the bottle to the top with cold water. Then add ½ tsp. chemically pure baking soda and close tightly. Shake briefly and serve immediately.

Half And Half

Mix equal parts whipping cream and milk or water. Boil and chill.

Buttermilk-C

Stir 1 tsp. vitamin C powder into a glass of milk. Add a pinch of potassium chloride. Additional seasoning may be pepper and herbs. Stir and enjoy.

Food Recipes

Despite the presence of aflatoxins, benzopyrenes, and solvents in many foods, it is possible to have a delicious and safe diet. Many persons need to gain weight, and with the emphasis in today's society on losing weight, consider yourself lucky in this respect. Help yourself to lots of butter, whipping cream, whole milk, avocados, and olive oil. Make your own preserves and baked goods, including breads. Remember, when you are recovering from a major illness it is essential not to diet to lose weight. You must wait two years after you are recovered to try to lose weight.

Daily Foods

Dairy products should contain at least 2% fat to enable you to absorb the calcium in them.

All milk should be sterilized

by boiling it for 10 seconds. If it makes mucous, you already have a chronic respiratory infection. Try to clear this up.

Change brands every time you shop to prevent the same pollutants from building up in your body.

If frying or cooking with fat, use <u>only</u> olive oil, butter or lard (the BHT and BHA preservatives in lard are OK except for seizure sufferers). Mix them for added flavor in your dishes. <u>Never use margarine, Crisco™ or other hydrogenated fats. Do not cook over flames or grill, even when electric.</u>

Eat lots of **fresh fruits and vegetables.** Wash them off <u>only</u> with cold tap water, not commercial food "wash". Scrub hard with a stiff bristled brush. Then cut away blemishes. Always peel potatoes, apples, and carrots. Modern dirt is full of chemicals and is toxic to you.

Be sure to drink plenty of **plain water** from your cold faucet throughout the day, especially if it is difficult for you to drink it with your meals. If you don't like the taste of your own tap water, try to get it from a friend with newer plumbing. Use a polyethylene (opaque) water jug from a grocery store to transport it. Never drink water that has been run through a water softener or copper plumbing or has traveled through a long plastic hose. Don't drink water that has stood in a container for a day. Dump it and sterilize the container. To further improve flavor and to dechlorinate attach a small faucet filter made of carbon only. Or buy a filter pitcher (see *Sources*). Don't drink water that has stood in the filter pitcher very long, either.

Because commercial **cold cereals** are very convenient, but have solvents, here are two replacements.

Two Granolas

7 cups rolled oats (old fashioned, not quick)
1 tsp. salt
1 cup wheat germ (fresh, not defatted)
½ cup honey
½ cup sunflower seeds, immaculate quality
½ cup milk (no need to sterilize, it is being baked)
½ cup melted butter
1 cup raisins, rinsed in vitamin C water

Mix dry ingredients together. Mix liquid ingredients and add gradually, while tossing until thoroughly mixed. Place in large ungreased pans and bake in slow (250°) oven. Stir occasionally, baking until brown and dry, usually 1-2 hours. Store in airtight container in freezer.

6 cups rolled oats
½ cup raw wheat germ
1 cup sesame seeds
1 cup sunflower seeds (raw, unsalted)
1 tsp. cinnamon
½ cup melted butter
½ cup honey

Preheat oven to 250°. Toss all ingredients in mixing bowl. Spread thinly on a baking sheet and bake 20-25 minutes. Stir often in order to brown evenly. When golden, remove and let cool. Makes 12 cups.

If you would like to add nuts to your granola recipes, rinse them in cold tap water first, to which vitamin C powder has been added (¼ tsp. per pint). This removes aflatoxins.

Peanut Butter

Use fresh unsalted roasted peanuts—they will be white on the first day they arrive at the health food store from the distributor. (Ask when they will arrive.) Or shell fresh roasted peanuts yourself, throwing away all shriveled or darkened nuts. Grind, adding salt and vitamin C (¼ tsp. per pint) as you go. For spreadability, especially for children, grind an equal volume of cold butter along with the peanuts. This improves spreadability and digestibility of the hard nut particles. This will probably be the most heavenly peanut butter your mouth has ever experienced.

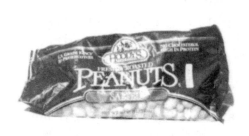

Fig. 87 Light colored, roasted peanuts in the shell had no aflatoxin.

Sweetening and Flavoring

Brown Sugar. Although I am prejudiced against all sugar from a health standpoint, my testing revealed no benzene, propyl alcohol, wood alcohol. However it does contain sorghum mold and must be treated with vitamin C to detoxify it. Add ¼ tsp. to a 1 pound package; knead until well mixed.

Maple syrup. Add vitamin C to newly opened bottle, ¼ tsp. to retard mold. Keep refrigerated and use promptly.

Flavoring. Use maple, vanilla (both natural and artificial), and any pure spice. They are free of molds and solvents.

Honeys. Get at least 4 flavors for variety: linden blossom, orange blossom, plain clover and local or wild flower honey

Add vitamin C to newly opened jar to detoxify ergot mold (¼ tsp. per pint).

Jams and jellies. They are not safe unless homemade.

Fruit syrup. Use one package frozen fruit, such as cherries, blueberries or raspberries. Let thaw and measure the amount in cups (it might say on the package). Add an equal amount of clover honey to the fruit. Also add ¼ tsp. vitamin C powder. Mix it all in a quart canning jar and store in the refrigerator. Use this on pancakes, cereal, plain yogurt and homemade ice cream too. Use to make your own flavored beverages in a seltzer maker or to make soda pop. If you wish to use fresh fruit, bring it to a boil to sterilize. Use it up in a few days or boil to sterilize it again.

Note for diabetics

Diabetics must not use artificial sweeteners. Nor can they use all the sweeteners listed. Try stevia powder instead.

Preserves

Keep 3 or 4 kinds on hand, such as peach, pineapple, and pear. Peel and chop the fruit. It should not have any bruises. If you use a metal knife, rinse the fruit lightly afterwards. Add just enough water to keep the fruit from sticking as it is cooked (usually a few tablespoons). Then add an equal amount of honey, or to taste and heat again to boiling. Put in sterile jars in refrigerator. Make marmalade the same way, slicing the fruit and peel thinly. Always add vitamin C powder to a partly used jar to inhibit mold. <u>Never</u> use up partly molded fruit by making preserves out of it. <u>Throw it out.</u>

C Dressing

½ cup olive oil
¼ cup fresh lemon juice or white distilled vinegar
1 tsp. thyme, fenugreek or both (capsules are freshest)
1 tsp. vitamin C powder
½ tsp. brown sugar

Combine the ingredients in a clean salad dressing bottle. Shake. Refrigerate. The basic recipe is the oil and vinegar in a 2:1 ratio. After mixing these, add any pure spice desired. Or add fresh tomato chunks for creaminess.

Cheese Sauce

Add milk to cheese in equal amounts. Gradually heat to boiling while stirring. Add more of either to obtain the desired consistency. Boil 10 seconds. Use immediately.

Sour Cream-C

2 cups heavy whipping cream, previously boiled
¼ tsp. citric acid
¼ tsp. vitamin C powder
1 tsp. fresh onion juice or other seasoning (optional)

Stir until smooth, refrigerate 2 hours.

Yogurt

Buy a yogurt maker. Be sure and use boiled milk.

Soups

All home made soups are nutritious and safe, provided you use no processed ingredients (like bouillon), or make them in metal pots. Use herbs and aluminum-free salt to season. Always add a dash of vitamin C or tomato juice or vinegar to draw out calcium from soup bones for you to absorb.

Fish and Seafood recipe

Any kind of fish or seafood is acceptable, provided it is well-cooked. Don't buy food that is already in batter. The simplest way to cook fish is to poach it in milk. It can be taken straight from the freezer, rinsed, and placed in ¼ inch of milk (unboiled is fine) in the frying pan. Heat until it is cooked. Turn over and repeat. Throw away the milk. Serve with fresh lemon and herbs.

Baked Apples

Peel and core carefully. Remove all bruises (this is where the patulin is). Cut in bite-sized pieces, add a minimum of water and cook or bake minimally. Add a squirt of lemon juice when done. Serve with cinnamon, whipping cream and honey.

Ice creams

from the grocery store are loaded with benzene and other solvents. Fortunately there are ice cream makers that do everything (no cranking)! Or try our recipe which uses a blender. Be sure not to add store bought flavors, except vanilla or maple.

5 Minute Ice Cream

(Strawberry) Use 2 half pints of whipping cream, previously boiled, 1 package of frozen strawberries (about 10 oz.), and ½ cup clover honey. Pour frozen strawberries into blender. Pour whipping cream and honey over them. Blend briefly (about 10 seconds), not long enough to make butter! Pour it all into a large plastic bowl. Cover with a close fitting plastic bag and place in freezer. Prepare it a day ahead. Try using other frozen fruits, such as blueberries and cherries. Keep a few berries out of the blender and stir them in quickly with a non-metal spoon before setting the bowl in the freezer. There are many ice cream recipes to be found in old cook books. Avoid those with raw eggs or processed foods as ingredients. You may add nuts if you rinse them in vitamin C water.

Cookies, cakes and pies

Bake them from scratch, using unprocessed ingredients. Use simple recipes from old cook books.

Seven Day Sample Menu

Because processed foods have many toxins, you must cook as much from scratch as possible. So for convenience sake, keep your meals simple in preparation. You may want to prepare ahead and refrigerate your dressings and toppings. Or you could make a hot soup for dinner, refrigerate, and eat the leftovers for lunch. Don't save leftovers more than two days. Make sure they are covered. Try baking several potatoes at one time, refrigerate and put them in a salad the next night. Variety is the spice of life, so combine the allowed foods in the most creative ways you can imagine. And don't forget herbs and spices; learn to use them from old cook books.

	Breakfast	Lunch	Dinner
Day 1	Granola and honey with milk, half n' half or whipping cream 1 cup fresh squeezed fruit juice Water Milk	Fresh ground peanut butter and preserve sandwich Soup Milk Water	Orange roughy fish Fresh green beans with butter Baked potato with Sour Cream-C topping or fresh chives Pie (homemade) Milk 1 cup fresh squeezed or frozen vegetable juice Water

Day 2	Egg (limit is 2) Fried potatoes 1 glass milk Peppermint herb tea Fresh orange juice	Bagel (from bakery) Sour Cream-C Tomato 1 cup vegetable juice Water Milk	Homemade bean or lentil soup Sardines Dinner roll and butter Salad Homemade dressing Ice cream (homemade) Water
Day 3	Cream of Wheat™ cooked with raisins and milk Banana Peppermint herb tea ½ cup milk Water	Tuna sandwich with olives and butter Soup Milk Water	Baked sweet potato with butter and sweetening. Fresh broccoli with cheese sauce Bread and butter Chopped, peeled pear and whipping cream 1 cup vegetable juice Milk Water
Day 4	French toast with maple syrup Egg Homemade grapefruit juice Milk Water	Avocado and sour cream sandwich ½ cup vegetable juice Bread and butter Water	Lobster or sautéed shrimp Fresh asparagus Potatoes, any style ½ cup vegetable juice Water Milk
Day 5	Cooked cereal 1 glass milk Sliced banana with whipping cream and honey 1 glass water	Cold potato salad with C Dressing Soup ½ cup vegetable juice Custard Water Milk	1 can sardines or salmon in easy-open can (can openers shed metal) Salad of lettuce, tomato, olives, avocado with homemade dressing Bread with butter Ice-cream (optional) ½ cup vegetable juice Water Milk
Day 6	Egg and homemade biscuit with honey and butter Milk Fruit juice (homemade) Water	Homemade peanut butter sandwich ½ cup vegetable juice Milk Water	Gourmet pizza: home baked bread topped with olive oil, sliced tomato or homemade sauce, grated cheese, sardines or anchovies, chopped vegetables, garlic and onion Salad Milk Water

Day 7	Pancakes Banana or chopped fruit with cream Milk Water	Salmon sandwich (from flip top can) ½ cup vegetable juice Milk Water	Stir-fry vegetables: broccoli, carrots, cab- bage, in olive oil and butter Bread and butter Pie (optional) Milk Water

Remember, take vitamin C and B-complex with each meal.

Too Sick To Cook, Too Tired To Eat

Pick three meals from the sample menu that need no cooking and eat them every day.

Recipes for Natural Body Products

You can use just borax (like 20 Mule Team Borax™) and washing soda (like Arm & Hammer Super Washing Soda™) for all types of cleaning including your body, laundry, dishes and your house! You don't need all of those products you see in commercials for each special task!

Even if you have dry skin, difficult hair or some other unique requirement, just pure borax will satisfy these needs. A part of every skin problem is due to the toxic elements found in the soaps themselves. For instance aluminum is commonly added as a "skin moisturizer". It does this by impregnating the skin and attracting water, giving the illusion of moist skin. In fact you simply have moist aluminum stuck in your skin which your immune system must remove. While borax won't directly heal your skin or complexion, it does replace the agents that are causing damage, so that healing can occur.

Borax Liquid Soap

Empty 1 gallon jug
1/8 cup borax powder
Plastic funnel

Funnel the borax into the jug, fill with cold tap water. Shake a few times. Let settle. In a few minutes you can pour off the clear part into dispenser bottles. This is the soap!

Easier way: use any bottle, pour borax powder to a depth of a ½ inch or so. Add water. Shake. When you have used it down to the undissolved granules, add more water and shake again. Add more borax when the undissolved granules get low.

Keep a dispenser by the kitchen sink, bathroom sink, and shower. It does not contain aluminum as regular detergents and soaps do, and which probably contribute to Alzheimer's disease. It does not contain PCBs as many commercial and health food varieties do. It does not contain cobalt (the blue or green granules) which causes heart disease and draws cancer parasites to the skin. Commercial detergents and non-soaps are simply not safe. Switch to homemade bar soap and borax for all your tasks! Borax inhibits the bacterial enzyme *urease* and is therefore antibacterial. It may even clear your skin of blemishes and stop your scalp from itching.

For Laundry

Borax (½ cup per load). It is the main ingredient of non-chlorine bleach and has excellent cleaning power without fading colors. Your regular laundry soap may contain PCBs, aluminum, cobalt and other chemicals. These get rubbed into your skin constantly as you wear your clothing. For bleaching (only do this occasionally) use original chlorine bleach (not "new improved" or "with special brighteners", and so forth). Don't use chlorine if there is an ill person in the house. For getting out stubborn dirt at collars, scrub with homemade bar soap first; for stains, try grain alcohol, vinegar, baking soda.

For Dishes

Don't believe your eyes when you see the commercials where the smiling person pulls a shining dish out of greasy suds. Any dish soap that you use should be safe enough to eat because <u>nothing</u> rinses off clean. Regular dish detergents, <u>including health brands</u>, are now polluted with PCBs. They also contain harmful chemicals. Use borax for your dishes. Or use paper plates and plastic (not styrofoam) cups.

In The Dishwasher

Use 2 tsp. borax powder pre-dissolved in water. If you use too much it will leave a film on your dishes. Use vinegar in the rinse cycle.

In The Sink

Use a dishpan in the sink. Use ¼ cup borax and add a minimum of water. Also keep a bit of dry borax in a saucer by the sink for scouring. <u>Don't use any soap at all for dishes that aren't greasy and can be washed under the faucet with nothing but running water.</u> Throw away your old sponge or brush or cloth because it may be PCB contaminated. Start each day by sterilizing your sponge (it harbors Salmonella) or with a new one while the used one dries for three full days. Clean greasy pots and pans with a paper towel first. Then use homemade bar soap.

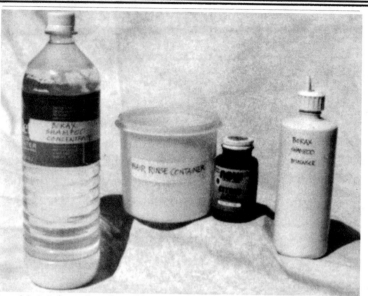

Fig. 88 Make a bottle of borax liquid to fill your soap dispensers and shampoo bottle. Use citric acid to rinse and condition.

Shampoo

Borax liquid is ready to use as shampoo, too. It does not lather but goes right to work removing sweat and soil without stripping your color or natural oils. It inhibits scalp bacteria and stops flaking and itching. Hair gets squeaky clean so quickly (just a few squirts does it) that you might think nothing has happened! You will soon be accustomed to non-lathery soap. Rinse very thoroughly because you should leave your scalp slightly acidic. Take a pint container to the shower with you. Put ¼ tsp. citric (not ascorbic) acid crystals (see *Sources*) in it. For long hair use a quart of rinse. Only **citric acid** is strong enough to get the borax out, lemon juice and vinegar are not. After shampooing, fill the container with water and rinse. Rinse your whole body, too, since citric acid is also anti-bacterial. All hair shampoo penetrates the eye lids and gets into the eyes although you do not feel it. It is important to use this natural rinse to neutralize the shampoo in your eyes. (Some people have stated that citric acid makes their hair curlier or reddens it. If this is undesirable, use only half as much citric acid.) Citric acid also conditions and gives body and sheen to hair.

Hair Spray

I don't have a recipe that holds your hair as well as the bottle of chemicals you can buy at the store. Remarkably a little lemon juice (not from a bottle) has some holding power and no odor! Buy a 1 cup spray bottle. Squeeze part of a lemon, letting only the clear juice run into the bottle. Fill with water. Keep it in the refrigerator. Make it fresh every week. Spraying with just plain water is nearly as good! For shinier hair, drop a bit of lemon peel into the bottle.

Homemade Soap

A small plastic dishpan, about 10" x 12"
A glass or enamel 2-quart sauce pan
1 can of lye (sodium hydroxide), 12 ounces
3 pounds of lard (BHT and BHA are OK here)
Plastic gloves
Water

1. Pour 3 cups of very cold water (refrigerate water overnight first) into the 2-quart saucepan.
2. Slowly and carefully add the lye, a little bit at a time, stirring it with a wooden or plastic utensil. (Use plastic gloves for this; test them for holes first.) Do not breathe the vapor or lean over the container or have children nearby. Above all <u>use no metal</u>. The mixture will get very hot. In olden days, a sassafras branch was used to stir, imparting a fragrance and insect deterrent for mosquitoes, lice, fleas, ticks.

3. Let cool at least one hour in a safe place. Meanwhile, the unwrapped lard should be warming up to room temperature in the plastic dishpan.
4. Slowly and carefully, pour the lye solution into the dishpan with the lard. The lard will melt. Mix thoroughly, at least 15 minutes, until it looks like thick pudding.
5. Let it set until the next morning; then cut it into bars. It will get harder after a few days. Then package.

If you wish to make soap based on olive oil, use about 48 ounces. It may need to harden for a week.

Liquid Soap

Make chips from your homemade soap cake. Add enough hot water to dissolve. Add citric acid to balance the pH (7 to 8). If you do not, this soap may be too harsh for your skin.

Skin Sanitizer

Make up a 5 to 10% solution of food grade alcohol. Food grade alcohols are grain (ethyl) alcohol or vodka. Find a suitable dispenser bottle. Mark it with a pen at about one tenth of the way up from the bottom. Pour 95% grain alcohol (190 proof) to this mark (for 50% grain alcohol or vodka make your mark one fifth of the way up). Add water to the top. Keep shut. You may add a chip of lemon peel for fragrance.

Use this for general sanitizing purposes: bathroom fixtures, knobs, handles, canes, walkers, and for personal cleanliness (but use chlorine bleach for the toilet bowl once a week). Always clean up after a bowel movement with <u>wet</u> toilet paper. This is not clean enough, though. Follow with a stronger damp paper towel. This is still not clean enough; use a final damp paper towel with skin sanitizer added. After washing hands, sanitize them too, pouring a bit on one palm and put finger tips of the other hand in it, scratch to get under nails, repeat on other hand. Rinse with water.

> Do not use this recipe, nor keep any bottles of alcohol in the house of a recovering alcoholic.

Deodorant

Your sweat is odorless. It is the entrenched bacteria feeding on it that make smells. You can never completely rid yourself of these bacteria, although they may temporarily be gone after zapping. The strategy is to control their numbers. Here are several deodorants to try. Find one that works best for you:

Vitamin C water. Mix ¼ tsp. to a pint of water and dab it on. Then dab on cornstarch.

Citric Acid water. Mix ¼ tsp. to a pint of water and dab it on. Then dab on cornstarch.

Only a few drops of these acids under each armpit are necessary. If these acids burn the skin, dilute them more. Never apply anything to skin that has just been shaved!

Corn starch. Many people need only this. Dab it on.

> Use only unpolluted **cornstarch** (see *Sources*).

Baking soda has been deleted as a deodorant because benzene was found in some boxes.

Lemon juice. This acid is not as strong, use what you need.

Pure alcohol (never rubbing alcohol). The food grade alcohols are grain alcohol and vodka. Dab a bit under each arm and/or on your shirt or blouse, then dab on cornstarch. If the alcohol burns, dilute it with water. Be very careful not to leave the bottle where a child or alcoholic person could find it. Pour it into a different bottle!

Pure zinc oxide. You may ask your pharmacist to order this for you. She or he may wish to make it up for you too, but do not let them add <u>anything</u> else to it. It should be about 1 part zinc oxide powder to 3 parts water. It does not dissolve. Just shake it up to use it. After you get it home, you can add corn-starch to it to give it a creamy texture. Heat 3 tsp. cornstarch in 1 cup of water, to boiling, until dissolved and clear. Cool and add some to the zinc oxide mixture (about equal parts). Store unused starch mixture in the refrigerator. Only make up enough for a month.

Alcohol and zinc oxide. This is the most powerful deodor-ant. Apply alcohol first, then the zinc oxide, then dab on corn-starch.

Remember that you need to sweat! Sweating excretes toxic substances, especially from the upper body. Don't use deodorant on weekends. Go to the sink and wipe clean the armpits like our grandparents did. Often, just plain cornstarch is enough! These homemade deodorants are not as powerful as the commercial varieties–this is to your advantage.

Brushing Teeth

Buy a new toothbrush. Your old one is soaked with toxins from your old toothpaste. Use only water or chemically pure baking soda if you have any metal fillings. Put a pinch in a glass, add water to dissolve it. Use food-grade hydrogen perox-ide (see *Sources)* if you have only plastic fillings. Dilute it from 35% to 17½% by adding water (equal parts). Store hydrogen peroxide only in polyethylene or the original plastic bottle. Use 4 or 5 drops on your toothbrush. It should fizz nicely as oxygen is produced in your mouth. Your teeth will whiten noticeably in 6 months. Before brushing teeth, floss with 4 or 2 pound monofilament fish line. Double it and twist for extra strength. Rinse before use. Floss and brush only once a day. If this leaves you uncomfortable, brush the extra times with plain water and a second "water-only" toothbrush. Make sure that nothing solid, like powder, is on your toothbrush; it will scour the enamel and give you sensitive teeth, especially as you get older and the enamel softens. Salt is corrosive—don't use it for brushing metal teeth. Plain water is just as good.

For Dentures

Use salt water. It kills all germs and is inexpensive. Salt water plus grain alcohol or food-grade hydrogen peroxide makes a good denture-soak.

Mouthwash

A few drops of food grade hydrogen peroxide added to a little water in a glass should be enough to make your mouth foam and cleanse. Don't use hydrogen peroxide, though, if you have metal fillings, because they react. Don't use regular drug store variety hydrogen peroxide because it contains toxic additives. Health food store varieties contain solvents from the bottling process. See *Sources*. Never purchase hydrogen peroxide in a bottle with a metal cap.

For persons with metal tooth fillings, use chemically pure baking soda or just plain hot water. A healthy mouth has no odor! You shouldn't need a mouthwash! If you have breath odor, search for a hidden tooth infection or cavitation.

Contact Lens Solution

A scant cup of cold tap water brought to a boil in glass saucepan. After adding ¼ tsp. aluminum free salt and boiling again, pour into a sterile canning jar. Refrigerate. Freeze some of it.

Lip Soother

For dry, burning lips. Heat 1 level tsp. sodium alginate plus 1 cup water until dissolved. After cooling, pour it into a small bottle to carry in your purse or pocket (refrigerate the remainder). Dab it on whenever needed. If the consistency isn't right for you, add water or boil it down further. You can make a better lip soother by adding some lysine from a crushed tablet, vitamin C powder, and a vitamin E capsule to the alginate mix. If you have a persistent problem with chapped lips, try going off citrus juice.

Foot Powder

Use a mixture of cornstarch and zinc oxide poured into a salt shaker with a lid. Add long rice grains to fight humidity. You may also try arrow root or potato starch. If you don't have zinc oxide use plain cornstarch.

Skin Healer Moisturizer Lotion

1 tsp. sodium alginate
1 cup water

Make the base first by heating these together in a covered, non-metal pan until completely dissolved. Use low heat–it will take over an hour. Use a wooden spoon handle to stir. Set aside. Then make the following mixture:

¼ tsp. Vitamin C (ascorbic acid) (You may crush tablets)
¼ tsp. lysine (crush tablets)
2 tbs. pure vegetable glycerin
2 vitamin E capsules (400 units or more, each)
1 tsp. apricot kernel oil (olive oil will do)

1 tbs. lemon juice from a lemon or ¼ tsp citric acid (this is optional)
1 cup water

Heat the water to steaming in a non-metal pan. Add vitamin C and lysine first and then everything else. Pour into a pint jar and shake to mix. Then add the sodium alginate base to the desired thickness (about equal amounts) and shake. Pour some into a small bottle to use as lip soother. Pour some into a larger bottle to dispense on skin. Store remainder in refrigerator. (See *Sources* for sodium alginate, vegetable glycerin and apricot kernel oil. Sodium alginate is also available in capsule form at some health food stores.)

Other Skin Healers

Vitamin C powder (ascorbic acid, not the same as citric acid). Put a large pinch into the palm of your hand. With your other hand pick up a few drops of water from the faucet. Rub hands together until all the powder is dissolved and dispensed. It may sting briefly. Do this at bedtime, especially for cracked, chapped hands. Include lips if they need it.

Vitamin E oil. Vitamin E oil from Now Foods was not polluted at the time of this writing, but for the future it would be safer to rely on capsules. Snip open a capsule and rub into skin.

50% Glycerin. Dilute 100% vegetable glycerin with an equal amount of water. This is useful as an after shave lotion.

Vitamin C liquid. Mix ¼ tsp. vitamin C powder in one pint water (crushed tablets will do). This is useful as an after shave lotion and general skin treatment.

Apricot Kernel Oil. This is a very light oil, useful as an after shave lotion and general skin treatment.

Cornstarch (see *Sources*). Use on rashes, fungus, moist or irritated areas and to prevent chafe.

Combining several of these makes them more effective.

Dry skin has several causes: too much water contact, too much soap contact (switch to borax), low body temperature, not enough fat in the diet, or parasites.

Massage Oil

Use olive oil. It comes in very light to heavy textures. Pick the right one for your purpose. Alginate mixtures can be used instead of, or added to, oil. Starch solutions are good, too.

Sunscreen Lotion

Purchase PABA (see *Sources*) in 500 mg tablet form. Dissolve 1 tablet in grain alcohol or vodka. Grind the tablet first by putting it in a plastic bag and rolling over it with a glass jar. It will not completely dissolve even if you use a tablespoon of the alcohol. Pour the whole mixture into a 4 ounce bottle of homemade skin softener. Be careful not to get the lotion into your eyes when applying it. A better solution is to wear a hat or stay out of the sun. Remember to *take* PABA as a supplement, too (500 mg, one a day).

Nose Salve

(When the inside of the nose is dry, cracked and bleeding.)

Pour ½ tsp. pure vegetable glycerin into a bottle cap. Add ½ tsp. of water.

Applicator: use a plastic coffee stirrer or straw; cut a slit in the end to catch some cotton wool salvaged from a vitamin bottle and twist (cotton swabs, cotton balls and wooden toothpicks are sterilized with mercury which in turn is polluted with thallium). Dip it into the glycerin mixture and apply inside the nose with a rotating motion. Do each nostril with a new applicator.

Quick Corn Starch Skin Softener

4 tsp. corn starch (see *Sources*)
1 cup water
    Boil starch and water until clear, about one minute.

Cornstarch Skin Softener

1 tsp. lysine powder or 8 tablets, 500 mg each
1 tsp. Vitamin C powder (ascorbic acid); or 8 tablets, 500 mg each
3 tsp. cornstarch (see *Sources*)
Vitamin E, 1 capsule 400 mg
¼ tsp. apricot kernel oil (optional)
1 cup water
    Boil starch and water until clear, about one minute. Add other ingredients and stir until dissolved. Cool. Pour into dispenser bottle. Keep refrigerated when not in use. Apply after washing dishes and after showering.

After Shaves

    Vitamin C. ¼ tsp. vitamin C powder, dissolved in 1 pint water.

    Apricot kernel oil.

    Vegetable glycerin. Equal parts glycerin and water or to suit your need.

Personal Lubricants

    Heat these together: 1 level tsp. sodium alginate and 1 cup water in a covered non-metal pan until completely dissolved. Use very low heat and stir with a wooden spoon handle. It takes a fairly long time to get it perfectly smooth. After cooling, pour into a small dispenser bottle. Keep the remainder refrigerated.

    Or, mix and heat 4 tsp. cornstarch and 1 cup water until completely dissolved in a covered saucepan. Use non-metal

537

dishes and a non-metal stirring spoon. Cool. Pour some into dispenser bottle. Refrigerate remainder. This is many person's favorite recipe.

Baby Wipes

Cut paper towels in quarters and stack in a closable plastic box. Run tap water over them, drain the excess. Add 1 tsp. grain alcohol and/or borax liquid on top. Close. Put a dab of the Quick Cornstarch Softener recipe on top of each wipe as you use it.

People Wipes

¼ tsp. powdered lysine (you may crush tablets)
¼ tsp. Vitamin C powder (you may crush tablets)
¼ cup vegetable glycerin
1 cup water

Prepare wipes by cutting paper towels in quarters. Use white, unfragranced towels that are strong enough to hold up for this use. Fold each piece in quarters again and stack in a plastic zippered baggy. Pour the fluid mixture over the stack and zip. Store a bag full in the freezer to take on car trips. If you want to keep them a month or more, add 1 tbs. grain alcohol or vodka to the recipe.

For bathroom use, dampen a roll of paper towels under the cold tap first. Then pour about ¼ cup of the mixture over the towel roll around the middle. Store in plastic shopping bag or stand in plastic waste basket.

Recipes For Natural Cosmetics

Eye liner and Eyebrow Pencil

Get a pure charcoal pencil (black only) at an art supply store. Try several on yourself (bring a small mirror) in the store to see what hardness suits you. You may need to wet it with water or a vitamin E perle first. Don't put any chemicals on your *eyelids*, since this penetrates into your eye. To check this out for yourself, close your eye tightly and then dab lemon juice on your eyelid. It will soon burn! Everything that is put on skin penetrates. Otherwise the nicotine patch and estrogen patch wouldn't work. Not even soap belongs on your eyelids! Charcoal pencils are cheap. Get yourself half a dozen different kinds so you can do different things.

You could also use a capsule of activated charcoal. Empty it into a saucer. Mix glycerin and water, half and half, and add it to the charcoal powder until you get the consistency you like. Use a brush for eyelashes; use a finger for eyebrows.

Lipstick

Beet root powder (see *Sources*)
100% vegetable glycerin

Combine 1 tsp. vegetable glycerin and 1 tsp. beet root powder in a saucer. Stir until <u>perfectly</u> smooth. Then add ½ tsp. of vitamin E oil. Snip open vitamin E capsules or buy vitamin E oil (see *Sources*). Very thick olive oil can be substituted. Apply liberally with your finger or a lipstick brush. Do not purse or rub your lips together after application. To make the lipstick stay on longer, apply 1 layer of lipstick, then dab some corn starch over the lips, then apply another layer of lipstick. Store in a small glass or plastic container in the refrigerator, tightly covered in a plastic bag.

Face Powder

Use cornstarch from the original box. You may also try arrow root starch or potato starch. Use your fingers or a tissue to apply because applicators can carry bacteria.

Blush (face powder in a cake form)

Add 50% glycerin to cornstarch in a saucer to make a paste. Slowly add beet root powder to the desired color. Use part of a charcoal capsule to darken it, if desired. A drop of food grade alcohol will also darken it. To make 50% glycerin, add equal parts of glycerin and water. Try to make the consistency the same as your brand name product, and you can even put it back in your brand name container.

Recipes For Household Products

Floor Cleaner

Use washing soda from the grocery store. You may add borax and boric acid (to deter insects except ants). Use white distilled vinegar in your rinse water for a natural shine and ant repellent. Do not add bleach to this. For the bathroom floor use plain bleach water—follow the label. Never use chlorine bleach if anybody in the home is ill or suffers from depression. Use grain alcohol (1 pint to 3 quarts water) for germ killing action instead of chlorine.

Furniture Duster and Window Cleaner

Mix equal parts white distilled vinegar and water. Put it in a spray bottle.

Furniture Polish

A few drops of olive oil on a dampened cloth. Use filtered water to dampen.

Insect Killer

Boric acid powder (not borax). Throw liberal amounts behind stove, refrigerator, under carpets and in carpets. Since boric acid is white, you must be careful not to mistake it for sugar accidentally. Keep it far away from food and out of children's reach. Buy it at a farm supply or garden store (or see *Sources*). It will not kill ants.

Ant Repellent

Spray 50% white distilled vinegar on counter tops, window sills and shelves and wipe, leaving residue. Start early in spring before they arrive, because it takes a few weeks to rid yourself of them once they are established. If you want immediate action, get some lemons, cut the yellow outer peel off and cover with grain alcohol in a tightly closed jar. Let stand at least one hour. Use 1 part of this concentrate with 9 parts water in a spray bottle. Mix only as much as you will use because the diluted form loses potency. Spray walls, floors, carpets wherever you see them. The lemon solution even leaves a shine on your counters. Use both vinegar and lemon approaches to rid yourself of ants.

To treat the **whole house**, pour vinegar all around your foundation, close to the wall, using one gallon for every five feet. Expect to damage any foliage it touches. Reapply every six months.

Flower and Foliage Spray

Food-grade hydrogen peroxide. See instructions on bottle.

Moth Balls

I found this recipe in an old recipe book. Mix the following and scatter in trunks and bags containing furs and woolens: ½ lb. each rosemary and mint, ¼ lb. each tansy and thyme, 2 tbs. powdered cloves.

Carpet Cleaner

Whether you rent a machine or have a cleaning service, don't use the carpet shampoo they want to sell, even if they "guarantee" that it is all natural and safe. Instead add these to a bucket (about four gallons) of water and use it as the cleaning solution:

Wash water	Rinse water
1/3 cup borax	¼ cup grain alcohol
	2 tsp. boric acid
	¼ cup white distilled vinegar **or**
	4 tsp. citric acid

Borax does the cleaning; alcohol disinfects, boric acid leaves a pesticide residue, and the vinegar or citric acid give luster. If you are just making one pass on your carpet, use the borax, alcohol, and boric acid. Remember to test everything you use on an unnoticed piece of carpet first.

Health Improvement Recipes

Black Walnut Hull Tincture

This new recipe is four times as strong as the previous one, so it is called **Black Walnut Hull Tincture Extra Strength**.

Your largest enamel or ceramic (not stainless steel, not aluminum) cooking pot, preferably at least 10 quarts
Black walnuts, in the hull, each one still at least 50% green, enough to fill the pot to the top
Grain alcohol, about 50% strength, enough to cover the walnuts
½ tsp. vitamin C
Plastic wrap or cellophane
Glass jars or bottles

The black walnut tree produces large green balls in fall. The walnut is inside, but we will use the whole ball, uncracked, since the active ingredient is in the green outer hull.

Rinse the walnuts carefully, put them in the pot, and cover with the alcohol. Sprinkle on half the vitamin C. Seal with plastic wrap and cover. Let sit for three days. Pour into glass jars or bottles, discarding walnuts, and divide the remaining vitamin C amongst the jars. If the glass jar has a metal lid, first put plastic wrap over the top before screwing on the lid. Potency is strong for several years if unopened, <u>even if it darkens</u>.

You have just made <u>Extra Strength</u> Black Walnut Hull Tincture. It is stronger than the concentrate made with just a few black walnuts in a quart jar (my earlier recipe), because there are more walnuts per unit liquid. In addition, you will not dilute it before use (although when you take it, it will usually be in water).

543

When preparing the walnuts, rinse only with cold tap water. You may need to use a brush on areas with dirt. If you are not going to use all of them in this batch, you may freeze them in a resealable plastic bag. Simply refrigerating them does not keep them from turning black and useless. The pot of soaking walnuts should not be refrigerated. Nor does the final tincture need any refrigeration.

Exposure to air does cause the tincture to darken and lose potency. To reduce air exposure, fill the pot as much as possible, without touching the plastic wrap, while still keeping a snug fitting lid. Even more importantly, the glass jars or bottles you use to store your tincture should have as little air space as possible, without touching the plastic wrap on top. A large jar should be divided into smaller ones when you are ready to use it. The idea is not to have partial jars, with a lot of air space, sitting for longer than a month or so.

There are several ways to make a 50% grain alcohol solution. Some states have Everclear,™ 95% alcohol. Mix this half and half with water. Other states have Everclear that is 76.5% alcohol. Mix this three parts Everclear to one part water. Yet another method is to buy vodka that is 100 proof. This is already 50% alcohol.

Remember, never use any kind of purchased water to make tincture.

Black Walnut Hull Tincture (Regular Strength)

This is the potency I used originally. It is included here in case you prefer it or wish to treat a pet. The Extra Strength recipe is four times as potent as the original recipe, so it must be diluted in quarters. (Similarly, if you have a lot of the Regular Strength left and want to use it in place of Extra Strength, simply take four times as much.)

Black Walnut Hull Tincture Extra Strength
Grain Alcohol, about 10%

Mix one part extra strength tincture with three parts of the 10% alcohol. Store in glass containers same as described above.

There are several ways to make a 10% grain alcohol solution. Some states have Everclear,™ 95% alcohol. Mix this one part Everclear to nine parts water. Other states have Everclear that is 76.5% alcohol. Mix this one part Everclear to seven parts water. Yet another method is to buy vodka that is 100 proof (50% alcohol) and mix one part vodka with four parts water.

Black Walnut Hull Extract (Water Based)

Because you do not know how commercially available extracts were made, and may not be able to test for solvent pollution, it is wisest to make it yourself!

This recipe is intended for alcoholic persons: cover the green balls in the 10 quart (non-metal) pot with cold tap water. Heat to boiling, covered. Turn off heat. When cool, add vitamin C, cover with plastic wrap, and the lid. Let stand for 1 day. It will be darker than the tincture. Do not dilute. Pour into freezable containers. Refrigerate what you will use in two days and freeze the rest. Add vitamin C after thawing or during refrigeration (¼ tsp. per quart).

For use: in programs calling for Extra Strength Black Walnut Hull Tincture use four times as much of this water based recipe (8 tsp. instead of 2 tsp. Extra Strength).

Important Note: do not use bottled or purchased water to make this tincture or you could pollute it with benzene!

Quassia recipe

Add 1/8 cup quassia chips to 3 cups water. Simmer 20-30 minutes. Pour off 1/8 cup now and drink it fresh. Refrigerate remainder. Drink 1/8 cup 4 times/day, until a total of ½ cup of chips is consumed. Flavor with spices.

Emmenagogue (Menstrual Period Inducer)

Here are four herbs that can each bring on your period. They can be started anytime but the most effective time is before your next calculated period time (count days as if you never missed a period).

1 oz sassafras bark
1 oz rue (cut)
1 oz marjoram herb
1 oz blue cohosh root
4½ cups boiling water

Add the herbs to the boiling water and turn down to simmer, covered, for 20 minutes. Do not boil. Strain and refrigerate in sterile glass jar. Pour one cup for yourself in the morning. Let warm to room temperature, and sip between meals, making it last until supper.

Bowel Program

Bacteria are always at the root of bowel problems, such as pain, bloating and gassiness. They can not be killed by zapping, because the high frequency current does not penetrate the bowel contents.

Although most bowel bacteria are beneficial, the ones that are not, like *Salmonellas* and *Shigellas*, are extremely detrimental because they have the ability to invade the rest of your body and colonize a trauma site or weakened organ. These same bacteria colonize a cancer tumor and delay healing after the malignancy is stopped.

Another reason bowel bacteria are so hard to eradicate is that we are constantly reinfecting ourselves by keeping a reservoir on our hands and under our fingernails.

- So the first thing to do is **improve sanitation**. For a serious problem, use 50% grain alcohol (100 proof vodka) in a spray bottle at the bathroom sink. Sterilize your hands after bathroom use and before meals.
- Secondly use **turmeric** (2 capsules 3 times a day, this is the common spice) which I find helps against *Shigella*, as well as *E. coli*. Expect orange colored stool.
- Third use **fennel** (1 capsule 3 times a day).
- Fourth use **digestive enzyme tablets** with meals as directed on the bottle. (But only as long as necessary, because these frequently harbor molds.)
- Fifth use a single 2 tsp. dose of **Black Walnut Hull Tincture Extra Strength**. Add it to a ½ glass of water and sip over a 15 minute period. Stay seated until any side effect from the alcohol wears off.
- Sixth take **Cascara sagrada** capsules if constipated (start with one capsule a day, use up to maximum on label). Remember to drink a cup of hot water upon rising in the morning. This will begin to regulate your elimination.

It can take all six to get rid of a bad *Shigella* problem in a week. Afterward, you must continue to eat only sterile dairy products. Note that the Kidney Cleanse is often effective with bowel problems. Try it also.

You will know you succeeded when your tummy is flat, there is not a single gurgle, and your mood improves!

Constipation Tea

Constipation is often caused by *E. coli* and *Salmonella* from dairy foods, or from killing "good" bowel bacteria with antibiotics (killing a few by zapping actually <u>restores</u> good flora). Eat foods that restore the body's good bowel flora: vegetables, sterilized milk (the milk sugar is essential), lots of water.

There are a lot of remedies for constipation, but many people enjoy this tea:

1 tbs senna tea leaves
½ tsp. mint leaves

Boil for one minute in a quart of water, add a dash of vitamin C and brown sugar to taste. Sip through the day to avoid "belly-ache". It can take years for the body's flora to "right themselves" after an antibiotic session, be patient.

Weight Reduction

Here are two ancient herbal recipes for obesity. I have not personally determined their effectiveness.

Fucus
2 oz *Fucus vesiculosus*, cut (see *Sources*)
3 cups cold tap water
Boil for 15 minutes, covered. Cool. Dose: ¼ cup four times a day on an empty stomach. After one week increase dose to ½ cup. You may add any flavoring desired.

Watch the pot carefully as it comes to a boil. If it boils over, you will have a month of stove-cleaning to do. The odor of *Fucus* boiling is wretched. So is the taste. Maybe garlic (fresh) would improve it.

Fennel
1 oz fennel seed (crushed or powdered is fine)

3 cups cold tap water

Boil water, pour over herb. Steep 30 minutes. Strain. Add 4 oz honey (optional). Drink one cup each day.

You could take them both together, along with the Bowel Program, to be more successful, but the best single weight reducer is the Liver Cleanse.

Kidney Cleanse

½ cup dried Hydrangea root
½ cup Gravel root
½ cup Marshmallow root
4 bunches of fresh parsley
Goldenrod tincture (leave this out of the recipe if you are allergic to it)
Ginger capsules
Uva Ursi capsules
Vegetable glycerin
Black Cherry Concentrate, 8 oz
Vitamin B6, 250 mg
Magnesium oxide tablets, 300 mg

Measure ¼ cup of each root and set them to soak, together in 10 cups of cold tap water, using a non-metal container and a non-metal lid (a dinner plate will do). After four hours (or overnight) add 8 oz. black cherry concentrate, heat to boiling and simmer for 20 minutes. Drink ¼ cup as soon as it is cool enough. Pour the rest through a bamboo strainer into a sterile pint jar (glass) and several freezable containers. Refrigerate the glass jar.

Boil the fresh parsley, after rinsing, in 1 quart of water for 3 minutes. Drink ¼ cup when cool enough. Refrigerate a pint and freeze 1 pint. Throw away the parsley.

Dose: each morning, pour together ¾ cup of the root mixture and ½ cup parsley water, filling a large mug. Add 20 drops of goldenrod tincture and 1 tbs. of glycerin. Drink this mixture in divided doses throughout the day. Keep cold. <u>Do not drink it all at once</u> or you will get a stomach ache and feel pressure in your bladder. If your stomach is very sensitive, start on half this dose.

Save the roots after the first boiling, storing them in the freezer. After 13 days when your supply runs low, boil the same roots a second time, but add only 6 cups water and simmer only 10 minutes. This will last another 8 days, for a total of three weeks. You may cook the roots a third time if you wish, but the recipe gets less potent. If your problem is severe, only cook them twice.

After three weeks, repeat with fresh herbs. You need to do the Kidney Cleanse for six weeks to get good results, longer for severe problems.

Also take:

- Ginger capsules: one with each meal (3/day).
- Uva Ursi capsules: one with breakfast and two with supper.
- Vitamin B6 (250 mg): one a day.
- Magnesium oxide (300 mg): one a day.

Take these supplements just before your meal to avoid burping.

Some notes on this recipe: this herbal tea, as well as the parsley, can easily spoil. Heat it to boiling every fourth day if it is being stored in the refrigerator; this resterilizes it. If you sterilize it in the morning you may take it to work without refrigerating it (use a glass container).

When you order your herbs, be careful! Herb companies are not the same! These roots should have a strong fragrance. If the ones you buy are barely fragrant, they have lost their active ingredients; switch to a different supplier. Fresh roots can be used. Do not use powder.

- Hydrangea (*Hydrangea arborescens*) is a common flowering bush.
- Gravel root (*Eupatorium purpureum*) is a wild flower.
- Marshmallow root (*Althea officinallis*) is mucilaginous and kills pain.
- Fresh parsley can be bought at a grocery store. Parsley flakes and dried parsley herb do <u>not</u> work.
- Goldenrod herb works as well as the tincture but you may get an allergic reaction from smelling the herb. If you know you are allergic to this, leave this one out of your recipe.
- Ginger from the grocery store works fine; you may put it into capsules for yourself (size 0, 1 or 00).

There are probably dozens of herbs that can dissolve kidney crystals and stones. If you can only find several of those in the recipe, make the recipe anyway; it will just take longer to get results. Remember that vitamin B_6 and magnesium, taken daily, can prevent oxalate stones from forming. But only if you stop drinking tea. Tea has 15.6 mg oxalic acid per cup[37]. A tall glass of iced tea could give you over 20 mg oxalic acid. Switch to herb teas. Cocoa and chocolate, also, have too much oxalic acid to be used as beverages.

Remember, too, that phosphate crystals are made when you eat too much phosphate. Phosphate levels are high in meats, breads, cereals, pastas, and carbonated drinks. Eat less of these, and increase your milk (2%), fruits and vegetables. Drink at least 2 pints of water a day.

---

[37] Taken from *Food Values* 14ed by Pennington and Church 1985.

Cleanse your kidneys at least twice a year.

You can dissolve all your kidney stones in 3 weeks, but make new ones in 3 days if you are drinking tea and cocoa and phosphated beverages. None of the beverage recipes in this chapter are conducive to stone formation.

Liver Herbs

Don't confuse these liver herbs with the next recipe for the Liver Cleanse. This recipe contains herbs traditionally used to help the liver function, while the Liver Cleanse gets gallstones out.

6 parts comfrey root, *Symphytum officinale* (also called nipbone root)
6 parts tanner's oak bark, *Quercus alba* (white oak bark)
3 parts gravel root, *Eupatorium purpureum* (queen of the meadow)
3 parts Jacob's staff, *Verbascum thapsus* (mullein herb)
2 parts licorice root, *Glycyrrhiza glabra*
2 parts wild yam root, *Dioscorea villosa*
2 parts milk thistle herb, *Silybum marianum*
3 parts walnut bark, *Juglans nigra*, (black walnut bark)
3 parts marshmallow root, *Althea officinalis* (white mallow)
1 part lobelia plant, *Lobelia inflata* (bladder pod)
1 part skullcap, *Scutellaria lateriflora* (helmet flower)

Mix all the herbs. Add ½ cup of the mixture to 2 quarts of water. Bring to a boil. Put lid on. Let sit for six hours. Strain and drink 1½ cups per day. Put the strained herbs in the freezer and use them one more time.

Liver Cleanse

Cleansing the liver of gallstones dramatically improves digestion, which is the basis of your whole health. You can expect your allergies to disappear, too, more with each cleanse you do! Incredibly, it also eliminates shoulder, upper arm, and upper back pain. You have more energy and increased sense of well being.

Cleaning the liver bile ducts is the most powerful procedure that you can do to improve your body's health.

But it should not be done before the parasite program, and for best results should follow the kidney cleanse and any dental work you need.

It is the job of the liver to make bile, 1 to 1½ quarts in a day! The liver is full of tubes (*biliary tubing*) that deliver the bile to one large tube (the *common bile duct*). The gallbladder is attached to the common bile duct and acts as a storage reservoir. Eating fat or protein triggers the gallbladder to squeeze itself empty after about twenty minutes, and the stored bile finishes its trip down the common bile duct to the intestine.

For many persons, including children, the biliary tubing is choked with gallstones. Some develop allergies or hives but some have no symptoms. When the gallbladder is scanned or X-rayed nothing is seen. Typically, they are not in the gallbladder. Not only that, most are too small and not calcified, a prerequisite for visibility on X-ray. There are over half a dozen varieties of gallstones, most of which have cholesterol crystals in them. They can be black, red, white, green or tan colored. The green ones get their color from being coated with bile. Notice in the picture how many have imbedded unidentified objects. Are they fluke remains? Notice how many are shaped like corks with longitudinal grooves below the tops. We can visualize the blocked bile ducts from such shapes. Other stones are composites–made of many smaller ones–showing that they regrouped in the bile ducts some time after the last cleanse.

At the very center of each stone is found a clump of bacteria, according to scientists, suggesting a dead bit of parasite might have started the stone forming.

As the stones grow and become more numerous the back pressure on the liver causes it to make less bile. Imagine the situation if your garden hose had marbles in it. Much less water would flow, which in turn would decrease the ability of the hose to squirt out the marbles. <u>With gallstones, much less cholesterol leaves the body, and cholesterol levels may rise.</u>

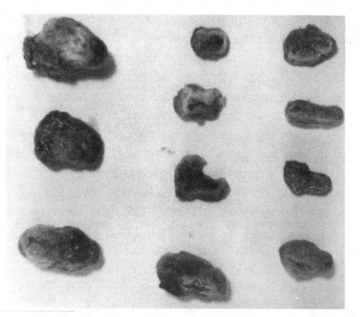

Fig. 89 These are gallstones.

Gallstones, being porous, can pick up all the bacteria, cysts, viruses and parasites that are passing through the liver. In this way "nests" of infection are formed, forever supplying the body with fresh bacteria. No stomach infection such as ulcers or intestinal bloating can be cured permanently without removing these gallstones from the liver.

Cleanse your liver twice a year.

Preparation.

- You can't clean a liver with living parasites in it. You won't get many stones, and you will feel quite sick. <u>Zap daily the week before, or get through the first three weeks of the parasite killing program before attempting a liver cleanse.</u> If you are on the maintenance parasite program, you are always ready to do the cleanse.

- Completing the kidney cleanse before cleansing the liver is also <u>highly recommended</u>. You want your kidneys, bladder and urinary tract in top working condition so they can efficiently remove any undesirable substances incidentally absorbed from the intestine as the bile is being excreted.

- Do any dental work first, if possible. Your mouth should be metal free and bacteria free (cavitations are cleaned). A toxic mouth can put a heavy load on the liver, burdening it immediately after cleansing. Eliminate that problem first for best results.

Ingredients

Epsom salts	4 tablespoons
Olive oil	half cup (light olive oil is easier to get down)
Fresh pink grapefruit	1 large or 2 small, enough to squeeze 2/3 to 3/4 cup juice

Ornithine	4 to 8, to be sure you can sleep. Don't skip this or you may have the worst night of your life!
Large plastic straw	To help drink potion.
Pint jar with lid	

Choose a day like Saturday for the cleanse, since you will be able to rest the next day.

Take no medicines, vitamins or pills that you can do without; they could prevent success. Stop the parasite program and kidney herbs, too, the day before.

Eat a no-fat breakfast and lunch such as cooked cereal with fruit, fruit juice, bread and preserves or honey (no butter or milk), baked potato or other vegetables with salt only. This allows the bile to build up and develop pressure in the liver. Higher pressure pushes out more stones.

2:00 PM. Do not eat or drink after 2 o'clock. If you break this rule you could feel quite ill later.

Get your Epsom salts ready. Mix 4 tbs. in 3 cups water and pour this into a jar. This makes four servings, ¾ cup each. Set the jar in the refrigerator to get ice cold (this is for convenience and taste only).

6:00 PM. Drink one serving (¾ cup) of the ice cold Epsom salts. If you did not prepare this ahead of time, mix 1 tbs. in ¾ cup water now. You may add 1/8 tsp. vitamin C powder to improve the taste. You may also drink a few mouthfuls of water afterwards or rinse your mouth.

Get the olive oil and grapefruit out to warm up.

8:00 PM. Repeat by drinking another ¾ cup of Epsom salts.

You haven't eaten since two o'clock, but you won't feel hungry. Get your bedtime chores done. The timing is critical for success; don't be more than 10 minutes early or late.

9:45 PM. Pour ½ cup (measured) olive oil into the pint jar. Squeeze the grapefruit by hand into the measuring cup. Remove pulp with fork. You should have at least ½ cup, more (up to ¾ cup) is best. You may top it up with lemonade. Add this to the olive oil. Close the jar tightly with the lid and shake hard until watery (only fresh grapefruit juice does this).

Now visit the bathroom one or more times, even if it makes you late for your ten o'clock drink. Don't be more than 15 minutes late.

10:00 PM. Drink the potion you have mixed. Take 4 ornithine capsules with the first sips to make sure you will sleep through the night. Take 8 if you already suffer from insomnia. Drinking through a large plastic straw helps it go down easier. You may use ketchup, cinnamon, or brown sugar to chase it down between sips. Take it to your bedside if you want, but drink it standing up. Get it down within 5 minutes (fifteen minutes for very elderly or weak persons).

Lie down immediately. You might fail to get stones out if you don't. The sooner you lie down the more stones you will get out. Be ready for bed ahead of time. Don't clean up the kitchen. As soon as the drink is down walk to your bed and lie down flat on your back with your head up high on the pillow. Try to think about what is happening in the liver. Try to keep perfectly still for at least 20 minutes. You may feel a train of stones traveling along the bile ducts like marbles. There is no pain because the bile duct valves are open (thank you Epsom salts!). **Go to sleep,** you may fail to get stones out if you don't.

Next morning. Upon awakening take your third dose of Epsom salts. If you have indigestion or nausea wait until it is gone before drinking the Epsom salts. You may go back to bed. Don't take this potion before 6:00 am.

2 Hours Later. Take your fourth (the last) dose of Epsom salts. Drink ¾ cup of the mixture. You may go back to bed.

After 2 More Hours you may eat. Start with fruit juice. Half an hour later eat fruit. One hour later you may eat regular food but keep it light. By supper you should feel recovered.

How well did you do? Expect diarrhea in the morning. Use a flashlight to look for gallstones in the toilet with the bowel movement. Look for the green kind since this is <u>proof</u> that they are genuine gallstones, not food residue. Only bile from the liver is pea green. The bowel movement sinks but gallstones float because of the cholesterol inside. <u>Count them all roughly</u>, whether tan or green. You will need to total 2000 stones before the liver is clean enough to rid you of allergies or bursitis or upper back pains <u>permanently</u>. The first cleanse may rid you of them for a few days, but as the stones from the rear travel forward, they give you the same symptoms again. You may repeat cleanses at two week intervals. Never cleanse when you are ill.

Sometimes the bile ducts are full of cholesterol crystals that did not form into round stones. They appear as a "chaff" floating on top of the toilet bowl water. It may be tan colored, harboring millions of tiny white crystals. Cleansing this chaff is just as important as purging stones.

How safe is the liver cleanse? It is very safe. My opinion is based on over 500 cases, including many persons in their seventies and eighties. None went to the hospital; none even reported pain. However it can make you feel quite ill for one or two days afterwards, although in every one of these cases the maintenance parasite program had been neglected. This is why the instructions direct you to complete the parasite and kidney rinse programs first.

CONGRATULATIONS

You have taken out your gallstones <u>without surgery</u>! I like to think I have perfected this recipe, but I certainly can not take credit for its origin. It was invented hundreds, if not thousands, of years ago, THANK YOU, HERBALISTS!

This procedure contradicts many modern medical viewpoints. Gallstones are thought to be formed in the gallbladder, not the liver. They are thought to be few, not thousands. They are not linked to pains other than gallbladder attacks. It is easy to understand why this is thought: by the time you have acute pain attacks, some stones <u>are</u> in the gallbladder, <u>are</u> big enough and sufficiently calcified to see on X-ray, and <u>have</u> caused inflammation there. When the gallbladder is removed the acute attacks are gone, but the bursitis and other pains and digestive problems remain.

The truth is self-evident. People who have had their gallbladder surgically removed still get plenty of green, bile-coated stones, and anyone who cares to dissect their stones can see that the concentric circles and crystals of cholesterol match textbook pictures of "gallstones" exactly.

Lugol's Iodine Solution

It is too dangerous to buy a commercially prepared solution. It is certain to be polluted with propyl alcohol or wood alcohol. Make it yourself or ask your pharmacist to make it up for you. The recipe to make 1 liter (quart) is:

44 gm (1½ ounces) iodine, granular
88 gm (3 ounces) potassium iodide, granular

Dissolve the potassium iodide in about a pint of the water. Then add the iodine crystals and fill to the liter mark with water. It takes about 1 day to dissolve completely. Shake it from time to time. Keep out of sight and reach of children. <u>Do not use if allergic to iodine.</u> Be careful to avoid bottled water for preparation.

Vitamin D Drops

1 gram cholecalciferol (see Sources)
10 cups olive oil

Mix in a non-metal container. It may take a day of standing to dissolve fully. Refrigerate. Ten <u>drops</u> contain 40,000 iu. Use within a year.

Pathogen Frequencies

Living creatures emit a range of frequencies, also called *bandwidth*. As they age, the bandwidth shrinks. When they die, sometimes all that is left is a single frequency.

Most of the organisms listed below are dead on commercially available and prepared slides (see *Sources* for biological supply companies). However they still exhibit a 5 KHz bandwidth, probably due to testing with a frequency generator that was only accurate to 100 Hz, and also due to using more voltage than necessary (like when a powerful radio station comes in at its own frequencies and ones nearby, too). Some testing was done with a more accurate frequency generator at a lower power level so some bandwidths are reported much more narrowly.

If the same person retests the same specimens with the same equipment within a few days, the results will be absolutely identical (within 1 Hz) 90% of the time. Why a few of the results will not be identical is not known. However different people, and even the same person at different times of the year, can notice that the perceived frequencies shift by as much as 3 KHz (still less than 1% change).

Some specimens have more than one range listed; this may be characteristic of the organism or may be due to having an undocumented organism on the same microscope slide.

Blank locations represent organisms for whom there are prepared slides available, but whose bandwidth has not been determined.

Bandwidth Of Organism Families

In general, the smaller the organism the lower the frequency and narrower the bandwidth. This chart shows the major families studied and where they fall in the spectrum.

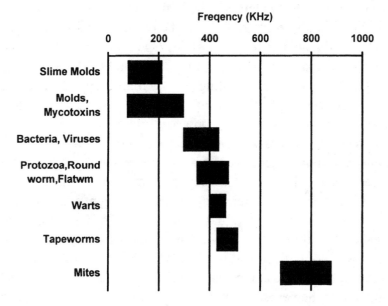

Fig. 90 Chart of bandwidths for organism families.

Mold, Mold Toxin Frequencies

Other molds and mold toxins	KHz
Aflatoxin	177,188
Cytochalasin B	77,91
Ergot	295
Griseofulvin	288
Sorghum syrup	277
Sterigmatocystin	88,96,133,126
Zearalenone	100

Slime Molds	KHz
Argyria	81
Lycogala	126
Stemonitis	211

Bacteria and Viruses

Including locations where I commonly found them.

	Low Freq (KHz)	High Freq (KHz)	Use freq gen for 3 min @
Acetobacter aceti			
Adenovirus	393	393	393
Adenovirus (2nd range)	371.45	386.90	
Agrobacterium tumefaciens			
Alcaligenes faecalis			
Alpha streptococcus	369.75	385.4	380,375
Azobacter chroococcum			
Bacillus anthracis causes anthrax in cattle (tooth)	393.5	398.05	395,364,368
Bacillus anthracis (2nd range)	363.2	365.3	
Bacillus anthracis (3rd range)	359.4	370.5	
Bacillus anthracis spores	391.45	386.95	388
Bacillus cereus	373.65	375.85	374.5
Bacillus megaterium			
Bacillus sterothermophilus			
Bacillus subtilis spores			
Bacillus subtilis var. niger	371.85	387.1	385,380,375
Bacteria capsules (capsular strain)	416.05	418.75	417.5
Bacterial capsules	362.4	357.6	360
Bacteroides fragilis found with common roundworm Ascaris	324.3	325.0	325
Bacteroides fragilis (2nd range)	325.7	326.0	
Beta streptococcus (tooth)	380.6	387.4	385
Blepharisma	405.65	407.45	406.5
Bordetella pertussis "whooping cough" (tooth)	329.85	332.25	331
Borellia burgdorferi Lyme disease	378.95	382.0	380
Branhamella (Neisseria) catarrhalis (has hole at 398)	394.9	396.7	396
Brucella abortus			
Cabbage Black Rot			
Campylobacter fetus smear	365.3	370.6	368
Campylobacter pyloridis	352.0	357.2	355
Candida albicans (pure powder) common yeast	384.2	388.4	386
Caulobacter vibrioides			
Central spores (bacillus smear)	372.45	378.65	376
Chlamydia trachomatis	379.7	383.95	381
Clostridium acetobutylicum	382.8	391.15	389,384
Clostridium botulinum (tooth) causes food poisoning	361.0	364.55	362

Clostridium perfringens			
Clostridium perfringens spores	394.2	398.1	396
Clostridium septicum	362.05	365.6	364
Clostridium sporogenes			
Clostridium tetani (tooth) causes tetanus			
Corynebacterium diptheriae (tooth) causes diphtheria	340	344	342
Corynebacterium pseudodiphthericum			
Corynebacterium xerosis	315.65	316.8	316.0
Coxsackie virus B-1 found with Bacteroides fragilis	360.5	366.1	364
Coxsackie virus B-4 found with Bacteroides fragilis	361.45	363.7	362.5
Coxsackie virus B-4 (2nd range)	363.9	364.9	
Crithidia fasciculata			
Cytomegalovirus (CMV) antigen	408.35	410.75	409
Cytophaga rubra	428.1	432.2	430
Diplococcus diphtheriae	357.95	364.0	361
Diplococcus pneumoniae	351.65	368.45	365,360
Eikanella corrodens	379.5	384.3	382
Enterobacter aerogenes intestinal bacterium	374	374	374
Epstein Barre virus (EBV)	372.5	382.85	380,375
Erwinia amylovora	347.2	352.1	350
Erwinia carotovora	368.1	377.0	373
Escherichia coli (E. coli) intestinal bacterium	356	356	356,393
Escherichia coli (E. coli) (2nd range)	392	393	
Gaffkya tetragena causes respiratory infections	344.85	352.5	350
Gardnerella vaginalis ovarian and genital tract infection	338.0	342.55	340
Haemophilus influenzae bacterial meningitis, infects joints	336.41	336.41	336
Hepatitis B antigen	414.55	420.8	418
Herpes simplex 1	291.25	293.05	292,345.5
Herpes simplex 1 (2nd range)	345.35	345.75	
Herpes simplex 2 (fresh smear)	353.9	362.9	360,355
Herpes Zoster "shingles"	416.6	420.2	418
Histomonas meleagridis (liver)	376.55	378.7	377
Histoplasma capsulatum	298.3	304.85	302
HIV	365	365	365
Influenza A and B (flu shot)	313.35	323.9	320,315
Iron Bacterium Sphaerotilus			
Klebsiella pneumoniae causes pneumonia	398.45	404.65	401,419
Klebsiella pneumoniae (2nd range)	416.9	421.9	
Lactobacillus acidophilus (tooth)	346.05	351.65	349

Leptospira interrogans spirochete	397.05	401.1	399
Lumpy Jaw			
Measles antigen	369.5	373.0	371
Micrococcus luteus			
Micrococcus roseus			
Mumps antigen	377.6	384.65	382
Mycobacterium para TB			
Mycobacterium phlei	409.65	410.65	410.0
Mycobacterium smegmatis			
Mycobacterium tuberculosis (infec nodule) causes tuberculosis	430.55	434.2	432
Mycoplasma	322.85	323.9	323.5,346
Mycoplasma (range 2)	342.75	349.3	
Neisseria gonorrhea causes gonorrhea	333.85	336.5	334
Neisseria sicca			
Nocardia asteroides found in Parkinson's Disease	354.95	355.35	355.1,368
Norcardia asteroides (2nd range)	363.7	370	
Propionobacterium acnes	383.75	389.0	387
Proteus mirabilis	320.55	326.0	324,349
Proteus mirabilis (2nd range)	345.95	352.1	
Proteus vulgaris urinary tract pathogen	408.75	416.45	413,336,328
Proteus vulgaris (2nd range)	333.75	339.15	
Proteus vulgaris (3rd range)	327.2	329.5	
Pseudomonas aeruginosa found in open wounds	331.25	334.6	333
Pseudomonas fluorescens			
Respiratory syncytial virus	378.95	383.15	380
Rhizobium leguminosarum			
Salmonella enteriditis intestinal infection	329	329	329
Salmonella paratyphi	365.05	370.1	368,385
Salmonella typhimurium food poisoning, nervousness, apathy	382.3	386.55	355,386,390
Serratia marcescens	349.45	352.1	351
Shigella dysenteriae intestinal problems	390.089	390.089	390.089
Shigella flexneri depression	394	394	394
Shigella sonnei invades tumors	318	318	318
Sphaerotilus natans	388.4	393.45	391
Spirillum itersonil			
Spirillum serpens	378.35	382.8	380
Spirillum sinuosum			
Spirillum volutans			
Spores in bacteria spore stain			
Staphylococcus aureus (culture)	376.27	380.85	
Staphylococcus aureus (slide) source is tooth infection, causes abscesses, heart disease, invades tumors	381	381	378,381

Staphylococcus epidermidis infects skin and mucous membranes			
Streptococcus lactis occurs in milk	382	387	385
Streptococcus mitis lung infection, tooth infection, abscesses, causes stiff knees	313.8	321.1	318
Streptococcus pneumoniae causes pneumonia and inner ear disease	366.85	370.2	368
Streptococcus pyogenes (tooth)	360.5	375.3	373
Streptococcus sp. group G (tooth)	368.15	368.85	368
Sub terminal spores bac. smear	385.15	385.95	
Terminal spores bacillus smear			
Tobacco mosaic virus (tobacco)	427.15	429.55	428
Treponema pallidum causes syphilis	346.85	347.4	347
Troglodytella abrassari	377.75	385.2	383,419
Troglodytella abrassari (2nd range)	416.9	422.2	
Veillonella dispar	401.75	405.2	403
Vibrio (photobacterium) fischeri			

Roundworms, Flatworms, One-celled Animals

	Low Freq (KHz)	High Freq (KHz)	To kill, use freq. gen for 3 min. at these frequencies
Acanthamoeba culbertsoni			
Acanthocephala			
Anaplasma marginale	386.4	388.0	387,422
Anaplasma marginale (2nd range)	415.3	424	
Ancylostoma braziliense (adult)	397.6	403.25	401
Ancylostoma caninum	383.1	402.9	400,393,386
Ancylostoma duodenale male			
Anguillula aceti			
Ascaris larvae in lung common roundworm of cats and dogs	404.9	409.15	408
Ascaris lumbricoides (m and f)			same
Ascaris megalocephala (male)	403.85	409.7	408
Babesia bigemina			
Babesia canis smear			
Balantidium coli cysts	458.8	462.9	460
Balantidium sp. trophozoites (from guinea pig) parasitic ciliate			
Besnoitia (lung sect.) protozoan	352.8	361.4	358

Capillaria hepatica (liver sect.)	424.25	430.65	428
Chilomastix cysts (rat)	388.95	390.7	389,426
Chilomastix cysts (rat) (2nd range)	425.2	427.3	
Chilomastix mesnili (trophozoites)			same
Chilomonas, whole mount	393.75	400	398
Clinostomum metacercaria			
Clonorchis metacercariae			
Clonorchis sinensis	425.7	428.75	427
Clonorchis sinensis eggs			
Cryptocotyle lingua (adult)	409.95	416.0	414
Didinium			
Dientamoeba fragilis	401.35	406.05	404
Dipetalonema perstans (microfilaria human blood)			
Dirofilaria immitis dog heartworm	408.15	411.15	409
Echinoporyphium recurvatum	418.55	423.9	421
Echinostoma revolutum	425.5	429.65	428
Eimeria stiedae			
Eimeria tenella			
Endamoeba gingivalis trophozoite	433.8	441.0	438
Endolimax nana trophozoites and cysts	394.25	397.1	396,432
Endolimax nana trophozoites and cysts (2nd range)	430.5	433.35	
Entamoeba coli cysts			
Entamoeba coli trophozoites	397.0	400.35	398
Entamoeba histolytica trophozoite	381.1	387.8	385
Enterobius vermicularis	420.95	426.3	423
Eurytrema pancreaticum	420.35	422.3	421
Eurytrema pancreaticum stages			
Fasciola hepatica	421.35	427.3	425
Fasciola hepatica cercariae	423.8	430.6	427
Fasciola hepatica eggs	422.0	427.6	425
Fasciola hepatica metacercariae			
Fasciola hepatica miracidia	421.75	424.7	423
Fasciola hepatica rediae	420.6	427.5	425
Fasciolopsis buskii adult	427.7	435.1	434
Fasciolopsis buskii eggs	427.35	435.45	434
Fasciolopsis buskii eggs unincubated			
Fasciolopsis cercariae	429.5	436.25	434
Fasciolopsis miracidia	427.35	435.2	434
Fasciolopsis rediae	427.3	433.0	432
Fischoedrius elongatus	441.75	443.2	442
Gastrothylax elongatus	451.9	457.1	455
Giardia lamblia (trophozoites)	421.4	426.3	424
Giardia lamblia cysts			
Gyrodactylus	378.75	381.8	380
Haemonchus contortus	386.8	395.5	393
Haemoproteus			

Name			
Hasstile sig. tricolor (adult)	448.05	455.1	453
Heterakis			
Hypodereum conoideum	424.45	429.55	427
Iodamoeba butschlii trophozoites and cysts	437.85	448.5	445,402
Iodamoeba butschlii trophozoites and cysts (2nd range)	398.15	404.75	
Leishmania braziliensis	400.05	405.1	403
Leishmania donovani	398.0	402.65	400
Leishmania mexicana	400.2	403.8	402
Leishmania tropica	402.1	407.4	405
Leucocytozoon	397.45	402.55	400
Loa loa	360.551	360.551	361
Macracanthorhynchus	438.85	442.8	440
Metagonimus Yokogawai	437.35	442.1	440
Monocystis agilis			
Myxosoma	409.6	416.95	414
Naegleria fowleri	356.9	364.35	362
Naegleria fowleri (brain sec.)			
Necator americanus (infect larvae)			
Notocotylus quinqeserialis			
Onchocerca volvulus (tumor)	436.3	442.1	440
Paragonimus Westermanii adult	437.8	454.2	452,447
Passalurus ambiguus	428.8	444.15	441,437
Pelomyxa carolinensis			
Plasmodium cynomolgi	417.3	424.5	422
Plasmodium falciparum smear	372.3	373.8	373.0
Plasmodium vivax smear	438.15	445.1	442
Platynosomum fastosum adult			
Pneumocystis carnii (lung)	405.75	409.15	407
Prosthogonimus macrorchis(eggs)	396.85	404.75	401
Sarcina lutea			
Sarcocystis	450.55	454.95	452
Schistosoma haematobium	473	473	473
Schistosoma japonicum eggs			
Schistosoma mansoni	353	353	353
Stephanurus dentalus (ova)	457.35	463.1	461
Stigeoclonium	404.25	415.25	412,407
Strongyloides (filariform larva)	398.4	402.0	400
Strongyloides parasitic females			
Toxocara (eggs)			
Toxoplasma (human strain)	395.0	395.0	395
Trichinella spiralis (muscle)	403.85	405.57	404.5
Trichomonas muris			
Trichomonas vaginalis	378.0	383.6	381
Trichuris sp. (male)	388.3	408.9	406
Trypanosoma brucei	423.2	431.4	429
Trypanosoma cruzi (brain tissue)	460.2	465.65	463

Trypanosoma equiperdum	434.6	451.25	448,442,438
Trypanosoma gambiense	393.75	398.7	396
Trypanosoma lewisi (blood smear)	424.5	426.0	425
Trypanosoma rhodesiense	423.5	428.55	426
Urocleidus	442.35	450.0	447

Wart Frequencies

(Most of these are from homemade slides.)

	Low Freq	High Freq	Use freq gen for 3 min @
Wart BS	402	406	404
Wart CC	426	432.35	430
Wart FR	459.3	464.75	462
Wart HA	434.8	444.1	442,437
Wart HRCm	438.9	448.55	446,441
Wart human papilloma plantar	404.7	406.75	405
Wart human papilloma virus	402.85	410.7	407
Wart JB	418.75	422.4	420
Wart L arm	343.65	345.95	344
Wart papilloma cervix smear	404.05	404.6	404.3

Tapeworms

Tapeworms are segmented. The first segment is the head, called the *scolex*. Tapeworms grow by adding a new segment to their body.

Tapeworms can have very large bandwidths (range of frequencies), and it varies by the length of the specimen! It is as if each new segment has a unique, and slightly lower, frequency.

Do not use a frequency generator to kill tapeworms. If you accidentally kill middle segments instead of working your way up from the bottom, you may conceivably <u>promote</u> dispersion! Use only a zapper.

	Low Freq	High Freq
Cysticercus fasciolaris	436.4	440.05
Diphyllobothrium erinacei (Mansoni) (scolex)	467.25	487.55
Diphyllobothrium erinacei eggs		
Diphyllobothrium latum (scolex)	452.9	472.3
Dipylidium caninum (proglottid composite)	439.55	444.3
Dipylidium caninum (scolex)	451.95	472.15
Echinococcus granulosus	451.6	461.5
Echinococcus granulosus (cysts)	441.15	446.5
Echinococcus granulosus (eggs)		
Echinococcus multilocularis	455.85	458.35
Heterophyes heterophyes		
Hymenolepis cysticercoides	478.0	481.75
Hymenolepis diminuta	445	481.15
Hymenolepis diminuta ova		
Hymenolepis nana eggs		
Moniezia (scolex)	430.35	465.2
Moniezia expansa (composite)	430.35	465.2
Moniezia expansa eggs		
Multiceps serialis	453.6	457.8
Pigeon tapeworm		
Taenia pisiformis (cysticercus)	475.2	482.1
Taenia pisiformis eggs (ova)	465.2	469.7
Taenia saginata (cysticercus)	476.5	481.05
Taenia saginata eggs		
Taenia solium (cysticercus)	475	475
Taenia solium (scolex)	444.0	448.9
Taenia solium eggs		

Mite Frequencies

These are the organisms that cold viruses ride in with!

Mite	KHz
Demodex folliculorum folicle mite	682
Dermatophagoides dust mite	707
Meal mite	718
Ornithonyssus bird mite	877,878
Sarcoptes scabei itch	735

Miscellaneous Frequencies

	KHz
Blue-green Algae	256
Bryozoa cristatalla	396
Mucor mucedo	288
Rhizobium meliloti	330
Rotifer	1151

It's easy to make homemade slides when you or a family member is ill. Finding out the frequencies of these illnesses helps you identify them (use the Pathogen Frequency Chart) and also lets you know if you are chronically getting them back.

Unidentified pathogens	Low Freq	High Freq
A cold virus HRC	395.8	395.8
Fungus EW	362.0	364.9
Fungus JWB	397.2	400.75
Tooth decay	384.3	387.2
Tooth decay (N)	367.9	375.05
Tooth decay (N) (2nd range)	326.95	331.5
Tooth decay (N) (3rd range)	293.2	297.4
Tooth plaque I	378.8	383.05
Tooth plaque I (2nd range)	294.7	298.25
Tooth plaque I (3rd range)	233.1	238.2
Tooth plaque II	384.95	387.05
Tooth plaque II (2nd range)	278.75	284
Tooth plaque II (3rd range)	212.15	218
Tooth plaque II (4th range)	340.15	344.8
Tooth plaque II (5th range)	305.5	310.35

Toxic Elements

Although not living, solvents and toxins must exhibit characteristic frequencies, otherwise how could the Syncrometer detect specific ones? This needs further exploration.

Most of the toxic elements I use are metals, heavy metals and lanthanides. But some are not; examples are PCBs and formaldehyde.

Some important elements are missing, like iron, zinc and manganese. This is because I never could find them present in the white blood cells, and I finally gave up searching for them.

Below is a list of the 70 or so toxic elements I use. Most of them were obtained as Atomic Absorption Standard Solutions and are, therefore, very pure. This prevents mistakes in identifying a toxin. They were stored in ½ ounce amber glass bottles with bakelite caps and permanently sealed with plastic film since testing did not require them to be opened (they get close enough to the frequency field). The exact concentration and the solubility characteristics are not important in this qualitative test. The main sources of these substances in our environment are given beside each item.

Toxic Substance	Sources
Aflatoxin B	beer, bread, apple cider vinegar, moldy fruit, nuts
Aluminum	cookware, deodorant, lotions, soaps
Aluminum silicate	salt, water softener
Antimony	fragrance in lotions, colognes
Arsenic	pesticide, "treated" carpet, wallpaper
Asbestos	clothes dryer belt, hair blower, paint on radiators
Barium	lipstick, bus exhaust
Benzalkonium chloride	toothpaste
3,4 Benzopyrene	flame cooked foods, toast
4,5 Benzopyrene	flame cooked foods, toast
Beryllium	hurricane lamps, gasoline, dentures, kerosene
Bismuth	colognes, lotions, antacids
Boron	
Bromine	bleached "brominated" flour
Cadmium	galvanized water pipes, old tooth fillings
Cerium	tooth fillings
Cesium	clear plastic bottles used for beverages
Chlorine	from Chlorox™ bleach
Chromium	cosmetics, water softener
Cobalt	detergent, blue and green body products
Copper	tooth fillings, water pipes
Dysprosium	paint and varnish
Erbium	packaging for food, pollutant in pills
Europium	tooth fillings
Europium oxide	tooth fillings, catalytic converter

572

Fiberglass	dust from remodeling or building insulation
Formaldehyde	foam in mattresses and furniture, paneling
Gadolinium	tooth fillings
Gallium	tooth fillings
Germanium	with thallium in tooth fillings (pollutant)
Gold	tooth fillings
Hafnium	hair spray, nail polish, pollutant in pills
Holmium	usually found in presence of PCBs
Indium	tooth fillings
Iridium	tooth fillings
Lanthanum	computer and printing supplies
Lead	solder joints in water pipes
Lithium	printing supplies
Lutetium	paint and varnish
Mercury	tooth fillings
Molybdenum	auto supplies
Neodymium	pollutant in pills
Nickel	tooth fillings, metal glasses frames
Niobium	pollutant in pills, foil packaging for food
Palladium	tooth fillings
Platinum	tooth fillings
Polychlorinated biphenyl PCB	detergent, hair spray, salves
Polyvinyl chloride acetate (PVC)	glues, building supplies, leaking cooling system
Praseodymium	pollutant in pills
Radon	cracks in basement cement, water pipes
Rhenium	spray starch
Rhodium	tooth fillings
Rubidium	tooth fillings
Ruthenium	tooth fillings
Samarium	tooth fillings
Scandium	tooth fillings
Selenium	
Silver	tooth fillings
Sodium fluoride	toothpaste
Strontium	toothpaste, water softener
Tantalum	tooth fillings
Tellurium	tooth fillings
Terbium	pollutant in pills
Thallium acetate	pollutant in mercury tooth fillings
Thorium nitrate	earth (dust)
Thulium	pollutant in many brands of Vitamin C
Tin	toothpaste
Titanium	tooth fillings, body powder
Tungsten	electric water heater, toaster, hair curler
Uranium acetate	earth (dust)
Vanadium pentoxide	gas leak in home, candles (not necessarily lit)

Ytterbium	pollutant in pills
Yttrium	pollutant in pills
Zirconium	deodorant, toothpaste

Solvents

This is a list of all the solvents I use together with the main source of them in our environment. These are chemicals, very pure, obtained from chemical supply companies, unless otherwise stated. Those marked with an asterisk (*) were the subject of a recent book *The Neurotoxicity of Solvents* by Peter Arlien-Soburg, 1992, CRC Press.

Solvent	Source
1,1,1, Trichloro ethane* (TCE)	flavored foods
2, 5-Hexane dione*	flavored foods
2 Butanone* (methyl ethyl ketone)	flavored foods
2 Hexanone* (methyl butyl ketone)	flavored foods
2 Methyl propanol	
2 Propanol (propyl alcohol)	see the propyl alcohol list
Acetone	store-bought drinking water, cold cereals, pet food, animal feed
Acetonylacetone (2,5 hexanedione)	flavored foods
Benzene	see the benzene list (page 354)
Butyl nitrite	
Carbon tetrachloride	store-bought drinking water, cold cereals, pet food, animal feeds
Decane	health food cookies and cereals
Denatured alcohol	obtained from pharmacy
Dichloromethane* (methylene chloride)	store-bought orange juice, herb tea blends
Gasoline regular leaded	obtained at gasoline station
Grain alcohol	95% ethyl alcohol obtained at liquor store
Hexanes*	decaffeinated beverages
Isophorone	flavored foods
Kerosene	obtained at gasoline station
Methanol (wood alcohol)	colas, artificial sweeteners, infant formula
Mineral oil	lotions

Mineral spirits	obtained from paint store
Paradiclorobenzene	mothballs
Pentane	decaffeinated beverages
Petroleum ether	in some gasolines
Styrene*	styrofoam dishes
Toluene*	store-bought drinking water, cold cereals
Trichloroethylene* (TCEthylene)	flavored foods
Xylene*	store-bought drinking water, cold cereals

Pathogen Frequency Chart

Use this chart if you know the frequency and wonder what the pathogen might be.

KHz

Pathogen	Low	High	50	100	150	200	250	300	350
Cytochalasin B	77.00	77.00	m						
Arcyria	81.00	81.00	s						
Sterigmatocystin	88.00	88.00		m					
Cytochalasin B (2nd)	91.00	91.00		m					
Sterigmatocystin (2nd)	96.00	96.00		m					
Zearalenone	100.00	100.00		m					
Lycogala	126.00	126.00			s				
Sterigmatocystin (4th)	126.00	126.00			m				
Sterigmatocystin (3rd)	133.00	133.00			m				
Aflatoxin	177.19	177.19				m			
Stemonitis	211.00	211.00				s			
Sorghum syrup	277.00	277.00						m	
Griseofulvin	288.00	288.00						m	
Herpes simplex 1	291.25	293.05						v	
Ergot	295.00	295.00						m	
Histoplasma capsulatum	298.30	304.85						b b	
Corynebacterium xerosis	315.65	316.80							b
Shigella sonnei	318.00	318.00							b
Streptococcus mitis	313.80	321.10							b b
Influenza A and B (flu sho	313.35	323.90							v v
Mycoplasma	322.85	323.90							b
Bacteroides fragilis	324.30	325.00							b
Proteus mirabilis	320.55	326.00							b
Bacteroides fragilis (2nd)	325.70	326.00							b
Salmonella enteriditis	329.00	329.00							b
Proteus vulgaris (3rd)	327.20	329.50							b
Bordetella pertussis	329.85	332.25							b b
Pseudomonas aeruginos	331.25	334.60							b
Haemophilus influenzae	336.41	336.41							b
Neisseria gonorrhea	333.85	336.50							b
Proteus vulgaris (2nd)	333.75	339.15							b
Gardnerella vaginalis	338.00	342.55							b b
Corynebacterium diptheri	340.00	344.00							b
Herpes simplex 1 (2nd)	345.35	345.75							v
Wart L arm	343.65	345.95							w
Treponema pallidum	346.85	347.40							b
Mycoplasma (2nd)	342.75	349.30							b
Lactobacillus acidophilus	346.05	351.65							b b
Proteus mirabilis (2nd)	345.95	352.10							b b
Erwinia amylovora	347.20	352.10							b b
Serratia marcescens	349.45	352.10							b b
Gaffkya tetragena	344.85	352.50							b b
Schistosoma mansoni	353.00	353.00							p
Nocardia asteroides	354.95	355.35							b
Escherichia coli (E. coli)	356.00	356.00							b
Campylobacter pyloridis	352.00	357.20							b
Loa loa	360.55	360.55							p
Besnoitia (lung sect.) prot	352.80	361.40							p p
Bacterial c+B145apsules	357.60	362.40							b b
Herpes simplex 2 (fresh s	353.90	362.90							v v
Coxsackie virus B-4	361.45	363.70							v

s = slime mold, m = mold, b = bacteria, v = virus, y = yeast, p = parasite (one-celled animals), t = tapeworm, x = mite

KHZ

Pathogen	Low	High	350		400		450	500
Diplococcus diphtheriae	357.95	364.00	b	b				
Naegleria fowleri	356.90	364.35	p	p				
Clostridium botulinum	361.00	364.55		b				
Coxsackie virus B-4 (2nd)	363.90	364.90		v				
Bacillus anthracis (2nd)	363.20	365.30		b				
Clostridium septicum	362.05	365.60		b				
Coxsackie virus B-1	360.50	366.10		v				
Diplococcus pneumoniae	351.65	368.45	b	b				
Streptococcus sp. group	368.15	368.85		b				
Nocardia asteroides (2nd	363.70	370.00		b	b			
Salmonella paratyphi	365.05	370.10		b	b			
Streptococcus pneumoni	366.85	370.20		b	b			
Bacillus anthracis (3rd)	359.40	370.50	b	b	b			
Campylobacter fetus sme	365.30	370.60		b	b			
Measles antigen	369.50	373.00		v	v			
Plasmodium falciparum s	372.30	373.80			p			
Enterobacter aerogenes	374.00	374.00			b			
Streptococcus pyogenes	360.50	375.30		b	b			
Bacillus cereus	373.65	375.85			b			
Erwinia carotovora	368.10	377.00		b	b			
Central spores (bacillus s	372.45	378.65			b			
Histomonas meleagridis (I	376.55	378.70			b			
Staphylococcus aureus (c	376.27	380.85			b	b		
Staphylococcus aureus (s	381.00	381.00				b		
Gyrodactylus	378.75	381.80			p	p		
Borellia burgdorferi	378.95	382.00			v	v		
Spirillum serpens	378.35	382.80			b	b		
Epstein Barre Virus (EBV)	372.50	382.85			v	v		
Respiratory syncytial viru	378.95	383.15			v	v		
Trichomonas vaginalis	378.00	383.60			p	p		
Chlamydia trachomatis	379.70	383.95			b	b		
Eikanella corrodens	379.50	384.30			b	b		
Mumps antigen	377.60	384.65			v	v		
Troglodytella abrassari	377.75	385.20			b	b		
Alpha streptococcus	369.75	385.40		b	b	b		
Sub terminal spores bac.	385.15	385.95				b		
Salmonella typhimurium	382.30	386.55				b		
Adenovirus (2nd range)	371.45	386.90			v	v		
Streptococcus lactis	382.00	387.00				b		
Bacillus subtilis var. niger	371.85	387.10			b	b		
Beta streptococcus	380.60	387.40				b		
Entamoeba histolytica tro	381.10	387.80				p		
Anaplasma marginale	386.40	388.00				p		
Candida albicans	384.20	388.40				y		
Propionibacterium acnes	383.75	389.00				b		
Shigella dysenteriae	390.09	390.09					b	
Chilomastix cysts (rat)	388.95	390.70				p	p	
Clostridium acetobutylicu	382.80	391.15				b	b	
Bacillus anthracis spores	386.95	391.45				b	b	
Escherichia coli (E. coli)	392.00	393.00					b	
Adenovirus	393.00	393.00					v	
Sphaerotilus natans	388.40	393.45				b	b	
Shigella flexneri	394.00	394.00					b	
Toxoplasma (human strai	395.00	395.00					p	
Haemonchus contortus	386.80	395.50				p	p	
Branhamella (Neisseria)	394.90	396.70					b	
Endolimax nana trophozo	394.25	397.10					p	
Bacillus anthracis	393.50	398.05					b	
Clostridium perfringens s	394.20	398.10					b	

s = slime mold, m = mold, b = bacteria, v = virus, y = yeast, p = parasite (one-celled animals), t = tapeworm, x = mite

577

KHz

scale markers across top: 3 5 0 · · · 4 0 0 · · · 4 5 0 · · · 5 0 0

Pathogen	Low	High	Markers
Trypanosoma gambiense	393.75	398.70	p
Chilomonas, whole mount	393.75	400.00	p p
Entamoeba coli trophozoi	397.00	400.35	p p
Leptospira interrogans	397.05	401.10	b b
Strongyloides (filariform l	398.40	402.00	p p
Leucocytozoon	397.45	402.55	p p
Leishmania donovani	398.00	402.65	p p
Ancylostoma caninum	383.10	402.90	p p p
Ancylostoma braziliense (	397.60	403.25	p p
Leishmania mexicana	400.20	403.80	p p
Wart papilloma cervix sm	404.05	404.60	w
Klebsiella pneumoniae	398.45	404.65	b b
Prosthogonimus macrorc	396.85	404.75	p p
Iodamoeba butschlii (2nd)	398.15	404.75	p p
Leishmania braziliensis	400.05	405.10	p
Veillonella dispar	401.75	405.20	p
Trichinella spiralis (muscl	403.85	405.57	p
Wart BS	402.00	406.00	w
Dientamoeba fragilis	401.35	406.05	p
Wart human papilloma pl	404.70	406.75	w
Leishmania tropica	402.10	407.40	p
Blepharisma	405.65	407.45	b
Trichuris sp. (male)	388.30	408.90	p p p
Ascaris larvae in lung	404.90	409.15	p
Pneumocystis carnii (lung	405.75	409.15	p
Ascaris megalocephala (	403.85	409.70	p
Mycobacterium phlei	409.65	410.65	b b
Wart human papilloma vir	402.85	410.70	w w
Cytomegalovirus (CMV) a	408.35	410.75	v v
Dirofilaria immitis	408.15	411.15	p p
Stigeoclonium	404.25	415.25	p p
Cryptocotyle lingua (adult	409.95	416.00	p p
Proteus vulgaris	408.75	416.45	b b
Myxosoma	409.60	416.95	p b
Bacteria capsules (capsul	416.05	418.75	b
Herpes Zoster	416.60	420.20	v v
Hepatitis B antigen	414.55	420.80	v v
Klebsiella pneumoniae (2	416.90	421.90	b b
Troglodytella abrassari (2	416.90	422.20	b b
Eurytrema pancreaticum	420.35	422.30	p
Wart JB	418.75	422.40	w w
Echinoporyphium recurva	418.55	423.90	p p
Anaplasma marginale (2n	415.30	424.00	p p
Plasmodium cynomolgi	417.30	424.50	p p
Fasciola hepatica miracidi	421.75	424.70	p
Trypanosoma lewisi (bloo	424.50	426.00	p
Enterobius vermicularis	420.95	426.30	p
Giardia lamblia (trophozoi	421.40	426.30	p
Fasciola hepatica	421.35	427.30	p
Chilomastix cysts (rat) (2	425.20	427.30	p
Fasciola hepatica rediae	420.60	427.50	p
Fasciola hepatica eggs	422.00	427.60	p
Trypanosoma rhodesiens	423.50	428.55	p
Clonorchis sinensis	425.70	428.75	p
Hypodereum conoideum	424.45	429.55	p
Tobacco mosaic virus	427.15	429.55	v
Echinostoma revolutum	425.50	429.65	p
Fasciola hepatica cercari	423.80	430.60	p p
Capillaria hepatica (liver s	424.25	430.65	p p

s = slime mold, m = mold, b = bacteria, v = virus, y = yeast, p = parasite (one-celled animals), t = tapeworm, x = mite

KHz

Pathogen	Low	High	Markers
Trypanosoma brucei	423.20	431.40	p p
Cytophaga rubra	428.10	432.20	b b
Wart CC	426.00	432.35	w w
Fasciolopsis rediae	427.30	433.00	p p
Endolimax nana (2nd)	430.50	433.35	p
Mycobacterium tuberculo	430.55	434.20	b
Fasciolopsis buskii	427.70	435.10	p p
Fasciolopsis miracidia	427.35	435.20	p p
Fasciolopsis buskii eggs	427.35	435.45	p p
Fasciolopsis cercariae	429.50	436.25	p p
Cysticercus fasciolaris	436.40	440.05	t t
Endamoeba gingivalis tro	433.80	441.00	p p
Onchocerca volvulus (tu	436.30	442.10	p p
Metagonimus Yokogawai	437.35	442.10	p p
Macracanthorhynchus	438.85	442.80	p p
Fischoedrius elongatus	441.75	443.20	p
Wart HA	434.80	444.10	w w
Passalurus ambiguus	428.80	444.15	p p p
Dipylidium caninum	439.55	444.30	t t
Plasmodium vivax smear	438.15	445.10	p p
Echinococcus granulosus	441.15	446.50	t
Iodamoeba butschlii troph	437.85	448.50	p p
Wart HRCm	438.90	448.55	w w
Taenia solium (scolex)	444.00	448.90	t
Urocleidus	442.35	450.00	p p
Trypanosoma equiperdu	434.60	451.25	p p p
Paragonimus Westermani	437.80	454.20	p p p
Sarcocystis	450.55	454.95	p
Hasstile sig. tricolor (adult	448.05	455.10	p p
Gastrothylax elongatus	451.90	457.10	p
Multiceps serialis	453.60	457.80	t
Echinococcus multilocula	455.85	458.35	t
Echinococcus granulosus	451.60	461.50	t t
Balantidium coli cysts	458.80	462.90	p p
Stephanurus dentalus (ov	457.35	463.10	p p
Wart FR	459.30	464.75	w w
Moniezia (scolex)	430.35	465.20	t t t t
Moniezia expansa (comp	430.35	465.20	t t t t
Trypanosoma cruzi (brain	460.20	465.65	p
Taenia pisiformis eggs (o	465.20	469.70	p
Dipylidium caninum (scol	451.95	472.15	t t t
Diphyllobothrium latum (s	452.90	472.30	t t t
Schistosoma haematobiu	473.00	473.00	p
Taenia solium (cysticercu	475.00	475.00	t
Taenia saginata (cysticer	476.50	481.05	t t
Hymenolepis diminuta	445.00	481.15	t t t t t
Hymenolepis cysticercoid	478.00	481.75	t t
Taenia pisiformis (cystice	475.20	482.10	t t
Diphyllobothrium erinacei	467.25	487.55	t t t

s = slime mold, m = mold, b = bacteria, v = virus, y = yeast, p = parasite (one-celled animals), t = tapeworm, x = mite

		KHz	550	600	650	700	750	800	850
Pathogen	Low	High							
Demodex folliculorum foli	682.00	682.00				x			
Dermatophagoides dust	707.00	707.00				s			
Meal mite	718.00	718.00				x			
Sarcoptes scabei itch	735.00	735.00					x		
Ornithonyssus bird mite	877.00	878.00							

s = slime mold, m = mold, b = bacteria, v = virus, y = yeast, p = parasite (one-celled animals), t = tapeworm, x = mite

Sources

This list was accurate as this book went to press. <u>Only the vitamin sources listed were found to be pollution-free, and only the herb sources listed were found to be potent</u>, although there may be other good sources that have not been tested. The author has no financial interest in, or influence on any company listed, except for having family members in the Self Health Resource Center.

Note to readers outside the United States of America:

Sources listed are typically companies within the United States because they are the ones I am most familiar with. You may be tempted to try a more convenient manufacturer in your own country and hope for the best. <u>I must advise against this!</u> In my experience, an uninformed manufacturer <u>most likely</u> has a polluted product! Your health is worth the extra effort to obtain the products that make you well. One bad product can keep you from reaching that goal. This chapter will be updated as I become aware of acceptable sources outside the United States. Best of all is to learn to test products yourself.

Item	Source
Amber glass or polyethylene bottles, ½ ounce	Continental Packaging Solutions (large quantities); Self Health Resource Center; Drug store,
Apricot kernel oil	Starwest Botanicals, Inc.
Arginine	Spectrum Chemical Co.; Seltzer Chemicals, Inc.
Artemesia (wormwood) seed	R.H. Shumway
Baking soda (sodium bicarbonate)	Spectrum Chemical Co.

Beet root	San Francisco Herb & Natural Food Co.
Belts for clothes dryer	Three that tested negative to asbestos are: Maytag™ 3-12959 Poly-V belt, Whirlpool™ FSP 341241 Belt-Drum Dr. (replaces 660996), and Bando™ V-Belt A-65. Bando American makes other belts, some of which might be the right size for your dryer. Call for a dealer near you, make sure it says "Made In America", not all do.
Black cherry concentrate	Bernard Jensen Products; Health food store
Black Walnut Hull Tincture	New Action Products
Borax	Grocery store
Boric acid	Spectrum Chemical Co.; health food store; pharmacy; animal feed store
Cascara sagrada	San Francisco Herb & Natural Food Co.; Self Health Resource Center; Health food store
Chemical Supply Companies	Aldrich Chemical Co.; Spectrum Chemical Co.; ICN Pharmaceuticals, Inc. (research chemicals only, including genistein); Boehringer Mannheim Biochemicals (research only)
Cholecalciferol	Spectrum Chemical Co.
Citric acid	Univar
Cloves	San Francisco Herb & Natural Food Co. (ASK for fresh); Starwest Botanicals, Inc.
Cornstarch	Spectrum Chemical Co.; Lady Lee brand in the grocery store; Argo brand (25 lb. sack only); Unilever Best Foods
Dental bleach	Self Health Resource Center
EDTA	Spectrum Chemical Co.
Electronic parts	A Radio Shack near you; Mouser
Empty gelatin capsules, size 00	Capsugel; Health food store
Filters, coconut charcoal	Pure Water Products (pitchers), Seagull Distribution Co. (faucet, shower, whole house)
Flaxseed oil	Spectrum Chemical Co.
Fucus	San Francisco Herb & Natural Food Co.

Ginger capsules	San Francisco Herb & Natural Food Co. (bulk)
Goldenrod tincture	Blessed Herbs; Self Health Resource Center
Grain alcohol (ethyl alcohol)	Liquor store; search for the ¾ liter or 1 liter size of Everclear.
Gravel root (herb)	San Francisco Herb & Natural Food Co.; Starwest Botanicals, Inc.
Histidine	500 mg from Jomar Labs
Homeopathic remedies	Dolisos America, Inc., and others
Hydrangea (herb)	San Francisco Herb & Natural Food Co.
Hydrogen peroxide 35% (food grade)	Univar
Iodine	Spectrum Chemical Co.
Lugol's iodine	For slide staining (*not internal use*) from Spectrum Chemical Co.; or farm animal supply store. For internal use must be made from scratch. (For disinfecting food, *Veggie Wash* from Source of Health; New Action Products).
L-lysine powder	Spectrum Chemical Co.
Magnesium oxide	Spectrum Chemical Co.
Marshmallow root (herb)	San Francisco Herb & Natural Food Co.; Starwest Botanicals, Inc.
Microscopes, slides and equipment	Carolina Biological Supply Co.; Ward's Natural Science, Inc.; Southern Biological Supply Co.
Microscopes	Carolina Biological Supply Company, Ward's Natural Science, Inc., Edmund Scientific Co.
Milk Thistle	San Francisco Herb & Natural Food Co.
Mullein tea	San Francisco Herb & Natural Food Co.
Niacin	100 mg or 250 mg time release, Bronson Labs; Spectrum Chemical Co.
Ornithine	Spectrum Chemical Co.; Seltzer Chemicals, Inc.
Ortho-phospho-tyrosine	The Natural Health Choice, Ltd.
Ozonator	Superior Health Products (ask for non-black tubing)
P24 antigen sample	The Natural Health Choice, Ltd.
PABA (para amino benzoic acid)	Bronson Labs
Pantothenic acid	Spectrum Chemical Co.

Peroxy	See Hydrogen peroxide
Photo-micrographic camera and film	Ward's Natural Science, Inc.
Potassium bicarbonate	Spectrum Chemical Co., or pharmacy
Potassium chloride	Spectrum Chemical Co.
Potassium iodide	Spectrum Chemical Co.
Rascal	New Action Products (as Raz-Caps)
Salt (sodium chloride)	Spectrum Chemical Co.
Sodium alginate	Spectrum Chemical Co. or health food store
Stevia powder	Self Health Resource Center
Tea	San Francisco Herbs, buy in bulk, any single herb variety.
Thallium, homeopathic	Dolisos America, Inc.
Thioctic acid (also called lipoic acid)	Spectrum Chemical Co.
Uva Ursi, herb	San Francisco Herb & Natural Food Co.
Vanilla extract	Durkee's™ or Mexican brands
Vitamin B Complex	Spectrum Chemical Co.; Seltzer Chemicals, Inc.
Vitamin B_2	Spectrum Chemical Co.; Seltzer Chemicals, Inc.
Vitamin B_6	Spectrum Chemical Co.; Seltzer Chemicals, Inc.
Vitamin B_{12}	Spectrum Chemical Co
Vitamin C (ascorbic acid) synthetic	Roche Vitamins (all other sources I tested had either toxic selenium, yttrium, or thulium pollution!)
Vitamin D	See cholecalciferol
Vitamin E	Bronson Labs
Washing soda (sodium bicarbonate)	Spectrum Chemical Co.
Water filter pitchers	See filters
Wormwood capsules, mixture	New Action Products; Self Health Resource Center
Zinc	Spectrum Chemical Co.
Zinc oxide	Spectrum Chemical Co.

Aldrich Chemical Co.
P.O. Box 355
Milwaukee, WI 53201
(414) 273-3850

Bando American Inc.
1149 West Bryn Mawr
Itasca, IL 60143
(800) 829-6612
(708) 829-6612
www.bandoamerican.com

Bernard Jenson Products
535 Stevens Ave.
Solana Beach, CA 92075
(800) 755-4027

Blessed Herbs
109 Barre Plaines Road
Oakham, MA 01068
(508) 882-3839
(800) 489-4372
www.blessedherbs.com

Boehringer Mannheim Biochemicals
9115 Hague Road
P.O. Box 50414
Indianapolis, IN 46250
(800) 262-1640

Bronson Labs
350 South 400 West, Ste. 102
Lindon, UT 84042
(800) 235-3200 retail
(800) 610-4848 wholesale
www.bronsonlabs.com

Capsugel
P.O. Box 640091
Pittsburgh, PA 15264-0091
(888) 783-6361
(864) 223-2270
www.capsugel.com

Carolina Biological Supply Co.
2700 York Road
P.O. Box 6010
Burlington, NC 27216-6010
(800) 334-5551
(336) 584-0381
www.carolina.com

Continental Packaging Solutions
230 West Monroe St.,
Ste. 2400
Chicago, IL 60606
(312) 666-2050
www.cgppkg.com

Dolisos America, Inc.
3014 Rigel Avenue
Las Vegas, NV 89102
(800) 365-4767
(702) 871-7153
www.dolisosamerica.com

Edmund Scientific Co.
101 E. Gloucester Pike
Barrington, NJ 08007-1380
(609) 573-6250
www.edsci.com

ICN Pharmaceuticals, Inc.
Biomedical Division
3300 Hyland Avenue
Costa Mesa, CA 92626
(800) 854-0530
(714) 545-0113
www.biomed.com

Jomar Labs
583-B East Hacienda Avenue
Campbell, CA 95008
(800) 538-4545
(408) 374-5920
www.jomarlabs.com

Mouser
1000 North Main St.
Mansfield, TX 76063-1514
(800) 346-6873
www.mouser.com

The Natural Health Choice, Ltd.
44 292 055 4943
Fax 44 292 055 3779
www.the-natural-choice.co.uk

New Action Products (USA)
P.O. Box 540
Orchard Park, NY 14127
(800) 455-6459 (USA only)
(716) 662-8000
www.newactionproducts.com
New Action Products (CANADA)
P.O. Box 141
Grimsby, Ont Canada
(800) 541-3799
(716) 873-3738 (Canada)

Pure Water Products
10332 Parkview Avenue
Westminster, CA 92683
(800) 478-7987

Radio Shack
www.radioshack.com

R.H. Shumway
P.O. Box 1
Graniteville, SC 29829
(803) 663-9771

Roche Vitamins, Inc.
340 Kingsland St.
Nutley, NJ 07110-1199
(800) 892-6510
(no retail sales)

San Francisco Herb & Natural Food Co.
47444 Kato Road
Fremont, CA 94538
(800) 227-2830 wholesale
(510) 770-1215 retail
www.herbspicetea.com

Seagull Distribution Co.
3670 Clairemont Drive, Ste. 2
San Diego, CA 92117
(888) 558-4825
(858) 270-7532
www.seagulldistribution.com

Self Heath Resource Center
1055 Bay Blvd. Suite A
Chula Vista, CA 91911
(800) 873-1663
(619)409-9500
www.shrc.net

Seltzer Chemicals, Inc.
5927 Geiger Ct.
Carlsbad, CA 92008-7305
(760) 438-0089

Source Of Health
P.O. Box 161080
San Diego, CA 92176
(866) 372-5275
Fax (619) 795-0569
www.sourceofhealth.com

Southern Scientific, Inc.
83 Euclid Avenue
P.O. Box 368
McKenzie, TN 38201
(800) 748-8735
(901) 352-3337

Spectrum Chemical Co.
14422 South San Pedro
Street
Gardena, CA 90248
(800) 791-3210
(310) 516-8000
www.spectrumchemical.com

Starwest Botanicals, Inc.
11253 Trade Center Dr.
Rancho Cordova, CA 95742
(800) 273-4372
(916) 638-8100

Superior Health Products
13549 Ventura Blvd.
Sherman Oaks, CA 91403
(800) 700-1543
(818) 986-9456
www.superiorhealthproducts.com

Univar (wholesale only)
2100 Hafley Avenue
National City, CA 91950
(800) 888-4897
(619) 262-0711

Ward's Natural Science, Inc.
5100 West Henrietta Road
Rochester, NY 14692
(800) 962-2660
(716) 359-2502
www.wardsci.com

Finale

I hope you have come to the same happy conclusion that I did a few years ago! We humans don't have hundreds of different maladies and disturbances. **We only have two!** And that is things that crawl or climb into us. And toxins: unnatural chemicals that we unknowingly inhale or consume.

The living things are both large and small: from worms we can see, to microscopic bacteria, viruses and fungi. The non-living things are pollutants in our air, food, dental metal and body products. Taking in a lot of pollutants hampers the body's ability to kill and get rid of the invaders. And so, gradually, as we get older or sicker, the body's invaders get the upper hand and take over. Don't be discouraged if you have lupus, cerebral palsy, cirrhosis, or any complex-sounding disease. Every disease is an example of the same process.

The good news is that our body can reclaim its sovereignty by throwing the rascals out. We must assist by throwing the pollutants out. Fortunately we don't have to do the whole job ourselves, we only need to <u>assist</u>. Our body has miraculous powers to clean itself up.

By reducing chronic disease to two problems, it becomes manageable. Ill health, even aging, can be reversed. Health comes back and rewards you.

With the new electronic insights and technology, our parasitic invaders can be vanquished with the closing of a switch. Preventing reinfection is the bigger challenge. Similarly, pollutants can be uncovered in as short a time as days, short enough to turn any sick, even terminal, sufferer's verdict around before tragedy occurs.

The tragedies of surgery, organ replacements, radiation, chemotherapies, doses of drugs, even death can be avoided. Reversing illness and turning into a shining example of your former healthy self could be the most exciting adventure of your life.

Killing your invaders is an easy matter: you simply purchase or build the device that can do that and take the proper herbs. Cleaning up dentalware is under your control, too—a financial expense not beyond your reach, hopefully. Trading your body products for unpolluted varieties is a job but not insurmountable. Cleaning your environment may be the stumbling block. If you can't unpollute your air, water, carpets, furniture, move. Move to a healthier dwelling! Get rid of it all. Like a cat that moves her kittens to a safer place, just move.

The healthiest house is no house. If you have been quite ill, move far enough south to avoid heating and cooling. Sit outside in the shade all day. Use your new wisdom and sharp eye to choose a new dwelling as free of pollutants as you can. No refrigerator indoors. No window air conditioner. No fiberglass insulation. No fossil fuels. No attached garage. No carpets or stuffed furniture, no foam bedding, no fresh paint, no pesticide. Go primitive. Health is primitive. You were born primitive—with health. Even if you weren't, you can undo much of the "inherited" damage.

Don't listen to the new doomsayers, who persuade you nothing can be done unless a gene is replaced. Your genes have been reliable for millions of years. Genes are the most reliable of all biological chemicals in your body. They are not faulty. They are hampered in their tasks. They are commandeered by metals and other species' genes, those of parasites, bacteria, and viruses. They wouldn't be there if pollutants weren't there. They allow invaders into the most jealously guarded recess of your being: your genes. But now you can throw the rascals out and reclaim your territory. It is not new genes that you need. You simply need your own genes back on the job, directed by your own body, working for you.

Index

A

abdominal pain, 99, 203, 268, 299
abscess, 54, 79, 135, 153, 158, 159, 163, 164, 216, 231, 510, 565, 566
Acanthocephala, 138, 274, 566
acetic acid, 296
acetone, 122, 162, 208, 320
acetylcholine, 221, 238
acidophilus, 21, 100, 564
acne, 167, 192, 193, 194
acupuncture, 51, 465
Adenovirus, 13, 179, 199, 357, 358, 359, 360, 361, 363, 368, 563
adrenal gland, 60, 113, 114, 143, 210, 212, 217, 281, 291, 373
aflatoxin, 38, 177, 180, 186, 225, 261, 280, 348, 349, 381, 382, 383, 384, 386, 390, 392, 422, 483, 491, 493, 494, 519
AIDS, 11, 35, 36, 90, 119, 126, 131, 149, 252, 351, 352, 353, 356, 368, 372, 385, 442, 443, 458, 493, 500
air conditioner, 40, 284, 313, 323, 346, 403, 446, 590
air filter, 137, 284
albuminuria, 417
alcoholism, 227, 228, 229, 230, 386
alkaline phosphatase, 80, 217
alkaline tide, 57
allergy, 85, 102, 105, 107, 111, 126, 135, 139, 140, 163, 169, 175, 190, 191, 216, 222, 223, 224, 225, 226, 242, 246, 258, 386, 495, 553, 558
aluminum, 37, 112, 137, 141, 171, 180, 181, 187, 189, 212, 244, 247, 269, 271, 274, 305, 310, 311, 314, 415, 421, 423, 424, 430, 433, 434, 435, 436, 438, 439, 450, 461, 473, 484, 485, 486, 487, 514, 521, 525, 526, 533, 543
aluminum silicate, 37, 138, 141, 212, 271
alveolar cavitational osteopathosis, 410

Alzheimer's, 33, 219, 250, 252, 269, 270, 272, 372, 495, 526
amalgam, 37, 65, 71, 107, 115, 157, 180, 409, 410, 413, 414, 416, 417, 418, 475, 485
amalgam tattoo, 410
American Dental Association (ADA), 37, 409, 414, 416
amino acid, 85, 232, 244
ammonia, 125, 243, 244, 320, 326
amoeba, 106, 274
Ancylostoma, 256, 257, 262, 566
anemia, 76, 162, 279, 285, 286
anesthesia, 90
angina, 176, 417
animal dander, 104, 135
animal feed, 125, 347, 574
ankle swelling, 68
ant repellent, 540
antibiotic, 134, 141, 170, 181, 248, 548
antimony, 105, 112, 123, 128, 140, 187, 435
antiseptic, 98, 344, 399, 436, 449
aorta, 478
appendicitis, 101, 268
appendix, 97, 101, 128
appetite, 134, 240, 268, 275, 288, 292, 300, 306, 376, 379, 388, 417
apple cider vinegar, 277, 348, 423, 493, 572
apricot kernel oil, 534, 535, 537
arginine, 120, 137, 210, 212, 425
arm, 49, 51, 118, 153, 154, 254, 255, 282, 321, 481, 482, 488, 531, 553, 569
armpit, 143, 144, 193, 531
arsenic, 4, 40, 68, 96, 100, 103, 110, 132, 137, 138, 141, 150, 160, 162, 168, 171, 185, 186, 187, 193, 206, 236, 242, 259, 268, 271, 282, 313, 314, 361, 403, 448
arthralgia, 417
arthritis, 51, 78, 80, 81, 82, 83, 84, 85, 86, 117, 137, 146, 151, 155, 214, 268, 419

THE CURE FOR ALL DISEASES

eye, 3, 14, 76, 140, 160, 161, 162,
175, 186, 259, 478, 497, 498, 528,
539, 590
eye disease, 3, 161, 175
eye makeup, 140, 186
eyelid, 146, 539

F

face, 36, 123, 181, 192, 193, 194,
209, 220, 227, 231, 253, 258, 280,
283, 369, 400, 448, 469, 540
face powder, 231, 540
fallopian tube, 250
Fasciola, 43, 249, 567
Fasciolopsis buskii, 33, 150, 166, 250,
331, 371, 490, 567
fatigue, 2, 4, 73, 95, 111, 113, 134,
139, 176, 177, 182, 183, 184, 185,
186, 187, 204, 245, 289, 311, 368,
417
fennel, 444, 547, 548
fenugreek, 175, 176, 370, 422, 521
fetus, 258, 417, 563
fever, 78, 201, 203, 204, 234, 365,
369
fiberglass, 39, 40, 80, 91, 100, 110,
133, 137, 143, 147, 150, 160, 168,
177, 241, 282, 284, 314, 336, 349,
403, 405, 447, 590
fibromyalgia, 51, 75, 76, 78
fibromyositis, 75
filaria, 31, 318
finger, 86, 136, 155, 195, 253, 282,
308, 321, 463, 486, 487, 508, 530,
539
fingernail, 501
fireplace lighter, 165
fish line, 72, 95, 218, 248, 296, 438,
533
flatworm, 33, 331
flavoring, 304, 378, 428, 548
flaxseed, 127
floss, 70, 72, 95, 162, 218, 296, 438,
481, 532
flour, 298, 306, 310, 361, 362, 379,
385, 423, 474, 572
flu, 78, 134, 168, 176, 201, 202, 203,
275, 425, 564
fluke disease, 117, 219, 221, 249,
250, 252, 494, 495

fluke egg, 145, 332
fluoride, 82, 112, 206, 296, 573
foam, 40, 194, 284, 314, 337, 404,
447, 449, 533, 573, 590
foam bedding, 314, 337, 590
foam filter, 284
foam furniture, 40, 449
folic acid, 120
Food and Drug Administration (FDA),
436
foot, 51, 57, 59, 60, 68, 247, 248, 328,
419, 506
formaldehyde, 40, 100, 108, 110, 112,
133, 137, 150, 160, 165, 168, 193,
236, 241, 282, 314, 361, 448, 449,
499, 500, 571
fragrance, 105, 136, 166, 185, 247,
253, 259, 284, 529, 530, 550, 572
Freon, 100, 160, 336, 446, 469
Fucus, 239, 548, 583

G

gadolinium, 124, 140, 207
Gaffkya, 170, 564
gallbladder, 80, 128, 132, 191, 477,
553, 559
gallium, 123, 124, 146
gallstone, 81, 150
galvanized pipe, 70, 210, 211, 450
ganglia, 180
Gardnerella, 69, 91, 102, 110, 114,
115, 119, 564
garlic, 137, 376, 548
gas hot water heater, 431
gas leak, 105, 140, 141, 149, 165,
166, 170, 171, 175, 187, 241, 255,
260, 268, 279, 319, 450, 573
gas pipe, 96, 165
gas stove burner, 476
gas, household, 231
gasoline, 124, 127, 162, 208, 221,
224, 227, 316, 416, 445, 472, 572,
574
gene, 3, 46, 206, 207, 209, 590
genital tract, 116, 564
germanium, 417
Giardia, 9, 103, 160, 239, 399, 567
ginger, 205, 514, 515
ginseng, 259, 263
glaucoma, 146, 213, 214

Q

R

S